Prepublication Reviews

An excellent road map and tool kit to assist you in creating a longer, healthier, more joyful life. Read and learn how to be too busy to die, and become ageless by losing track of time.
  –**Bernie Siegel, MD**, Author of *Love, Medicine, and Miracles* and *Peace, Love and Healing*

People are living longer and healthier lives. *Defy Aging* shows us how to do it well. It's a visionary road map to help us live fuller and richer lives. I highly recommend everyone over 40 to read it!
  –**Betty Friedan**, founder of the National Organization of Women and author of *The Feminine Mystique* and *The Fountain of Age.*

Dr. Brickey's new book *Defy Aging* has successfully achieved the near impossible task of distilling thousands of scientific articles and hundreds of books in the field of health and longevity into one easy-to-read compendium of anti-aging science. This is a must-read review book of an emerging new field of anti-aging medical technology which promises many of its readers will see their 150th birthday with full mental and physical faculties intact. I recommend it.
  –**Ronald Klatz, M.D., D.O.**, Founder and President of the American Academy of Anti-Aging Medicine, author of *Stopping the Clock* and *Ten Weeks to a Younger You*

Defy Aging is a must read for anyone wanting to live long and well.
  –**Dharma Singh Khalsa, M.D.**, author of *Brain Longevity*

Starting their own lives trusting no one over thirty, Baby Boomers never expected to age. Now finding themselves well over fifty, they are desperately looking for perpetual youth in all the wrong places. But it is not too late. There is an antidote to aging: read this book!
  –Distinguished Professor **Nicholas A. Cummings, Ph.D., Sc.D.**, a past president of the American Psychological Association, President of the Nicholas & Dorothy Cummings Foundation, and author of *Focused Psychotherapy.*

Defy Aging is a refreshing new way of looking at life. Dr. Brickey brilliantly addresses the mental and emotional aspects of living that are 70% of health and longevity with a practical program. *Defy Aging* is a book worth reading and a guide worth having.

–Jack G. Wiggins, Ph.D., Psy.D.
A past president of the American Psychological Association

Most books about longevity are about pills and diets and say little about the mental and emotional aspects that drive 70% of longevity. *Defy Aging* is a unique, ground breaking book that leaves behind conventional thinking and gives a map for living longer, richer, fuller lives. It is a visionary manifesto for acquiring the beliefs, attitudes, and lifestyle to live longer, healthier, and happier.

–Stanley Graham, Ph.D., a past president of the American Psychological Association.

What an exceptional book! Doctor Brickey marshals the evidence to prove what many of us have always suspected: longevity is at least 70% mental! Those with the right beliefs, attitudes, coping skills and lifestyles will continue to live well while living long. Those who do not attend to the mental aspects of aging not only have shorter lives, they also have more health problems, more pain and more depression. Do not wait until you are over 50 to read this book. And, do not confuse its easy reading style with a lack of substance. Brickey knows his stuff and knows it well enough to refrain from having to show it off with torturous academic prose.

–Ron Fox, Ph.D., a past president of the American Psychological Association.

Defy Aging reminds us that "old age ain't for sissies" but it is a time for discovery, warmth and wisdom, if we follow the road map outlined in this empowering book. I would heartily recommend it for any of us who are aging.

–Ellen McGrath, Ph.D., Internationally acclaimed executive coach, author of *When Feeling Bad is Good,* and frequent expert commentator on ABC News, Good Morning America, Fox News and 20/20.

When Dr. Brickey initially talked to me about living a vital, healthy life for 150 years, I was very skeptical. *Defy Aging* built such a strong research-based case that I'm now convinced. I have used his materials in my women's groups and they loved them.

–**Carol Roche, Ph.D.**, President of LifeCycle Directions.
Dr. Roche has doctorates in both physiology and psychology.

Defy Aging coaches and mentors you skill by skill on living longer and taking your life to a higher level. Dr. Brickey, an exceptional life coach, has an astonishing range and depth of knowledge. *Defy Aging* is a well-written, illuminating, practical guide to living a good life and a long life. I highly recommend it for professional coaches, their clients, and anyone who seeks a long, fulfilling life.

–**Ben Dean, Ph.D.**, Founder and President of MentorCoach, The nation's preeminent training program for clinicians becoming professional coaches.

DEFY

AGING

DEFY AGING

Develop the mental and emotional vitality
to live longer, healthier, and happier
than you ever imagined

Michael Brickey, Ph.D.

New Resources Press

Publisher's Cataloging-in-Publication
(Provided by Quality Books)

Brickey, Michael.
    Defy aging : develop the mental and emotional vitality to live
    longer, healthier, and happier than you ever imagined / Michael
    Brickey. – 1st ed.
    p. cm.
    Includes bibliographical references and index.
    LCCN: 00-91404
    ISBN: 0-9701555-0-6

    1. Aging–Prevention. 2. Longevity. 3. Aging–Psychological
    aspects. 4. Health.   I. Title

    RA776.75.B75 2000   612.6'8
                                   QBI00-509

Contents

Acknowledgments

I'd like to thank several good friends who reviewed chapters and provided ideas and encouragement. They are: Dr. Carol Roche, Dr. James Shulman, Dr. Ben Dean, Michael Leahy, Dr. Jayne Speicher-Bocija, Dr. Robert Birch, Dr. Marty Williams, and my lovely wife Dr. Deborah Stutman-Brickey. My Mid-Day Toastmaster's group (#1802) also was very helpful in giving feedback as the concepts evolved. You have helped make a dream come true and have helped many people live longer, healthier, happier lives.

Chapter 1

You Are Going to Live Longer–
Will You Choose to Live Well?

You can't help getting older but you don't have to get old.
–George Burns

Why defy aging? Most people base their expectations about the future on the past. They look in the rear view mirror at how their parents are aging or aged and presume the same is in store for them. They hear phrases like "you're not as young (capable) as you used to be," and are seduced into conventional expectations about aging. To paraphrase an advertising slogan, "Aging is not your father's *Old*smobile."

Huge paradigm shifts in how long and how healthy people can live create the opportunity to live a vital healthy life for 150 years. I would estimate that at least 50,000 Baby Boomers will do this–maybe more. But you can't drive your parents' *Old*smobile. You need a vision of healthy aging focused on what is possible rather than what has been. You need a continually renewing sense of purpose all your life. You need attitudes, beliefs and a lifestyle that foster health and longevity. And you need to defy conventional thinking about aging.

You have a choice–to just go along with conventional thinking, or to defy aging and live a long vital life. As Robert Frost[1] put it:

Two roads diverged in a yellow wood. . . .
I took the one less traveled by,
And that has made all the difference.

The longevity paradigm shift

The twentieth century brought rapid and profound paradigm shifts in our culture. The Wright brothers flew the first airplane in 1903. Today commercial airlines serve more than a billion passengers a year. Henry Ford began producing Model-T Fords in 1908. Today the U.S. alone has 130 million registered automobiles. In 1950 commercial television was just getting started. Today 98% of U.S.

households have a color television. In 1950 there were only sixty computers in the world. These vacuum tube computers often filled a whole room. Now millions of hand-sized electronic personal organizers can process far more information and access the Internet without wires.

In the last century changes in longevity and health may not have been as obvious, but they are equally profound. From Christ's birth to the year 1900 mankind gained an average of 3 days a year in longevity. Since 1900 we have gained an average of 110 days a year in life expectancy.[2]

In the U.S. life expectancy increased 62% in the last century.[3] At the turn of the millennium the U.S. has about 72,000 centenarians. The U.S. Census Bureau predicts we will have 170,000 centenarians in 2010 and 1,208,000 in 2050.[4] The number of centenarians will then explode when the huge Baby Boomer generation starts turning 100 around 2050. On the *Today Show* Willard Scott often calls centenarians to wish them a happy birthday. In the year 2000 if he spent eight hours a day, every day of the year, calling centenarians, he could spend a couple of minutes per call. In 2050, he would have less than nine seconds per call, seven days a week, 365.25 days a year.

Chronic disability rates for citizens over 65 have been dropping 1-2% a year since the government started collecting statistics in 1982.[5] [6] [7] Many centenarians are physically healthy and mentally sharp. Researchers have been pleasantly surprised that an increasing number of centenarians are vital and healthy until the last year or two of their lives.[8]

Better educational, informational, and financial resources are making it easier to pursue and achieve excellent health and longevity. Sixty percent of current centenarians had less than an eighth grade education. Today, 80% of Americans over 25 are high school graduates and 33% are college graduates. Personal computers have put knowledge at our finger tips (and soon at our spoken command). Greater affluence allows greater access to resources.

Genetic engineering, destined to be the premier technology of the century, has increased the life spans of fruit flies by 30% and nematodes (worms) by 500%. Genetic engineers enabled mice to eat high fat diets and remain trim and healthy. Genetic engineers successfully inserted genes into humans to replace missing genes and to kill cancer cells. Medicine is using stem cells to grow blood, skin, and other human tissues, developing transplant organs from animals, and developing artificial organs. Scientists have immunized mice against Alzheimer's disease and are beginning clinical trials with humans. There is a good chance scientific advances will not only cure diseases like Alzheimer's, but also help us enhance our thinking skills and memories. Hormone therapies for men and women will soon help people look, feel, and function twenty years younger. Who would have believed that straight-laced former Senator Bob Dole would be promoting Viagra? Fifty isn't what it used to be and neither is 100.

What current centenarians can tell us

A good start in our quest for longevity is to ask, What is unique about today's centenarians? Besides apparently having "good genes," they have only three things in common physically: 1) they are physically active people, 2) few smoke, and 3) they have maintained a fairly constant weight all of their lives.[9] The primary distinguishing factors for centenarians is between their ears. Mental traits that distinguish current centenarians are that they:
1. are active mentally,
2. are self-reliant and independent,
3. are optimistic,
4. have a good sense of humor,
5. have good coping skills, and
6. don't hold on to losses or resentments.

These are pretty straightforward traits that you can choose to develop and hone.

Let me illustrate these traits by telling you a little about the Delany sisters–Sadie and Bessie. Their father was a former slave. Sadie became a high school teacher and Bessie a dentist in Harlem. Neither married. Bessie was outspoken and Sadie was diplomatic. Both cared a great deal about doing the right thing and doing a good job. When they eventually retired, they were still active in their community and active with friends–though they refused to have a phone or television in their home. As centenarians, they did yoga exercises daily at home. A newspaper reporter interviewed them when Sadie was 102 and Bessie had her hundredth birthday. The reporter found they were such delightful, vital people that she helped them write a best-selling book, *Having Our Say: The Delany Sisters' First Hundred Years*. Imagine writing your first book when you were a centenarian. Then came a Tony winning Broadway play based on the book and a second best-selling book. Bessie died at home in 1995 at 104. Sadie died at home in January 1999 at 109.

What it takes

What does it take to have a healthy, vital life for well over a hundred years? Current centenarians tend to be fairly ordinary people with an extraordinary psychological edge. Researchers estimate that 30% of longevity is due to heredity.[10] That percentage will decrease with the advent of genetic engineering. The 70+% is up to you. Science, medicine, and genetics only create the potential for longevity. Beliefs, attitudes, coping skills, and lifestyles are critical determinants for who will defy aging with long lives, good health, keen minds, and a passion for life.

There are many books on what pills to take, exercises to do, or diets to follow to be healthy and live long. Of the hundreds of published interviews with current centenarians, however, not one attributed his or her longevity to taking pills, eating blue-green algae, doing a particular exercise, or following a severe diet. As Dr. Dean Edell[11] has reported, newspapers, magazines and television's insatiable appetite for new and alarming stories yields a profusion of contradictory advice and diet-of-the-month fads. If you are physically active, eat reasonably, and are not terribly overweight, mental factors are far more important to vital longevity than finding the perfect pill, diet, or workout. The biggest mental factors in longevity are a continually renewing sense of purpose, dealing with family members and friends dying, resilient coping skills, and dealing with massive change.

A vision of the future and an ageless society

In his ... "I have a dream speech," ... Martin Luther King Jr. had a vision of racial equality and harmony. While there is still much to be done, much of his vision has been manifested. Let me share my vision of the future ageless society.

In this vision, the world has become an even more magnificent feast of information, activities, and ideas–a playground inviting us to gather some playmates and play. Americans have outgrown the youth cult culture and appreciate people of all ages. We have become an ageless society.[12] With hormone replacements, wrinkle removing, and other medical advances, it's often hard to tell how old someone is anyway. There are centenarians who look, move, and think like 30-year-olds. After childhood age has become meaningless. People are valued for their qualities and contributions rather than their age or color. One hundred is as common as 65 was at the turn of the century. With so much change, people increasingly appreciate the continuity and perspective that experienced people offer. The Mentors for Families Foundation has facilitated many older people "adopting" children and families to be surrogate grandparents and mentors for struggling families.

Many people pursue serial careers and their cross-pollinating of ideas has become one of the most generative sources of innovation. The very fluid job market rewards workers according to their skills, talent, character, and services. Many people are self-employed. Most older Americans are financially comfortable enough that they feel they can afford to invest in health, fitness, relationships, helping others, and making a contribution. Centenarians are valued members of society who share their talents and wisdom in profit, nonprofit, and volunteer settings. With so much change people find comfort in leadership by experienced people just as millions were comforted by hearing the evening news by Walter Cronkite, news analysis by Daniel Shore, or leadership by President Reagan.

As the hippie movement in the 1960s and the environmental movement of the 1980s produced a shift in values and consciousness, the whole person movement of the 2010s shifted the focus from materialism to integration of mental, physical, and spiritual health. Brain wave biofeedback devices help people better identify and choose their emotional states and moods. Like dentist visits, most doctor visits are for checkups, monitoring, early detection, and prophylaxis. Telehealth monitoring helps with early identification of problems. Checkups are proactive consultations on how to be as fit and healthy as possible (as opposed to just checking for diseases). Anti-aging medicine is the most common medical specialty. Hearing and vision problems are readily treatable. Genetic engineering corrects a lot of health problems before they are manifested. Cancer, heart problems, and diabetes are as manageable or treatable as tuberculosis. Physicians and the public have a much better understanding of how the mind and body are one system.

In the 1990s more and more college students were over thirty. Now half of college students are over fifty. Learning technologies have made it easier to learn information and to understand complex relationships. Brain wave biofeedback devices help people access optimal learning states. The world's best teachers use virtual reality demonstrations to aid learning. Computer chip implants help people supplement their brains with information and information processing skills. Campuses, neighborhoods, and organizations have more of a mix of ages than ever before. With most of the population over forty, television, radio, and the new forms of media are offering very diverse and more sophisticated programs at a wide variety of intellectual levels. Information and programs are available on demand 24 hours a day at home.

The plan for defying aging

Defy Aging begins with a self-test in Chapter 2 to see how well you are defying aging. Chapter 3 looks at the role of attitudes, beliefs, lifestyles, coping skills, and genetics in determining who will live long and healthy lives and who won't. Chapter 4 looks at the connection between what we believe and think and our physical and mental health. It examines 36 beliefs that distinguish people who defy aging. If you want to adopt these beliefs, Chapter 5 gives you powerful strategies for changing beliefs and metaphors. Chapter 6 examines four attitudes that are key to healthy longevity–optimism, gratitude, dealing with it, and embracing lifelong learning and change. Exercises help you develop these attitudes. With people living longer and massive societal changes, you need to continually renew your sense of purpose. Chapter 7 presents a process for continually renewing your sense of purpose.

Living longer presents new challenges. Are you going to be married for 100 years? Chapter 8 examines how to make a marriage work for a century and how to be resilient if you choose a different path. Many men tell me that living longer isn't really living if there is no sex. With aids like Viagra, men can have erections long past 100. Chapter 9 discusses men's fears women's concerns about sex.

Another challenge is dealing with outliving friends and family. Some people are resilient at dealing with loss and some people never get over losses. Chapter 10 examines what makes for resilient, healthy grieving and includes exercises to help you develop these skills. Dealing with time and change is a lot easier with a carefully considered self-concept and an understanding of time lines. Chapter 11 examines these issues and provides helpful exercises.

Every month the media present a new "miracle" diet. Chapter 12 examines the nutritional tower of Babel and how to decide what you should eat and drink. Vitamins, minerals, and hormonal supplements can be very helpful. Chapter 13 helps separate supplement help from supplement hype.

Fitness does not need to be an ordeal. It does need to address all the key aspects of fitness and your weakest area of health. Chapter 14 considers how an intelligent approach to fitness now can keep you fit for well over a hundred years. A realistic longevity plan also needs to assess and minimize risks without taking the zest out of life. Chapter 15 considers risks and includes a risk assessment quiz. Another key ingredient to longevity is effectively managing finances. Chapter 16 advocates earning money well past "retirement age" and living below your means so you will have resources to take sabbaticals, change careers, or deal with adversities.

The last chapter examines the evidence from the biological sciences for 150 years of healthy living. Advances in medicine, genetic engineering, hormonal therapies, and medications are helping people look, feel, and function younger. These scientific advances are truly exciting.

Just reading *Defy Aging* will give you many new ideas and perspectives for how to live longer, healthier and happier than you ever imagined. The greatest benefit, however, comes from doing the program's dozens of exercises and developing your comprehensive mission statement.

Why live so long?

Why live to 150? For me it's like asking a mountain climber why she wants to climb mountains. It's not just the challenge. And I don't seek to be in the *Guinness Book of World Records* or *Ripley's Believe It Or Not* as the oldest person. Living to 150 is uncharted territory and life is a work of art. I want to craft a life that is enjoyable and purposeful for 150 years. And I want to show you how you can too. There is another reason to defy aging and live a long vital life–the alterative. People who do not attend to the mental aspects of longevity have shorter lives, more health problems, more pain and more depression.

When you decide and believe that you will live to 150, it changes your perspective on life. Mid-life becomes 75 instead of 40. Hormone replacement, which is common for women and will soon be common for men, will delay the physical and emotional shifts and sexual decline that accompanies declining hormone levels. So you can postpone that mid-life crisis at 40 to 75. By then you should be mature enough to handle it with ease. Setbacks are easier to absorb as there is more time to succeed at other ventures. If you like, you will have the time to pursue several careers or interests.

The choice

Most people expect a car to last about eight years and then be ready for the junk yard. (That's 80 years in people years.) Go to a car show, however, and you will see cars almost a hundred years old that look great and run well. Those cars will soon be centenarian cars. If we show the same attention and love for our bodies, minds and spirits as those car owners have done, we can be in as excellent condition as those classic cars.

Look around and it is obvious that many people choose overeating, not exercising, excessive television, or heart attack lifestyles. Only 40% of Americans even take vitamins on a regular basis. Many faces show the ravages of depression and stress. They might say, as Eubie Blake said on his 100th birthday, "If I had known I was going to live so long I would have taken better care of myself." There is another choice–to defy aging.

Question: Who wants to live to be 150 anyway?
Answer: 149-year-olds.

Ten Warning Signs of Mental Longevity

1. Refuses to hold onto resentments
2. Refuses to conform to conventional thinking
3. Refuses to engage in pessimistic thinking
4. Refuses to brood over losses
5. Insists on always learning and growing
6. Insists on being physically active
7. Insists on being self-reliant
8. Frequently is totally absorbed in activities
9. Places an inordinate emphasis on humor
10. Doesn't get drunk on New Year's Eve

Chapter 2

Test Your Mental Longevity

Answer yes or no to the following 42 questions. Count the number of yes answers you give. The test is intentionally transparent (yes answers being healthier) to make scoring easy and to make the test more instructive. Rationales for the items follow the instructions for scoring and interpretation.

Mental vitality
1. Do you average at least half an hour a day reading things that you do not have to read?
2. Do you have a passionate interest in at least one special interest other than your job and family?

Optimism
3. When someone gives you a compliment, do you usually believe it and accept it graciously?
4. Do you think that most people are good?
5. Do you think that next year will be better than this year?

Self-reliance and independence
6. Do you consider your doctor's advice but regard yourself responsible for your health?
7. Do you seek solutions to health problems other than taking medications?
8. When deciding what to eat, do you use your own criteria for what agrees with you and keeps you healthy and energetic (as opposed to deferring to friends or experts)?

Sense of humor
9. Have you laughed out loud in the last 24 hours
10. Can you tell a joke or say something funny and get others to laugh?

Cheerfulness
11. Are you cheerful?
12. Do you smile a lot?

Resilient coping skills

13. When you think of family members, friends or pets that have died, do you usually think of them fondly?
14. When there is new technology, do you welcome the change?
15. When someone cuts in front of you in traffic or tailgates you, do you take it in stride?
16. Would you be willing to pursue a new career if your current career were no longer satisfying?
17. When someone disappoints you, are you able to let go of any resentments within a week?

Relaxation skills

18. Do you engage in an activity several times a week that gets you in a relaxed, meditative state (e.g., yoga, classical music, breathing exercises, prayer, fishing)?
19. When you get upset, do you have a reliable way to quickly get yourself into a resourceful state?

Finances

20. At the end of each month do you have more savings than the previous month?
21. If you chose to quit your job and took a sabbatical, could you live comfortably for six months?

Sense of purpose

22. Do you believe in God or some form of higher power or truth or purpose in life?
23. Do you have a sense of purpose for your life?

Friends

24. Aside from work, do you spend at least four hours a week with friends?
25. Do you spend at least four hours a week with family members (or friends who are like family)?
26. Do you spend at least an hour a week with friends who are chronologically younger than you are or with children?
27. Are most of your friends positive, optimistic people?

Self-talk
28. When you "talk to yourself," is most of the conversation positive?

Sex
29. Do you have sexual relations with someone you care about at least once a week?

Physical risk taking
30. Do you always wear a seatbelt and not drive more than 10 miles over the speed limit?
31. Have you been free of any serious sports injuries in the last 10 years?

Physical fitness
32. Do you get a 30-minute cardiovascular workout at least twice a week?
33. Do you engage in activities that keep you physically flexible at least twice a week?
34. Do you engage in exercises or sports that require physical strength at least twice a week?
35. Do you breathe deeply (from your abdomen rather than your chest) at least a few minutes each day?

Health practices
36. Do you take a daily multiple vitamin?
37. Do you floss and brush your teeth at least once a day?
38. Do you drink at least six glasses of filtered water a day?
39. Do you refuse to "go on a diet?"
40. Do you maintain a fairly constant body weight that is within 20 pounds of your "ideal body weight?"
41. Does your lifestyle not include smoking cigarettes, cigars, or marijuana?

Longevity expectation
42. Do you believe that you will live past 100?

SCORING: Give yourself one point for each yes answer.

37-42   You have excellent mental longevity skills. The concepts in *Defy Aging* will feel natural and comfortable and help you reinforce and sharpen your excellent skills.

31-36   You are off to a good start. *Defy Aging* should be very helpful in filling in some gaps and reinforcing and honing your mental longevity skills.

25-30   You are doing a number of things well. It would be prudent to focus first on being clear and vivid about why you want to live a long, vital life. Begin with the easiest changes and take on the more difficult ones as you make progress.

< 25   You need to seriously consider what your life will be like as you age. *Defy Aging* can be extremely helpful. Make a vivid mental image of what you could be like if you really take care of yourself mentally and physically. Notice how you exude energy and vitality. Now make a vivid mental image of what it probably would be like if you don't make changes in your attitudes, beliefs, coping skills, and lifestyle. Perhaps this image has you hunched over, bored, in pain, and in a wheelchair in a nursing home at 80. Keeping those images in mind, begin with the easiest changes and take on the more difficult ones as you make progress.

RATIONALE FOR THE ITEMS:

Active mentally

While centenarians are a diverse group, virtually all of them are very active mentally and cite being mentally active as vital to long life. Like physical skills, mental skills are "use them or lose them" faculties.

Optimism

Martin Seligman's research, summarized in his book, *Learned Optimism*, provides an abundance of data on how optimistic people have better physical health, are more successful, and experience less depression. Depression is the "common cold" of mental health and the incidence of depression is becoming epidemic. Although many centenarians have had difficult lives, including dealing with two World Wars, the Great Depression, loss of loved ones, and in many cases poverty, few centenarians have reported problems with depression. Depression impairs people's immune systems. A major difference between centenarians and people who die at younger ages appears to be that most centenarians avoid depression and its effects–impairing sleep, appetite, energy levels, the immune system and enjoying life. Most researchers report that in interviews and psychological testing the vast majority of centenarians are upbeat.

Self-reliant and independent

Self-reliance and independence are major traits distinguishing centenarians. Researchers reported that the older centenarians become, the more they make decisions on the basis of what they believe as opposed to what others expect. Most take few medications and many only see a doctor when they have to. (They would be wiser to see a doctor for annual checkups.) They place responsibility for their health with themselves and not their doctors. They "march to a different drummer."

Sense of humor

Humor is commonly cited in centenarian interviews and observed by centenarian researchers. Humor requires flexible thinking (to understand word plays, double entendres, etc.). Laughing stimulates a lot of movement in the body and stimulates the immune system. Unlike the heart, the lymph system does not have a pump and relies on breathing to force lymph to circulate. In his book, *Anatomy of an Illness,* Norman Cousins describes how he used laughter to overcome a usually fatal illness (ankylosing spondylitis).

Cheerfulness

While research data on cheerfulness are scarce, cheerfulness certainly appears to be a close relative of optimism. Research and interviews often cite centenarians as satisfied with life. In her autobiography, *Bubbles,* opera diva Beverly Sills says she was asked if she was happy. She has two children; one is deaf and the other is mentally retarded. Her singing career was shortened by cervical cancer. She replied that, in view of the tragedies in her life, she doesn't know if she would describe herself as happy, but she is cheerful. Happiness is a by-product of having purpose and passion. Cheerfulness is a trait that can be learned and practiced.

Resilient coping skills

Hans Selye's classic 1956 book, *The Stress of Life,* documented how stress prompts the body to respond with a general adaption syndrome. The syndrome begins with adrenalin and other hormones rallying for the crisis (the alarm stage), and continues into the resistance and exhaustion stages if the stress is prolonged and severe. Everyone experiences stress. A certain amount of stress, especially from desirable events like a promotion or getting married, is good. Prolonged stress, however, takes its toll on our bodies and makes us vulnerable to illnesses. Centenarians' skill at dealing with stress protects their bodies from becoming run down and vulnerable to illnesses.

One of the most difficult stresses centenarians face is dealing with the loss of loved ones. People who cope effectively with loss focus on what was good about the loved ones and remember them fondly. They often think of their loved ones as a resource that they can call on for support and guidance. People who do not cope effectively focus on the loss and how things will never be the same.

Change is inevitable and becoming more and more rapid in our society. If you see each change as an ordeal (e.g., dreading the newest computers and software), then change becomes one more stress and one more factor that can contribute to depression.

Perspective is also important. Treating minor events, such as being cut off in traffic, as no big deal prevents your body from triggering its stress response. Perspective on larger stressors, for example, losing a job, can minimize the body's stress response and vulnerability to depression. If pursuing a new career is an ordeal, it can be very stressful. If you see it primarily as an exciting challenge, most of the stress will be eustress (good stress).

Hanging onto disappointments, resentments, and should-have-beens prompts the body's stress response, ties up emotional energy, and distracts people from finding solutions. Often people hang onto resentments, thinking the resentments will protect them from getting hurt again. Instead it just prolongs the hurt. Most centenarians have excellent skills at letting go of painful events and resentments. They live in the present.

Relaxation skills

Relaxation skills are essential to keeping the body in a harmonious state and avoiding stress responses. Just as muscles need both challenges and relaxation, our conscious minds need challenges and time off so unconscious and meditative states can do their intuitive work. People who are deprived of dream sleep (REM or Rapid Eye Movement sleep), even if they obtain an adequate number of hours of sleep, become extremely irritable. After several days of REM sleep deprivation they become irrational. Even when awake we appear to need periodic meditative states to be relaxed, flexible, and function well.

Quickly and effectively getting yourself out of an upset state is a micro resilient coping skill. It short circuits the stress response and helps us problem-solve and relate to people better.

Finances

What do couples argue about the most? Money. For most people finances are one of the most stressful areas of their lives. Feeling financially secure and knowing that you have some financial reserves helps you feel better emotionally and physically. If you are saving money (or paying off mortgages and debts) it is easier to feel optimistic about the future. The issue isn't how much money you have in absolute terms but living within your means, or better yet, living below your means and having the security of savings.

Sense of purpose

While it might be partially a generational phenomenon, most current centenarians profess a strong belief in God. It is possible to have a sense of purpose without literally believing in God. We all know people who do not believe in God but whose commitment to truth, justice, morality, or a cause makes them spiritual people and gives them a sense of purpose. When people lose their sense of purpose, they become vulnerable to depression and their immune systems become compromised and vulnerable to illness.

Friends

In his book, *Real Age,* Michael Roizen calculates how different factors affect one's life expectancy. For socialization he cites three factors: 1) being married, 2) seeing at least six friends at least monthly, and 3) participating in social groups. The "real age" for a 55-year-old man who meets all three criteria is 46, two criteria 49, one criterion 53, and no criterion 60. For a 55-year-old woman the real ages are 49, 53, 59, and 61. Presumably the effect is a little stronger for men because women in our culture are better at social networking. When a partner's spouse dies, his or her risk of illness or death skyrockets for the first year. Retirement also changes social networks and can be very stressful.

We become like the people with whom we socialize. A natural part of forming rapport with people is sharing interests and values. If most of our friends are older, we get pulled into their lifestyles and beliefs about aging. If many of our friends are younger, we get pulled into their younger lifestyles and beliefs about aging. If we associate with grumpy people, we are likely to develop negative banter. If we associate with positive, optimistic people, we are likely to develop upbeat thinking and conversations.

Self-talk

If you find yourself saying, "You stupid idiot, why did you say such a dumb thing," it is time to reprogram your self-talk. Motivational speaker and author Anthony Robbins makes a strong case that the quality of our lives depends on the quality of questions we ask ourselves, e.g., How can I make this better? What blessings am I grateful for? How can I make this a great day?

Sex

Sex enhances emotional intimacy, relaxes us, decreases stress, and is one of life's great pleasures. Michael Roizen in *Real Age* reports that women who are unsatisfied with the quality or quantity of their sexual relations have a life expectancy ½ a year less than is average for their age while women who are satisfied with both the quality and quantity have a life expectancy 1½ years longer than average. For men, fewer than five orgasms a year shortens life expectancy by 2½ years while more than 300 orgasms a year adds three years to their life expectancy.

Physical risk taking

There are many things people can do to lessen their physical risks. Driving a safe car, wearing seat belts, and not speeding are some of the easiest. Sports can be a great way to have fun, have a network of friends, and stay fit. Quite a few people become addicted to sports, however, and continue sports even when their bodies are telling them to change to a safer sport or exercise. A common example is runners who develop knee problems but "have to" continue running.

Physical fitness

Fitness does not need to be an obsession. It does need to include cardiovascular, strength, and flexibility activities. One of the things that often causes elderly people's health to deteriorate is falls. Many falls are due to weak muscles, poor balance, a lack of flexibility, and slow reflexes. Minor miracles have been performed in nursing homes just by getting residents to do some physical fitness exercises.

Many physically healthy people become addicted to sports and pursue the sport even when the pursuit is harming their bodies. For example, they may continue running despite knee problems or a cessation of menstrual periods. Longevity requires that we listen to our body's feedback and do something different if our physical activities are causing injuries or health problems.

Most people in our society have very constricted breathing. They breathe primarily from their chest cavity instead of their abdomens. Even a few minutes a day of deep breathing helps enormously. Unlike our hearts, our lymph system does not have a pump and is dependent on our breathing to circulate lymph.

Health practices

Most Americans do not receive all the vitamins and minerals they need from what they eat. Soil depletion has resulted in some of our fruits, vegetables, and grains no longer containing micronutrients such as copper, zinc, sulphur, iron, and magnesium. A daily multiple vitamin is an easy way to make sure you receive all the vitamins and minerals you need. (Note: Most men and many women should not have iron in their vitamins as it fosters free radical damage.) Taking individual vitamins and minerals can create imbalances between vitamins and minerals and needs to be carefully thought out. High doses of some vitamins or minerals can cause health problems.

Flossing and brushing your teeth not only promotes good dental hygiene and helps teeth and gums last a lifetime, but poor dental hygiene is linked to cardiovascular disease, strokes, and infections. Apparently the same bacteria that cause periodontal disease prompt an immune response which causes arteries to swell. Michael Roizen in *Real Age* reports that the absence of periodontal diseases can add 6.4 years to your life expectancy. Thus, daily flossing and brushing are extremely time and cost-effective health practices.

Most city tap water is probably OK but we would be healthier without the chlorine. Our bodies are 80% water and water is the primary vehicle for our bodies to circulate blood, lymph, hormones, cerebral spinal fluid, etc. and to eliminate wastes. Filtering water is easy and inexpensive. It removes chlorine and other chemicals but leaves in the minerals. Filtered water also tastes better than chlorinated water. Distilled water leaches chemicals from our bodies (and tastes flat). The Natural Resources Defense Council tested 103 brands of bottled water and found that one-third of them did not meet California standards and guidelines for bottled water.

When people reduce their calorie consumption, the body adapts by reducing its metabolism. When they go off a diet, the metabolism bounces back. There is a substantial body of research indicating that "yo-yo dieting" is hard on our body's systems, rarely works, and is worse than being overweight. Losing weight needs to be gradual and the result of ongoing health practices. The easiest way to lose weight, for most people, is to increase the muscle-to-fat ratio and metabolism by exercising. One of the few physical factors that distinguish centenarians is that they maintain a fairly constant body weight their whole adult lives.

The research on the health problems caused by cigarette smoking is overwhelming. Cigar smoking is associated with mouth cancers and some smoke is inhaled. Marijuana has 50% more carcinogens and 400% more tar than cigarettes. Prolonged use of marijuana also affects motivation, which in turn leads to less physical and mental activity.

Longevity expectation

Our minds try very hard to fulfill our beliefs and expectations. Just believing something does not make it happen, but if you believe you will live past 100, it is more likely to happen. To build this belief, study the supporting data, e.g., medical advances, the increasing number of centenarians, increasing resources, and the generally good health of many centenarians.

Chapter 3

Who Will Live to 150 or Longer?

With a little luck, there's no reason why you can't live to be one hundred. Once you've done that, you've got it made, because very few people die over one hundred. –George Burns

"The race is not always to the swift."
(Moral to *Aesop's Fable* of the *Tortoise and the Hare*)

In the fable of the tortoise and the hare, the tortoise is clearly the winner. The tortoise had a clear sense of purpose and a natural sense of pacing. The hare had impressive speed but poor planning. Not everyone will be able to live to 150 or longer. The challenge is to manage our resources well by changing what we can change and making the best of what we cannot change–that is, learning to adapt and cope well.

As with many complex systems, just one thing going wrong, however, can be fatal. Longevity requires giving special attention to "the weakest link in the chain." Most people only expect their cars to last five to ten years and their bodies to last about eighty years. If the car you have now were the only car you would ever have, what would you be willing to do to take care of it and make it last a lifetime? There are people who take very good care of Model T cars and they run and look as good as new. If you take good care of your mind and body, you have a good chance to live a healthy, vital life for 150 years or more.

Here are the four variables that will determine who will live to 150 or longer:

• Beliefs, attitudes, and coping skills–discussed in the chapters on:
  – beliefs that foster longevity
  – how to change beliefs
  – attitudes that foster longevity and change
  – mission and purpose
  – marriage
  – sex
  – outliving friends and family

  – time and change
- Lifestyle choices–discussed in the chapters on:
  – eating and drinking
  – supplements
  – fitness
  – managing risk
  – finances for a lifetime
- Heredity–discussed in this chapter
- Luck–which is in part due to attitudes, beliefs, coping skills, and lifestyle choices

Note that lifestyle choices are mental factors in that you choose your lifestyle. Even luck is to some extent mental in that your attitudes, beliefs, coping skills, and lifestyle choices have a lot to do with your luck. Heredity is currently 30% of the equation. Genetic engineering, however, is destined to reduce that percentage in the next few decades. Thus, 70% or more of longevity depends on your mental choices and paths.

When 2,032 adults were asked how long they want to live, 63% cited an age less than 100.[1] Respondents who were between 18 and 24 saw "old" as 58 while those over 65 said old starts at 75. Respondents feared living longer because of:

46% declining health
38% lack of money
13% losing mental faculties
11% becoming a burden on family
 9% being isolated or alone
 8% living in a nursing home or "old age" home

Let's look at each concern:

Declining health: As previously noted, people who take good care of themselves mentally and physically are living a lot healthier, as well as a lot longer. Many centenarians are in good health and have sharp minds until their last few years of life. People who die before 100 are more likely to have had prolonged illnesses than people who live past 100.

Lack of money: For most people, having enough money to live for well over 100 years means not retiring at the arbitrary age of 65, but continuing to work, at least part-time, for many more years. Healthy longevity requires productivity and a sense of purpose. Just playing golf for several decades would get pretty dull.

Losing mental faculties: Most centenarians are sharp mentally. To stay sharp mentally, you do have to continually learn and use your mind. It's a "use it or lose it" proposition. Scientists have prevented and cured Alzheimer's disease in mice and appear likely to find a prevention and cure for Alzheimer's disease for humans within a few decades. It is likely that genetic engineering and supplements will enhance our thinking and memories at all ages.

Becoming a burden on family: If you maintain good health and earn income after 65, it is unlikely that you would be a burden on your family.

Being isolated or alone: If you have no friends, it is your own doing–make some.

Living in a nursing home: You can just say no to nursing homes. There are many alternatives.

The survey responses appear to have been based on what respondents saw their parents' generation experience rather than considering what the future is likely to bring. For most people their quality of life as they age is the result of the choices they have made. True, some people are blessed with better health than others and accidents happen, but we can all make the best of our circumstances.

American society is very youth-oriented and there is a lot of mythology about older people. The research indicates that centenarians are very independent people and often in good health. But there is a trick. You have to stay healthy most of your life to get to 100.

Attitudes, beliefs and coping skills

> *Ask and you will receive.*
> *Seek and you will find.*
> *Knock, and it will be opened to you.* –Matthew 7:7

> *If you haven't the strength to impose your own terms upon life,*
> *you must accept the terms it offers you.*
> –T. S. Eliot, *The Confidential Clerk*

> *Once you are physically capable of winning a gold medal,*
> *the rest is 90% mental.* –Patti Johnson

Give your mind a vision and it sets out to fulfill it. Develop the attitudes, beliefs, and coping skills for longevity and you have the tools. With the vision, mental skills, and spirit of a pioneer, you can fulfill the dream. This is not to say that just wishing something makes it so. It is to say that:

- There is a large amount of evidence that living to 150 or longer is possible for tens, perhaps hundreds of thousands of people in our lifetime. The evidence is discussed in Chapter 17.
- There is a large amount of research that shows that people who have a mission, purpose, optimism, and good coping skills live a lot longer, happier lives.
- These longevity traits can be learned and *Defy Aging* will show you how.
- The default for not taking charge and seeking vital, healthy longevity as a goal is being sucked into conventional wisdom and lifestyles, e.g., "Act your age." "Well, what do you expect when you get to be your age?" or "Of course you can't, you're not as young as you used to be."

When you believe you can live to 150 or longer, your mind makes it a part of your identity and becomes alert to ideas and information on how to do it. It's like buying a new car and suddenly noticing that model everywhere. Most of us have worked at an organization that was bureaucratic, lifeless, and demoralizing. It saps your energy and spirit. If you have been fortunate enough to work for an organization that has a real sense of vision, you know how going to work can be exciting and give you energy. The same is true for your life.

Fifty years ago people often worked for the same employer their whole career. Today most people have had at least several jobs, and careers are full of ups and downs and soul searching. Consequently, having exceptional coping skills, a clear sense of who you are, and a mission have become more vital to mental health and longevity.

Just below the surface level with all its to-do lists are the programs that run our lives. There are metaphors, admonitions, self-talk, and self-expectations. Most computer users only know how to use the word processor, E-mail, and perhaps a spreadsheet. Those who are sophisticated, however, can change the settings and even the programs to do incredible things. The user and software are more important than the hardware as long as the hardware is adequate. A sophisticated computer user with an "archaic" 5-year-old computer can run circles around an unsophisticated user with the newest and fastest computer. This book is about the settings and software that enable you to program your life to live a vital life for 150 years or longer. It doesn't require an extraordinary IQ. It does require imagination, flexibility, desire, and self-discipline. The rewards will last you a very long lifetime.

No one believed a human could break the 4-minute mile. It was like a limit set by God. Roger Bannister[2] believed it could be done and used different training regimens, strategies, and beliefs than others runners used. Within months of his breaking the 4-minute mile barrier in 1954, he and another runner broke his record. Since 1954, there have been 17 official new record times for the mile. The current record is now 3 minutes and 44.39 seconds. Today, dozens of high school students can run a mile in less than 4 minutes.

Just wishing something doesn't make it so and just wishing for a long, vital life doesn't make it happen. Beliefs about what invariably happens to people as they age, however, can become a self-fulfilling prophecy that limits our longevity. Like Roger Bannister, we need to believe it is possible to do something most people don't think can be done–to live to 150 or longer. Like Roger Bannister we need to develop strategies to achieve new milestones. Longevity experts said the limit of human longevity is 115 years or possibly 120. In 1998 a French woman, Jeanne Calment, lived to 122. (She probably would have lived longer if she hadn't smoked cigarettes most of her life and if she had agreed to cataract surgery.) Now that the longevity limit mystique has been shattered, several new records will probably be set in the next 10 to 15 years. Within a few decades genetic engineering will enable physicians to turn on or turn off many of the genes that control diseases and aging.

While *Defy Aging* stretches your mind, the principles are research-based. By research-based I don't mean a knee jerk reaction to the latest study but a careful consideration of the context of research, the preponderance of evidence, and the biases and perspectives of the researchers. For example, Martin Seligman[3] conducted extensive research on optimism and found that:

- Thirty-five percent of third and fourth graders experience at least one episode of severe depression. Optimistic children were far less likely to experience depression or stay depressed. Pessimistic children were far more likely to become depressed and have their depression worsen or recur. Needless to say depressed children's school performance deteriorates.
- Pennsylvania State University (Penn State) freshmen who were optimists were more likely to have better first semester grades than their high school grades and SAT aptitude tests suggested. Pessimistic freshmen were more likely to have lower grades than expected.
- At West Point each year about one hundred freshman quit within the first two months. Seligman found that those who quit were more likely to have been pessimists. As at Penn State, the optimists outperformed their high school grades and SATs while the pessimists underperformed them.
- When Metropolitan Life Insurance Company included optimism in their selection process for life insurance agents, their new agents sold more insurance and stayed with the company longer.
- Male Harvard graduates were in reasonably good health until age 45 when the men who were pessimistic at 25 began having significantly more health problems than the men who were optimistic at 25. The difference became even more pronounced at 60. While the Harvard research looked at many factors, optimism was the strongest predictor of health after 45.
- Optimists are less likely to get sick.

- Optimists are more likely to survive cancer and less likely to have recurrences of cancer.
- When baseball players made optimistic remarks to the press, their team's winning percentages tended to increase. When players made pessimistic remarks, their team's winning percentages tended to decline.
- Basketball teams whose players' statements in newspaper sports columns reflected optimism outperformed the point spreads.

The good news is that optimism can be learned.

From 1940 to 1970 gerontologist Belle Boone Beard gathered data on 12,000 centenarians. She administered questionnaires to 3,000 of them, personally interviewed several hundred, and conducted projective psychological testing with 200 of them. She summarized the "substance" of their longevity as their "thinking, feeling, believing, and doing while surviving successfully."[4]

Research that follows people over long periods of time is rare and especially valuable. One of these studies followed male Harvard undergraduates from their freshman year to their sixties.[5] It included extensive health and psychological testing and interviews every few years. The study found that the most successful subjects had better "adaptive" skills, including:[6]

- altruism
- humor
- self-discipline and optimism
- goal-directed planning
- channeling aggression, desires, and impulses into healthy outlets

Each of these adaptive skills can be learned and cultivated.

Intelligence gives you the ability to adapt to changes. While there are many high IQ people who don't make good use of their intelligence, intelligence is a big advantage in dealing with the massive changes in the 21st century. Lifelong learners will be at a distinct advantage in earning money and appreciating health and lifestyle issues.

The current generation of centenarians often were independent, self-reliant individuals who had little use for doctors. Future centenarians are likely to be people who conscientiously monitor their health, make considerable use of preventive healthcare, and are quite sophisticated about health and risk issues. Like current centenarians they will consider themselves responsible for their own health and see doctors as consultants. These factors change the equation for longevity, making intelligence and lifelong learning more important and genetics less important to longevity.

Lifestyle choices

"Society expects older people to be sedentary, and many expect it of themselves. Only 10% of Americans over 65 jog, play tennis, cross-country ski, or engage in other vigorous exercise on a regular basis. The inactive majority lose about 30% of their strength and 40% of their muscle mass between ages 20 and 70 . . . remaining athletic for life can halt much of the debilitation that was once thought to be an inevitable part of aging.[7]

Lifestyle issues are critical to longevity. Some of the most critical choices are:
- being active and physically fit
- maintaining a healthy weight
- practicing preventive health care
- attending to your "weakest links"
- pursuing a job or activities that give you a sense of purpose and meaning
- having good friends
- balancing work and other pursuits
- moderating your use of alcohol
- avoiding drugs and nicotine
- avoiding risky sexual behaviors
- driving safe cars safely
- living within or below your financial means (which effects less stress and more financial resources)

Some people will have health problems that will limit their chances of living a long life. Certainly people who are grossly overweight will have difficulty passing 100. Some disabilities fit well with Judge Oliver Wendell Holmes Sr.'s admonition that the key to a long life is to have a low level chronic illness that you have to take care of. Some disabilities like diabetes, however, wear out the body prematurely. Hopefully, medical advances will help with such diseases.

You can have a long, happy life without being particularly achievement oriented. If we look at current centenarians, some, like the Delany sisters, were accomplished professionals. Others had more modest work histories and achievements. Current centenarians were born before 1900 and averaged less than an eighth grade education. Now 80% of Americans over 25 have a high school degree and one-third have a college education. Today's complex world favors lifelong learners. Having money to spend on taking care of yourself helps as well. People who can achieve a good income without killing themselves in the process also have an advantage. They will worry less about finances and be able to afford health care, education, and other resources to foster their longevity.

Luck

Finally, there is just plain luck. In 150 years everyone experiences difficulties and tragedies. Some people, however, experience more tragedies than others. In some cases this is random luck. In many cases our life choices increase or decrease risks.

Let me make an analogy between these factors and automobiles. Yes, some of us are Chevys, some Camrys, and some of us are lucky enough to be Lexuses (i.e., our heredity defines our physical capabilities and hardiness). A well-maintained Chevy, however, will outlast an abused Lexus. Some cars are more "intelligent" than others and self-diagnose problems and give you a warning when fluid levels are low or other problems have developed. These cars have an advantage in prompting the maintenance they need just as intelligent people are more resourceful than less intelligent people. Cars have lifestyles–where and how they are driven, whether they are kept in a garage, etc. Mental factors include having an owner who practices preventive maintenance and attends to updates and recalls. The car's health management includes oil changes, car washes, washing off salt, and early identification and correction of problems. Finally, there is the luck factor of not being in the wrong place at the wrong time and being in an accident. There are Chevys that are almost a hundred years old now because they were treated with tender loving care.

Genetics and its declining role in longevity

There are no such things as incurable, there are only things for which man has not found a cure. –Bernard Baruch[8]

Height is 65% hereditary and IQ is 60% hereditary.[9] Longevity, however, is only 30% hereditary. The most respected research concerning heredity and longevity comes from Danish studies of twins.[10] It is no accident that the research came from Denmark. They keep extraordinarily good vital statistics and are able to track data for decades. The twins study compared the longevity of identical twins with the longevity of fraternal twins. Since identical twins come from one egg that divided after conception, each child has identical genes. Fraternal twins, on the other hand, come from two eggs fertilized by two different sperm resulting in children who differ as siblings normally differ.

The life spans of identical twins varied by an average of 14.5 years–suggesting a large environmental influence. Life spans of fraternal twins varied by an average of 18.7 years–indicating that genetics did play a role as well. To simplify some complicated methodological analysis, the researchers determined that 30% of longevity is attributable to heredity. No subsequent research has seriously challenged its 30% figure. Albert Jacquard, a population expert, concluded that knowing how long your parents lived would increase your ability to predict your life span by a mere 2.6% compared to the expected life span for your age.[11]

There are several studies currently underway studying centenarians. One of the most sophisticated centenarian studies is the New England Centenarian Study directed by Thomas Perls and Associate Director Margery Silver.[12] Their data suggest that centenarians are distinguished by the mental traits that are the focus of this book and by not getting sick. The centenarians they studied typically were exceptionally healthy physically and mentally virtually all of their lives. The centenarians averaged only one medication each. In interviewing family members about deceased centenarians, Perls and

Silver found that most had a disability only during the last four years of their lives.

What most people fear about aging is becoming disabled, demented, and vegetating at a nursing home. The Perls and Silver centenarians certainly did not present such a picture. Rather they illustrated a phenomenon called "compressed morbidity" in which disability is "compressed" into the last few years of life.[13] Studies of aging and disability have shown a 1-2% decline in disability rates each year since the U.S. government started keeping statistics in1982.[14]

Perls and Silver also found that their centenarians had a disproportionate number of close relatives with long life spans. They concluded that while the Danish studies probably apply to most people, centenarians might be drawn from a different pool of genes with extraordinary longevity. The theory is intriguing and might have merit. Certainly collaborating studies are needed. Even if they are right, it is not clear whether their findings will generalize beyond the current generation of centenarians. Life was less complex for that generation and many of the diseases they had to survive have been cured. Also, the advent of genetic engineering and other medical advances is destined to lessen the importance of genetics.

It is not possible to predict exactly how much of longevity is due to genetics because it is a moving target. Let me illustrate with a personal example. As a young child, my son had a lot of ear infections. Without antibiotics (which came into common use in the 1950s) and/or tubes in his ears (which became common in the 1980s), he probably would have become deaf or died before he reached puberty unless we isolated him from other children. Because of medical advances, the genetics that gave him a high susceptibility to ear infections did not affect his longevity. When he was 10 years old, he became very sick and visits to the pediatricians and the hospital emergency room were fruitless. My wife and mother-in-law, however, remembered that a week before his illness he had visited a part of the country in which Lyme disease was a problem. After some Internet research, we returned to the hospital emergency room and told the doctor what the illness was and insisted on an antibiotic right away. The symptoms cleared within twenty-four hours. The antibiotic, parental detective work, and readily accessible consumer information prevented a long-term disability.

One of the most powerful genetic factors in who dies before 70 is susceptibility to infectious diseases.[15] Some diseases, like smallpox, have been eradicated. Polio is well on its way to a similar fate. Tetanus, tuberculosis, and hundreds of other disabling or fatal diseases are now treatable. Genetic traits that previously limited longevity might favor longevity for other diseases. For example, sickle cell anemia is resistant to malaria. Today we can easily cure malaria but we do not have a cure for sickle cell anemia yet. AIDS only became common in the 1980s. Who gets AIDS will be determined mostly by lifestyles, general levels of health, and genetic resistance to AIDS. As scientists learn how to treat and cure AIDS, genetic susceptibility to AIDS becomes less important to longevity. For diabetes, cancer, and many other diseases, medicine is making considerable inroads in better managing, treating or curing the disease. In short, advances in health care affect whether a genetic trait will affect longevity.

Consider how different the world was for current centenarians vs. Baby Boomers. Prior to 1920 most meats were heavily salted or smoked to preserve them because refrigerators were uncommon. Antibiotics were not commonly used until the 1950s. The sun's ozone layer did not become a serious problem until the 1980s. In the current centenarians' generation promiscuity and divorce were rare and most adults had one or only a few sexual partners in their lifetimes. With our society's premium on jobs with intellectual skills, genetic traits that cause severe disabilities don't necessarily impair one's ability to earn a substantial living, but intellectual deficits often limit a person to a minimum wage job.

Culture plays a factor. When our society glamorized smoking cigarettes, secondary smoke was unavoidable in urban settings. Genes that resist lung cancer were more critical to longevity. Our diets have changed. On the one hand fresh produce is readily available. On the other hand highly processed foods and fast foods have become prevalent. While we have a lot more resources and knowledge for staying fit, there are a lot of couch potatoes and obese people. These factors all influence what genes will be critical to longevity.

Longevity often runs in families. While some of the longevity might be due to heredity, some is due to similar values and lifestyles. If, for example, the parents and relatives abuse alcohol, smoke cigarettes, or overeat, the children are likely to do the same.

Finally, genetic engineering will enable people to turn genes on or off or insert them. Mapping of all human genes is ahead of schedule and should be completed by 2003. Genetic engineering will yield one breakthrough after another in the first two decades of the new millennium.

Thus 70% or more of your longevity is up to you and the choices you make. The choices are about what you think, what you believe, and the lifestyle you choose.

The choice

In his last oration, Moses told the Israelites, "I put before you life and death, blessing and curse. Choose life."[16] We have a similar choice:

Passive Aging

Those who choose passive aging don't give much thought to aging. It just happens. Over the years they add weight, develop health problems, and take medications. They tend to their jobs and responsibilities but do little to feed their minds and spirits. They assume that their aging will resemble aging in their parents' generation. While they might enjoy their current age, they assume the rest of life is downhill. They are prime candidates for chronic illnesses and nursing homes.

Successful Aging

Full of enthusiasm for life, those who choose successful aging see life as an adventure and steer their own destiny. They are independent and yet well connected to family and friends. They are optimistic and have a good sense of humor. They pursue passions and constantly learn and experience new ideas and activities. They take responsibility for their health and monitor their health. They exercise several times a week for anaerobic, aerobic, and flexibility benefits and find exercise gives them energy, vitality, and confidence. They are fit, healthy, and most don't take medications other than vitamins and hormonal supplements. They experience aging as giving them a clear sense of who they are and what is important in life–qualities that outweigh any disadvantages of aging. As they age, they become more direct, uninhibited, bold, powerful, generous, happy, and wise.

Chapter 4

36 Beliefs That Foster Your Longevity

The mind and the soul are like muscles,
if you use them they get stronger,
if you don't use them, they atrophy
or to use the popular phrase, use it or lose it.

Humans are still too death-oriented too guilt ridden too sub-
missive and fatalistic to demand immortality. To even hope for it.
–F. M. Esfandiary[1]

How beliefs profoundly affect our mental and physical health

Age is a question of mind or matter.
If you don't mind, age don't matter. –Satchel Paige

Our beliefs about aging are culturally programmed. Once we adopt beliefs about ourselves and our world, we filter information to support these beliefs. Smokers minimize and rationalize the deleterious effects of smoking. A staunch Democrat or Republican filters news to support his or her party and find fault with the other party. Parents might quickly defend their child and assume their child is right and the other party is wrong. Even parents whose children have committed atrocious crimes are often heard saying, "but he's a good kid." If you believe "people are no damn good," you will find plenty of evidence to support your view. If you believe people are wonderful, you will find plenty of evidence to support your view. Beliefs about ourselves can be some of the most persistent beliefs. If you believe you are "no good at math" you won't give math a chance. People who were shy teenagers and have outgrown their shyness might still believe they are shy.

Psychologists use the term *cognitive dissonance* to describe the conflict and discomfort people experience when confronted with information that contradicts their beliefs.[2] People try to relieve the discomfort by:

- denying the existence, credibility, or importance of the event, e.g., denying the existence of the Holocaust

- rationalizing the differences, e.g., an alcoholic who says he really doesn't have a drinking problem because he only drinks beer
- altering or distorting the evidence, e.g., conveniently forgetting or underreporting how much you ate or drank already
- insisting on more information, e.g., smokers who say the evidence that smoking causes lung cancer is inconclusive

Thus, people try to maintain consistent beliefs and self-concepts to feel a sense of control and stability in their lives and avoid the discomfort of conflicting information.

French psychologist Jean Piaget studied children's intellectual development and how they deal with cognitive dissonance. Piaget showed 4-year-old children a tall, thin container of water and a short, fat container of water (both containing the same amount of water). The children told him the taller container had more water. Even when he poured the water back and forth between the containers, 4-year-olds insisted the taller container held more. At age 5 and 6, children were likely to show confusion and possibly reorganize their thinking with a new rule about the amount of liquid being constant or height and breadth both being factors in determining the quantity. By age 7 or 8 children consistently understood the principles involved. Adults can go through the same kind of belief changes when confronted with compelling evidence or a compelling reason to change their beliefs.

Norman Cousins[3] describes research with medical students that illustrates how our beliefs affect our physical functioning. Half of the medical students took a red stimulant and half took a blue tranquilizer—or so it seemed. The researcher switched the pills so students who took the red pills and thought they were taking stimulants were actually taking tranquilizers and vice versa. Half of the medical students in each group reported symptoms consistent with their beliefs about the medication, as opposed to the symptoms that the medication actually produces. In another experiment cancer patients were given medication and advised of its side effects including hair loss. Half of the patients, however, were given a placebo ("sugar pill") and half of the patients receiving placebo medications reported hair loss.

Cousins[4] describes how when he was 10 years old and in a tuberculosis hospital, there were kids who viewed their tuberculosis as a death sentence and were resigned to the sentence. Other children, however, acted as if they were in a prison and could not wait to get out and live free again. He found that the kids who believed it was a death sentence typically fulfilled the belief and died within a few years, while those who fought it typically got better and were discharged. Cousins also describes how, at 49, he was told he had at best 18 months to live if he got plenty of bed rest and avoided physical and mental stress. His book, *Anatomy of an Illness*, chronicles how he refused to accept the death sentence, stayed active, and watched a lot of comedy films to "laugh himself back to health."

In alcohol research, people were given drinks that smelled and tasted like vodka but had no alcohol. They soon slurred their speech and showed other signs of inebriation. Similar experiments have been done with marijuana.

Research with antidepressant medications, e.g., Prozac, found that 75% of the benefit of the medication was from the placebo effect–i.e., patients who took the placebo showed 75% as much benefit as the patients who took the antidepressant medication. When patients were given a medication that they thought was an antidepressant *and the medication had side effects but was not an antidepressant,* they achieved about 90% as much success as patients who were actually taking an antidepressant.[5] This study wasn't just a single study but a meta analysis of studies of antidepressant medications vs. placebos.

This is not to say that all of health is mind over matter, but that the mind does play a major role in health, illness, and recovery. It plays this role in several ways:

- **Our beliefs set up self-fulfilling prophecies and behaviors.** As cognitive dissonance theory indicates, we often think and behave in ways that preserve our beliefs and self-concept rather than undergo the discomfort of confusion, not knowing, and going outside our "comfort zone."

- **Our beliefs about the efficacy of treatment.** With medications and with many treatments, placebo effects (the expectation that the drug or treatment is potent) account for an average of one-third of the benefits. For this reason, medication research is not considered credible unless there is a control group taking placebo medications. The control group's response is compared to the treatment group's response to determine how much of the benefit and side effects are due to placebo effects as opposed to ingredients in the medication.

- **The lifestyles we choose have a profound influence on our health.** If you love your work; enjoy relationships with your family, friends, and coworkers; exercise; and have a sense of purpose in life, you are far more likely to experience good mental and physical health.

- **The meanings we attach to events.** One person is devastated by mom's death and becomes severely depressed. Another person is happy that mom is in heaven and relieved from her suffering. When a driver cuts in front of their car, some people become incensed at the "affront," and go into a rage while others take it in stride. Every year thousands of teenage girls feel their life is over and overdose on pills because their boyfriends "broke up" with them. The stress of an event is determined primarily by the meaning we attach to the event.

- **Our minds and bodies are an apothecary.** Our thinking and behavior produce chemicals in our bodies. If you exercise and have a good outlook on life, your body naturally produces chemicals that help you feel good and have a healthy immune system. If you are sedentary and have a poor outlook, you are far more likely to take antidepressant medications or self-medicate with alcohol, cigarettes, street drugs, or addictive behaviors.

Our conscious minds are only able to focus on about seven things at once. Consequently, most of our thinking and actions are performed unconsciously. Like a computer, the programs we have developed take care of an enormous number of functions. Our conscious minds monitor a few events and redirect our activities if necessary. Initially, we put a lot of time and effort into developing new skills or beliefs. Once we learn them, they function automatically most of the time. It is possible, however, to identify and change our mental programs so they support our longevity goals.

Abraham Lincoln was once supposed to appoint a cabinet member and declined. When his staff asked why, Lincoln replied that he did not like the man's face. His staff objected to his reason and Lincoln replied, "By the time a man is thirty, he is responsible for his face." Lincoln also was quoted as saying, "Most people are about as happy as they make up their minds to be." While most people merely respond to life's choices as they come up, some people choose to sculpt who they want to be. The principle sculpting materials are beliefs.

Beliefs that promote aging and beliefs that promote longevity

The greatest discovery of my generation is that human beings can alter their lives by altering their attitudes of mind.
–William James

You often hear people say things like: "When you get to be my age . . . " or talk about "growing old gracefully," "acting your age," or "being over the hill." Many people believe that 65 means slowing down, giving up sex, and coasting the rest of their lives. These beliefs are deadly. Just as people take antioxidant vitamins to prevent free radical damage, people need to discard their aging beliefs and take "mental anti-aging vitamins." Here are some beliefs that are excellent mental anti-aging vitamins:

1. MY MIND IS A MUSCLE AND I KEEP IT STRONG AND FIT MY WHOLE LIFE.

Fitness requires mental and physical exercise, good nutrition, and taking advantage of medical advances. In the 1950s researchers reported that we lose 100,000 brain cells a day and that senility is inevitable if we live to an old age. Our brains have about a trillion neurons. Even if the 100,000 neurons a day were true, at 150 we would still have 99% of our brain's neurons. More precise research methodology and the use of computers, however, have discredited the dying cell research and yielded a more optimistic picture of aging.[6]

Proof that it is theoretically possible for adults to grow new brain cells came from a curious source. Male canaries sing but the females do not. Unscrupulous pet store owners injected female canaries with the male sex hormone, testosterone. The testosterone enabled them to sing temporarily–long enough to sell them. Researchers eventually found that the testosterone caused brain cell growth. Considerable research is addressing testosterone and Human Growth Hormone supplements in humans. Research on stem cells, infant brain tissue, and spinal cord injuries is closing in on how to grow brain cells in adult human brains. But we don't have to grow new cells to become smarter. We make new connections with other neurons (dendrite growth) continuously as we think and behave.

Aging does bring some decrease in the speed of mental processing, which in turn somewhat limits the complexity of new material that can be processed. Simple associative learning (pairing of ideas or events) shows only a modest decline in healthy elderly people. Older people can perform very complex thinking in areas in which they have developed competencies because they have "chunked" much of the information. Also, they might have developed compensatory strategies. For example, research indicates that older, experienced typists read further ahead in a document they are typing to compensate for slower mental processing. To make an analogy with computers, older individuals experience some decline in the processing speed (megahertz) and have more files on the hard drive. They still have a very capable computer and a computer with a lot more information and programs. This allows that older computer to make more sophisticated operations (as in human judgment).

Epidemiologist David Snowden[7] studied the Sisters of Notre Dame. Since about age twenty, the sisters lived in the same dormitories, ate the same food, and had access to the same health care. Thus, they basically had the same environmental influences. At every age, from 20 to 95, sisters with less than a bachelor's degree had higher mortality rates than sisters with a bachelor's degree. Those who had good vocabularies or improved their vocabularies as they grew older had better mental functioning in their older ages.

A research project with 191 nuns 80 and older studied their mental acuity over time and conducted autopsies on their brains when they died.[8] Many of the nuns did well on cognitive tests and had essentially normal brains when autopsied. Nuns who showed declines on the psychological tests or who had brain abnormalities at autopsy often had genes with ApoE Epsilon alleles that put them at risk for Alzheimer's disease. These gene alleles are receiving extensive research attention as candidates for gene therapy.

Psychologist Becca Levy's experiments demonstrated that when elderly people heard comments about mental faculties declining, they showed poorer thinking and memory than when they hear comments about benefits from wisdom, experience, and integrating accumulated knowledge.[9]

2. I CAN HAVE A SEXUALLY FULFILLING LIFE MY WHOLE LIFE.

A roll in the hay keeps the doctor away.[10]

Women who maintain good health, exercise, and take hormone supplements if needed, can have responsive and enjoyable sexual functioning in their hundreds. With men still tending to seek younger women and women tending to outlive men, one of the biggest difficulties for centenarian women is finding male partners.

Healthy testosterone levels (the principle male sex hormone), good health, and good cardiovascular circulation can keep men functioning well sexually for many, many years. With aids like Viagra, men can have erections long past 100.

Exercise and good nutrition can keep the circulatory system functioning well and prevent atherosclerosis (the biggest obstacle to engorging the penis or clitoris and vagina with blood). Exercise and nutrition promote good health and stimulate production of sex hormones. If that is not sufficient, hormone supplements can bring sex hormones to healthy levels.

Senator Strom Thurmond had the first of his four children at 69. Now in his late 90s he is an influential U.S. senator, tireless campaigner, and third in line to succeed the president. Decades ago Art Linkletter held a contest to see who was the oldest new father. He was 104. He also had twins when he was 100.[11] Linkletter also tells an amusing story of a 78-year-old widow who married a 79-year-old man and after six months she obtained a divorce and complained to a psychologist: "[Sex] That's all he wanted. Twenty-four hours a day . . . sex, sex, sex. I just couldn't take it anymore."[12]

3.   I PRACTICE CONTINUOUS QUALITY IMPROVEMENT WITH MY MENTAL AND PHYSICAL HEALTH.

It's a matter of periodically asking yourself, "If there were one thing I could do to improve my mental and physical health, what would it be?" While some people can work on several self-improvement efforts simultaneously, most people can only focus on one or two things at a time. Trying to do everything at once may dilute the effort. The same continuous quality improvement philosophy that resulted in automobiles and other consumer products lasting longer and functioning better can result in our functioning closer to our optimal levels. Mahoney and Restak[13] describe setting 10% goals, e.g., increase exercise 10%, increase fruits and vegetables 10%, drink 10% more water, increase reading 10%, decrease alcohol consumption 10%, decrease fat consumption 10%. When you achieve one 10% goal, you could increase it another 10% or pursue another 10% goal. Over time the cumulative changes become profound.

Once an improvement is soundly installed, it becomes a habit. As Nathaniel Emmons said, "Habit is either the best of servants or the worst of masters."

One key to improvement is finding role models, coaches, and mentors. There are people who already know and do what we want to learn and do. Why spend a lot of time reinventing the wheel? Another key is seeing criticism as a gift that helps you. As the Sufi poet Rumi put it, "Your criticism polishes my mirror."[14]

4. I LISTEN TO MY BODY AND PROACTIVELY FOSTER GOOD HEALTH.

Having harmony between mind and body involves "listening" to what your body tells you. Your environment and your body are filled with viruses and bacteria. When you catch a cold, the question isn't why you caught a cold, but why now? Colds are usually associated with feeling discouraged, overwhelmed, and run down. Some people have more vulnerable sinuses and respiratory systems than others. Catching a cold should prompt a scan for whether you are feeling discouraged or overstressed and consideration of what might promote a healthier sinus or respiratory system. A chain is only as strong as its weakest link. Most people have one body system that is more problematic than others. Listening to that system should prompt you to search for ways to help that system and strengthen your "weak link."

5. I ALWAYS HAVE A MISSION.

I promise to keep on living as though I expected to live forever.
Nobody grows old by merely living a number of years.
People grow old only by deserting their ideals.
Years may wrinkle the skin,
but to give up interest wrinkles the soul.
–General Douglas MacArthur

Having a mission or purpose in life is essential to our physical and mental health. Research suggests that diseases like cancer are far more likely to occur following depression or loss (e.g., death of a spouse). It's not surprising that major stressors can compromise your sense of purpose and impair your immune system. Conversely, research also indicates that people who have a strong sense of purpose often surprise their doctors by living despite "terminal illnesses."

Even quadriplegics and paraplegics can develop a zest for life as evidenced by individuals like W. Mitchell and Christopher Reeve. W. Mitchell[15] was hit by a drunk driver and suffered massive burns over his whole body and loss of much of his face, hands and feet. He went on to start a business and become a millionaire. He then became paraplegic due to injuries from an airplane crash. He bounced back and became a very successful motivational speaker, author, and even obtained 46% of the votes when he ran for Congress. Christopher Reeve played Superman in films and became quadriplegic when he sustained injuries from a horse riding accident. He has been a very active inspirational speaker, author,[16] and fund-raiser.

Mary Fasano graduated from Harvard at 89. U.S. Senator John Glenn was 77 when he became an astronaut again. Strom Thurmond, who is in his late 90s, is a U.S. senator and third in line to succeed the president of the United States. The Delany sisters wrote their first book, *Having Our Say,* when both were over 100 years old. It became a best-seller and a Broadway play. They also wrote a second best-selling book, *The Delany Sisters' Book of Everyday Wisdom.*

Americans tend to focus on happiness as their ultimate goal. It is in the Declaration of Independence–a God given right to life, liberty, and the pursuit of happiness. But you cannot pursue happiness. It is a by-product of having a purpose and loving and being engrossed in what you do. Focusing on happiness is like going to an amusement park–the rides are fun but when it's over, what's next? Of course not everyone who pursues a purpose will be happy and there are people who, at least consciously, don't have a purpose but are happy. Overall, however, having a mission and pursuing it is the most fruitful path to happiness.

Many people think of happiness as something that happens to you as opposed to something you make happen (by pursuing a mission). As Csikszentmihalyi found, "People are not happy because of what they do but because of how they do it."[17] His research emphasizes that getting fully involved in life and activities (a "flow" state) is vital to happiness. While taxable personal income in the U.S. has doubled between 1960 and 1990, even when adjusted for inflation, the percentage of Americans describing themselves as "very happy" has stayed at 30%.[18]

6. I SEARCH FOR THE SMART WAY TO DO THINGS.

Name virtually any skill and there are thousands of people who have spent a lifetime studying it and thousands of people who are masters at the skill. When I studied famous therapists and hypnotists, their early work was brilliant at the time but looks primitive now. Skills that took them decades to learn, we can now learn in weeks or months. For most skills, there is usually someone with expertise in the skill who has written about how to do it or who can teach it. Often change or learning can happen in an instant when you know how. The trick is learning from other people's experience.

To illustrate, consider the television program, *Inside the Actor's Studio.* In each two-hour program the host interviews one famous actor, actress, or director in depth and illustrates his or her work with movies clips. The guests often generously bare their souls and share their secrets on how they do their craft. The program ends with questions from the audience of acting and directing students. For the price of a monthly cable television bill, an aspiring actor, actress, or director can learn from the masters. If the session was profound, a videotape allows reviewing the program. There are hundreds of television and radio programs that offer high quality learning in other areas. The opportunities to learn from the masters today is incredible. You can even borrow cassette tapes from the library and learn while you are driving in your car.

7. MY MIND, BODY, AND SPIRIT ARE CONSTANTLY RENEWING THEMSELVES.

With reasonable health and nutrition practices, 85% of illnesses cure themselves without medications or a doctor's care. Your mind, body, and spirit have a miraculous capacity to heal and renew if given a chance. The starting point is believing in the process, respecting the process, and providing an environment for the process to work. As a psychologist I never cease to be amazed at how many people who have had miserable and brutal childhoods or challenging lives can turn out to be extraordinarily sensitive, successful, and admirable people. Authors like Bernie Siegel and Norman Cousins document case after case of people who were given a death sentence by their doctors only to have tumors disappear. In *Ageless Body, Timeless Mind,* Deepak Chopra describes how virtually all of the atoms in your body are replaced at least once a year.

8. I CULTIVATE MY SENSE OF HUMOR.

You don't stop laughing because you grow old;
you grow old because you stop laughing.
–Michael Pritchard

He who laughs lasts.

Humor helps you develop perspective and not take yourself too seriously. Want to stay "mentally fit?" Read a cartoon or listen to some jokes. These might seem like frivolous pleasures, but mentally they are extremely complex tasks. Humor requires appreciating other perspectives and understanding cultural norms and expectations. It is no accident that one of the eleven tests on the world's most respected IQ test asks people to arrange cartoon pictures to tell a story. For people who are learning a language or culture, understanding the culture's humor is one of the last skills they master. Humor requires great judgment and insight in knowing whether someone is likely to find something funny. What is funny to one person might be dumb or even offensive to another person.

Just as physical fitness is a "use it or lose it" proposition, your ability to understand humor declines with age *unless* you exercise your sense of humor on a regular basis. The phrase "someday you'll laugh at this" illustrates how humor also helps us put pain in perspective. Cartoons like *Peanuts* (Charlie Brown) and *Ziggy* prompt us to not take ourselves too seriously. *Dilbert's* satire assures us that we're not crazy but sometimes our jobs are. *The Family Circus* helps us appreciate how children perceive the world, enabling us to be more sensitive to their needs and nourish our childlike sides. *Doonesbury* and political cartoons lampoon our political processes and help us see when "the emperor has no clothes." Humor's ability to get us to appreciate others' perspectives is a great antidote for racial, political, and international problems.

Personal challenges for humor might be: 1) remembering even two jokes when a stand-up comedian fires one after another and has you in stitches, 2) telling a joke yourself and getting a laugh, and 3) developing your own jokes. Joking with young children provides a great opportunity to exercise humor and not worry about looking foolish or blowing a punch line. Of course you do have to hear a lot of knock knock jokes–over and over. When you listen to young children trying to make up their own jokes, you realize how much a person has to understand for humor to work.

In short, humor is an art form that exercises our minds. Appreciating humor can keep you "mentally fit" and add fun and enjoyment to your life. It is a great stress reliever.

9. I CULTIVATE A POSITIVE VOCABULARY.

Some words seduce people into unresourceful states. Examples that are best deleted from your vocabulary include: victim, pain, dysfunctional, and failure. This is not to suggest that you sanitize your vocabulary with euphemisms, but that you reframe issues with positive, hopeful terms. People often use metaphors such as you are breaking my heart, you are killing me, you give me a headache. Popular music uses a lot of these metaphors. The problem is that your body may believe you. Such phrases need to be replaced with more positive ways of expressing yourself.

Tony Robbins tells a fascinating story of how he was in a meeting and he became upset about a business deal. His business partner was unflappable. Robbins asked his partner why he wasn't upset. His partner explained that he taught himself not to get upset because doing so would place him at a disadvantage in negotiating business deals. Robbins pushed the issue by asking whether he wasn't outraged when the IRS audited them and withheld millions of dollars for years until Robbins eventually prevailed. His partner replied that he had been "a little perturbed."

If someone asks your age, you can be evasive, like Satchel Paige who responded, "How old would you be if you didn't know how old you was?" Or you can say "I'm *only* __years old."

Exercise 4-1: "Bad words"

When our kids were in elementary school they would periodically say, "aw, he said a bad word." They were referring to "four letter" words. The worst bad words, however, are words that prompt us to think negatively, pessimistically, and powerlessly. Make a list of these words that you tend to say and ask your spouse, friends, or colleagues to tease you with an "aw, you said a bad word" when you say them. Want to put some teeth into it? Offer to pay them a dollar every time they do it.

10. I CULTIVATE FOND MEMORIES AND LET BAD MEMORIES WITHER.

Belle Boone Beard's research[19] with centenarians found that they related twice as many positive memories as negative memories. She found that even when people's lives had a lot of tragedy, they often focused on the positive, such as how kind people were to them. She observed, "In general centenarians can recall so many more pleasant memories that I wonder whether they may deliberately have repressed unhappy memories."[20] Cultivating memories is like gardening–you need to nourish the good memories and weed out the bad ones.

11. ANY SUGGESTIONS OF SURGERY PROMPT AN INTENSE SEARCH FOR ALTERNATIVE SOLUTIONS.

Alternative therapies, e.g., meditation, spiritual practices, exercise, massage, better nutrition, and herbal treatments often can effect healing without surgery. Caution is certainly indicated as alternative therapies include a lot of silliness and quackery. Fortunately, physicians have started some rapprochement with alternative therapies and scientists are conducting more research on alternative therapies. Seventy-five medical schools now offer courses in alternative medicine. Authors like Andrew Weil, Herbert Benson, and Deepak Chopra offer the public research-oriented, integrative, balanced, and pragmatic approaches to considering alternative therapies.

I mean no disrespect to the good work surgeons do. Their focus, however, is on how surgery would help. Unless the surgery is urgent, it is wise to explore alternatives for several reasons:[21]

- Every year millions of unnecessary surgeries are performed. U.S. estimates are that between six and ten million surgeries a year are unnecessary (which is 20% of all U.S. surgeries). For example, the cesarean section ("C-section") rate in the U.S. was 5% in 1970. In the first half of the 1990s the rate was 23% in the U.S. but only 11% in England. Physicians and insurance companies became alarmed about these high rates and began a campaign to lower the rates to a target of 5.5%. Other very common surgeries that are unnecessary include 22% of hysterectomies and 30% of coronary bypasses.

- The mortality rate for major surgeries in the U.S. is 1.33%. With six to ten million unnecessary surgeries each year, there are tens of thousands of unnecessary surgery deaths a year. There are also complications from surgeries. Ten percent of hospital patients acquire an infection from their hospital stay. Twenty percent of hospital patients leave with a condition they didn't have when they entered the hospital.[22]

- Surgery that cuts muscles or fascia often disrupts posture and the relative position of organs. Consequently, it is not unusual for people to "recover normally" from surgery only to develop serious health problems several months later. There are therapists who know how to identify these problems and re-educate muscles to compensate. Most medical practitioners, however, are not familiar with the problems or the solutions. Surgeries for back problems and quite a few other body pains might be unnecessary with muscle reeducation. Surgeries for gastrointestinal problems, e.g., colostomies, could be unnecessary if treated with nutritional therapies, massage, relaxation, and/or colonics.

- Medical practitioners are in the business of providing medical treatments and are not likely to have expertise in alternative treatments or to promote alternative treatments. The number of surgeons in the U.S. has been increasing by 15% a year while the population is only increasing 4% a year. Thus, there is likely to be more "marketing" of surgery. Consumers must take responsibility for exploring alternatives.

- With most surgical expenses paid for by insurance, Medicare or Medicaid, consumers have been shielded from comparison information about different hospitals and surgeons. In the 1990s managed care has paid a lot of attention to these data, but many of their decisions appear to be based on costs as opposed to outcomes. Comparison information on surgery success rates is still difficult for the public to access.

- Some surgeries have a generally poor satisfaction rate. The literature on back disc surgeries and laminectomies, for example, found that 3.3.% of patients report increased pain, 2% report other complications, and 29% of patients report poor results. The "complete cure" rate is only about 50%. Certainly, alternative therapies such as Egoscue,[23] chiropractic, massage, and others are worth exploring first. (Egoscue is a system of exercises for aligning posture and movement. The exercises can be done at home.)

12. I MOVE LIKE A 20-YEAR-OLD.

Your body needs movement to function well–it's a "use it or lose it" system. One reason that people age physically is that they don't move as much as young people. There is no law saying they can't. "Acting one's age" is a death sentence. Moving keeps your muscles and bones strong. The lymph system, unlike the circulatory system, has no pump. The only way to get lymph to circulate is through body movement and breathing. Even emotions come from motion (hence the Latin derivation e[from]-motion). If playing music makes you feel like dancing and helps you move like a 20-year-old or even a teenager, do it.

Interestingly some of the leaders in the movement therapies developed their therapies because they were in pain. Physicist Moshe Feldenkris developed his system of movement therapy to overcome knee injuries that left him crippled. Peter Egoscue developed his system to help him recover from injuries he sustained in the Vietnam War. Callan Pinckney developed Callanetics to help her misaligned back, damaged knees, and failing health. Shakespearian actor Frederick Alexander developed his posture system to resolve his difficulty projecting his voice on stage. They demonstrate that even people who have poor posture or disabilities often can learn to move and function youthfully.

13. I EXERCISE MY EYES TO IMPROVE MY VISION.

With reading, computer screens, and indoor lighting, our lifestyles can be hard on our vision. The Bates system and variations of it provide exercises and visual hygiene practices that help people see better.[24] The Bates literature reports often reversing visual losses. Even if the program only prevents or slows loss, it is worth considering. Exercises can be slipped in while waiting at a traffic light, waiting in a line, or other down times. Simple exercises include:

- moving your eyes in counterclockwise and clockwise directions
- focusing your eyes progressively further away and then closer
- visualizing pictures in your mind's eye
- rubbing the palms of your hands together and placing them over your eyes (palming)
- relaxing your shoulder and head muscles
- yawning

Just as people who believe they can't do something subtly give themselves "hypnotic" self-defeating messages, your beliefs about your vision affects your vision. Visual histories of family members might lead you to expect similar visual problems. People who have painful memories might experience distortion in their vision and avoid visualizing in their mind's eye. People who do not like interacting with other people might obtain secondary benefits from being nearsighted. If you think the world is beautiful and you are delighted to see people, you are more likely to be giving your brain positive suggestions about seeing well. A sparkling mind and spirit show with eyes that sparkle.

I recall noticing that many scholarly people wear reading glasses and came to associate reading glasses with scholarship. I revere scholarship but dropped associating it with glasses. Now when I see reading glasses, they prompt me to do some eye exercises and reduce my need for reading glasses (or at least needing stronger ones).

It's no accident that the word vision not only connotes seeing but also imagination and foresight.

14. I AM A LIFELONG LEARNER.

Lifelong learning keeps you mentally sharp and fit. It helps you know how to take care of your health and finances, succeed at jobs, and enhance your relationships. It nurtures your sense of purpose and mission in life. With today's incredible pace of change, lifelong learning is essential to prospering and living to 150. Alvin Toffler in *Future Shock* observed that the pace of change is so rapid, most people will experience several careers in their lifetimes.

Universities are attracting increasing numbers of older students. Television, which used to just be three networks, now includes many high quality programs. The Internet and libraries give us incredible access to information. Virtual realities are in their infancy and will offer fantastic learning opportunities. We have unparalleled resources for lifelong learning. Our minds are like muscles—we can let them wither or we can use them and strengthen them.

When I was young I was amazed at Plutarch's statement that the elder Cato began at the age of 80 to learn Greek. I am amazed no longer. Old age is ready to undertake tasks that youth shirked because they would take too long. –William Somerset Maugham[25]

15. EVERY AGE HAS ITS BENEFITS.

*One way to look at getting older is to say "Whatever age I am is the **best** age." To that I add, "The age we **live in** is the best age."*
–Helen Hayes[26]

The antithesis of this belief is saying, wait until I'm old enough to drive, until I get married, until the kids are grown, until I retire . . . then I'll enjoy life. The trick is to focus on the benefits of your current age and experience your current age as the best of times. It's similar to what optimists do–putting the positives in the foreground and the negatives in the background. While "reality" has positives and negatives, optimists are happier, healthier, and live longer. Feminist Germaine Greer[27] believes menopause can be a very liberating experience in which many women hit a new stride of serenity, power, and productivity. Gail Sheehy in *New Passages* relates how "older" women and men are embracing a second adulthood with deeper meaning, renewed playfulness, and renewed creativity. She refers to the second adulthood as occurring between 45-85+ and the Age of Integrity occurring at 65-85+. I'm delighted to see her put the pluses on the end but she is still far from anticipating 150 and what to call the years from 85 to 150. When Ronald Reagan was campaigning for the presidency and his age was questioned, he quipped, "I won't hold my opponent's inexperience against him." Psychologists have found that older adults regulate their emotions better and are happier.[28]

16. I EXPECT TO HAVE AN ENJOYABLE, EXCITING LIFE AT 150.

*We are what and where we are
because we have first imagined it.* –Donald Curtis

There are two sources of support for this expectation: One comes from seeking data to support it. Information on advances in medicine, nutrition, and fitness, and centenarian role models, support a belief in increasing longevity and health and provide knowledge on how to do it. The second source is doing the things you need to do to make it happen. Just wanting it doesn't mean you will achieve it. Exercising, eating well, learning, and following the beliefs in this chapter make it happen and give you the evidence.

The more you imagine yourself having an exciting life in your hundreds and "script yourself" to do it, the more likely it is to happen. When your mind "plays movies" of what you will be doing in your hundreds, it sets out to make those movies happen. Your mind conceives it and then achieves it. The "writing your obituary" exercise in Chapter 7 can be very helpful in imaging and scripting your future for longevity. To illustrate I have included my obituary (sometime after 2095) in the Appendix.

17. I AM A TRAILBLAZER WHO LEAVES BEHIND CONVENTIONAL THINKING ABOUT LONGEVITY.

There are no Casper Milquetoasts among centenarians. . . .
they express themselves in bold and unconventional ways.
–Professor Belle Boone Beard[29]
who studied thousands of centenarians

What would you do if you were ten times bolder?
–Laurie Beth Jones, *The Path*

People are expected to "act their age" and "we all know" that "older people just can't do what they used to do." Unless you consciously and unconsciously have clear, strong beliefs to the contrary, you will get sucked into the conventional beliefs and expectations. Consequently, you need to think of yourself as following a different drummer and being out of step with what most people believe about aging. You are a pioneer, charting unmapped territory in time.

18. I HAVE A SERENITY ABOUT OUTLIVING MOST PEOPLE I KNOW.

If every death is traumatic for you, you will wear yourself out before you get to 150. It is important to have a sense of perspective and the big picture. You can care and feel without feeling every death is tragic. Most deaths aren't a tragedy. A tragedy is not living life fully, a list of what ifs, and not connecting with life. For many people the tragedy occurred years ago when they numbed themselves to experiencing life fully. As poet Stephen Vincent Benet put it, "Life is not lost by dying; life is lost minute by minute, day by dragging day, in all the thousand small uncaring ways." For those who have lived a full life but disease has greatly compromised their lives, death can be a relief.

When one of my children's classmates died of leukemia, I cried, imagining how I would feel if it had happened to one of my children. While the family suffered immense grief, they also became profoundly close and appreciated each other and appreciated life at a depth that few experience. They experienced an outpouring of love and support from friends and neighbors. Even lives cut short can prompt us to spiritual growth. Napoleon Hill expressed this with his belief that every adversity carries the seed of an equal or greater reward. Consider the example of Candy Lightner. Her 13-year-old daughter was walking home, on the sidewalk, and was killed by a repeat offender drunk driver. To prevent this from happening to other families, Ms. Lightner founded Mothers Against Drunk Driving (MADD). MADD's three million members have prevented tens of thousands of deaths from drunken driving. Another example of making the best of a premature death is in Rabbi Harold Kushner's wonderful book, *When Bad Things Happen to Good People.* Kushner describes his spiritual crisis when his son died of a rare disease and how he came to terms with the loss. Briefly he said God created a wonderful world with exquisite laws of nature and does not intervene in the laws of nature. Nevertheless, God is a powerful resource for finding meaning and coping.

People who believe in heaven or in reincarnation often find it easier to have perspective on death as they don't see death as the end. Chapter 10 discusses outliving friends and family in more detail.

19. I MAKE NEW FRIENDS ALL MY LIFE.

Make new friends and keep the old.
One is silver and the other gold .–a Girl Scout song

If you are going to live well past 100, you are going to outlive many of your friends and family members. Longevity requires good skills at dealing with losses (and *Defy Aging* devotes a whole chapter to the issue). Since you will be losing friends, it is essential that you keep making new friends all of your life.

"Socioemotional selective theory" has found that as people age most people narrow their social networks and focus on a smaller number of friends.[30] Emphasizing quality and depth is fine. To live to 150, however, you have to reject this conventional path and choose to make new friends all your life. Early in our careers we tend to focus on doing things–getting an education, job achievements, child rearing. By age 50 many people experience a values shift and begin placing more emphasis on relationships and friendships. Those who don't make this shift often find their later years are lonely years.

20. I'M REALLY YOUNGER THAN MY CHRONOLOGICAL AGE.

People are forever being told to "act their age,"
but the role no longer comes with stage directions.
                    –Joan Rivers[31]

How old would you be if you didn't know how old you was?
                    –Satchel Paige

We tend to become like the people we spend the most time with and the people we admire and want as friends. Thus, having friends who are young or have the freshness and passion of youth helps us stay young.

You could just look at your healthy body and lifestyle and know you are healthier than other people your chronological age. You could view yourself as blessed with a youthful mind and body. You could attribute your youthfulness to the things you do to stay youthful (exercise, movement, nutrition, beliefs, etc.). However you do it, you need to consciously and unconsciously think of yourself as prematurely young. As actress Betty White put it, "If you are a vital person, inside your head, that same person is still going on [as you age]. If you were a dull young person, you probably entered old age at thirty."[32] Comedian Phyllis Diller said of her face lifts, "It's done wonders for me...absolute wonders and I'm all for it!...you feel young inside and you get a boost from it every day. The best thing about it is that when I look in the mirror, my face matches what I feel inside–young."[33] Bob Hope says he doesn't consider himself old but a combination of all ages.[34]

21. I PACE MYSELF–I'M GOING TO BE AROUND A LONG TIME.

It's easy to take ourselves too seriously or become stressed. Pacing reminds you to keep perspective and not burn out or take undue risks. Most National Football League athletes don't live to 65 (and they started as some of the healthiest people in the country). As Aesop moralized in the story of the *Tortoise and the Hare*, "The race is not always to the swift." Turtles and tortoises appear to have the longest longevity in the animal kingdom. They get older and wiser but they don't show physiological signs of aging. Because they are well protected from predators, they have little stress in their lives. Few turtles or tortoises have birth certificates but scientists can count the rings on their shell the way they count rings on a tree. One giant tortoise that was captured in 1768 near the island of Mauritius lived for 150 years. He was still spry when he accidently fell off a ledge and died in the fall. In the plant kingdom, some trees have lived for over 5,000 years.

Contrast the lives of tortoises with the lives of opossums. Out of a litter of thirty, only five to ten babies live to be weaned. They lack speed or effective fighting skills and don't have a shell to protect them. Indeed one of their defenses is to pretend to be dead. They try to find their prey at night to evade their many predators. Their perilous life contributes to a maximum life span of only 2½ years and frequent problems with arthritis, cataracts, and weight loss.

Opossum researcher Steven Austad[35] found that on Sapelo island, a barrier island five miles off the Georgia coast, opossums had no predators. There opossums weren't timid and ventured out during the day. Tissue samples showed they aged more slowly than their mainland relatives. They also lived 25% longer. The longest living island opossum has lived 50% longer than any recorded mainland opossum. Apparently their less stressful lives resulted in their bodies producing fewer glucocorticoids for fight/flight responses and their bodies were better able to heal and repair when relaxed.

Pacific Salmon give another interesting example of the effect of stress. They swim and leap upstream in a frenzied pilgrimage to their spawning grounds to mate. Within a few weeks of mating, they die with bulging adrenal glands, stomach ulcers, kidney lesions, and a collapsed immune system. When a salmon's adrenal glands are removed shortly after mating, however, the salmon lives for another twelve months instead of two weeks.

The human parallels are obvious. Living a "Type A" lifestyle causes faster aging. The goal is not to live a stress-free life, but to have enough stress to make life interesting and challenging, but not so much as to tax your mind and body's health.

When you decide and believe that you can live to 150, it changes your perspective on life. You can skip that mid-life crisis at 40. You have time to pursue several careers or interests before mid-life at 75. Hormone replacement, which is common for women and will soon be common for men, will delay the physical and emotional shifts and sexual decline that used to occur with declining hormone levels. You would have an extra 35 years to rebound from setbacks and try new things before your mid-life crisis at 75, if you still want to have one.

22. I CHOOSE LIFE ENHANCING RISKS AND REDUCE RISKS WITH LITTLE BENEFIT.

Living 150 years gives you lots of opportunities to take risks. Taking risks (that don't kill or maim you) make life exciting and challenging. If we don't succeed at a venture, it can still be a learning and growth experience. Taking risks allows us to, as Joseph Campbell put it, "follow our bliss."

The other side of the coin are risks that have little payoff. For example, as teenagers many of us drove too fast and took other risks with fleeting benefits. Teenagers often act as if they were immortal. Many things we did as teenagers seem foolish in retrospect. You can make the same use of perspective to discern what things you do now that will seem unwise in the future. Living 150 years exposes you to a lot of risks such as automobile accidents, crime, and health hazards. Reducing these risks can be critical to living to 150.

23. I USE THE SERENITY PRAYER TO GIVE ME PERSPECTIVE.

God give us grace to accept with serenity the things that cannot be changed, courage to change the things which should be changed, and the wisdom to distinguish one from another.
–Reinhold Niebuhr

Theologian Reinhold Niebuhr put the serenity prayer in his church bulletin in 1934 and published it in the *Bulletin of the Federal Council of Churches* in 1943. Neibuhr is a good role model for the principle. He espoused pacifism and socialism in the 1930s but dropped both to oppose Hitler and Stalin. He was an early opponent of the Vietnam war and a founding member of the (liberal) Americans for Democratic Action. Dubbed "American politicians' favorite theologian" and a favorite of the Kennedy administration, he advocated "Christian realism." He wrote several books and taught at Union Theological Seminar for thirty years. Niebuhr, however, in turn attributed the prayer to 18th century Lutheran theologian Friedrich Oetinger.[36]

AA (Alcoholics Anonymous) adopted and immortalized the prayer. AA's version is stated more simply: *God grant me the serenity to accept the things I cannot change, the courage to change the things I can, and the wisdom to know the difference.*

Those who have difficulty relating to "God," address the prayer to their "Higher Power."

Consider how some survivors of Nazi concentration camps have a bright outlook and how some individuals who have a very comfortable life "worry themselves to death." It's not the amount of stress you have in life that ages you; it's how you handle it. Serenity helps you have confidence in following your beliefs and goals and confidence that the universe or God will help by providing what you need (if not always what you want).

Worry is like a rocking chair–it gives you something to do,
    but it doesn't get you anywhere. –Dorothy Galyean

Worry is just about the worst form of mental activity there is . . .
Worry is pointless. It is wasted mental energy. It also creates bio-
chemical reactions which harm the body, producing everything
from indigestion to coronary arrest, and a multitude of things in
between . . . Worry, hate, fear–together with its offshoots . . . all
attack the body at the cellular level. It is impossible to have a
healthy body under these conditions.
–Neale Donald Walsh, *Conversations with God,* Book 1, p. 188.

Even counting sheep is no good. I counted 10,000 in my sleep,
sheared them, combed and spun the wool, made them into coats,
took them to market, and lost $50. I haven't slept for a week.

Worry tries to cross the bridge before you come to it.

Worry makes the world go round, and round, and round.

24. I AM CHEERFUL.

Opera diva Beverly Sills has had a number of tragedies in her life. She has two children–one has mental retardation and the other is deaf. Her singing career was shortened by cancer. In her autobiography, *Bubbles,* she said she has been asked if she is happy and responded that with all of the tragedies in her life, she wouldn't say she was happy but she is cheerful. Happiness comes from having a mission and having some success in pursuing that mission. It is a process which many people find elusive. Cheerfulness, however, is more concrete. You know how to be cheerful. Even if you have to act it, it often becomes natural after a while. Like the song in *The King and I,* "make believe you're brave (or in this case cheerful) and the trick will take you far, you may be as brave (cheerful) as you make believe you are." Cheerfulness helps people feel good, enhances the immune system, and enhances relationships with others. It doesn't cost anything. Making cheerfulness part of your self-concept makes cheerfulness more likely to be a frequent emotional state and even your default emotional state.

25. I HAVE A CONTINGENCY FUND.

Following a different drummer requires rejecting a living from paycheck to paycheck mentality. Instead you need to save funds for career changes, hard times, health needs, or just taking a sabbatical. Stocks, bonds, and mutual funds often are good for contingency funds because they tend to have higher earnings than bank accounts and they are liquid. With such a fund, education, retraining, a sabbatical, or just taking some time off is a planned, funded expense–not a wish or fantasy. Knowing you have funds in case of unemployment or hard times can help you worry less and sleep better. It leaves you prepared for adversity.

26. I OBSERVE AND FOLLOW WHAT WORKS FOR ME RATHER THAN BLINDLY FOLLOWING GENERIC OR EXPERT ADVICE.

Most people who give advice promote what worked for them. It might not be what works for you. The best course is to choose what advice makes the most sense but regard it as a hypothesis that you need to test and validate or reject. The diet that works splendidly for a friend or celebrity might be terrible for you.

27. THE RESOURCES FOR LIVING LONGER ARE IMPROVING EVERY YEAR.

Chapter 17 discusses some of the incredible scientific advances that are changing our lives and extending our longevity. You can follow scientific advances in newspapers, magazines, newsletters, journals, the Internet, and even carefully selected radio and television programs. Knowing that resources are constantly improving and new resources are continually in the pipeline fosters justified optimism about longevity. That doesn't mean you need to be the first one to try every new product or procedure. It's usually wiser to wait until the bugs are worked out and the research is clear that it is safe.

28. THERE ARE NO ACCIDENTS IN LIFE.

This is perhaps the ultimate in optimism and faith. (I have to admit that I'm still struggling with adopting this one.) People who believe that everything happens for a purpose and that God is helping them are happier, healthier people. An extreme variation of the belief is Clement Stone's belief that the universe is conspiring to help him. Even if there were no God, believing in God prompts a lot of people to live a richer, happier life. Likewise, believing there are no accidents in life tends to prompt a richer, happier life whether the premise is true or not.

29. I DON'T NEED MANY MATERIAL THINGS TO MAKE ME HAPPY AND SUCCESSFUL.

For Americans in particular, it seems that we would be happy if only we had 50% more income. Of course, if we had that 50% more we would feel that our initial statement wasn't quite accurate but we would be happy if only we had another 50%. There is nothing wrong with material possessions. Beyond a basic level, however, they are not essential for a happy, fulfilling life.

Money gives you the ability to access lots of resources and help lots of people. If it puts you on a stressful, unfulfilling treadmill, however, it is not worth the price. The issue is whether pursuing more money fits with your mission and whether it interferes with other important values such as health, family, and friends. The U.S., Germany, and Japan are wealthy nations but surveys find that citizens of several less affluent countries score higher on measures of happiness. Within countries the relationship between money and happiness is a weak one. A study of lottery winners found they were no happier than people who had disabilities such as paraplegia or blindness (after a period of time for both to adjust to their circumstances).[37]

The antidote is to live below your means. If you need role models, *The Millionaire Next Door* cites many millionaires, including Sam Walton of Wal-Mart fame, who chooses a modest lifestyle and drives an old pickup truck. The belief does not imply that it is wrong to invest everything you have in pursuing a dream. Doing so, however, is a tough call and the criteria include both whether it really is a dream (vs. just making more money) and whether it has a chance at success.

If you love collecting art, antiques, or collectibles, keep in mind that you can choose to pay money to acquire them, house them, maintain them, and insure them or you can allow museums and shops to do this for you.

30. IF I INTELLIGENTLY PURSUE WHAT I LOVE, THE MONEY WILL COME.

When you love what you are doing, extraordinary effort, study, and practice are a labor of love. If you love what you do, you will become very good at it and people will sense your love and expertise and seek your services. When you don't like what you do, it takes a toll on you physically and mentally. I have met taxi drivers who love what they do and "make people's day" with their cheerfulness, friendliness, and their joy of life. The trick is seeing the larger picture and becoming engrossed in what you are doing (what Csikszentmihalyi calls flow). Flow involves doing something that is complex enough to be challenging but not so complex as to be overwhelming or impossible. Achieving this optimal balance often leads to becoming totally absorbed in the activity. Assuming the activity is a healthy one, you want to have a lot of "flow" in your life. Even with flow states, however, you need to apply two other criteria. One is Aristotle's admonition for all things in moderation. Thus you need to ask whether a particular pursuit compromises your health, family relations, or other important areas of your life. The second criterion involves ruling out addictions. I would functionally define an addiction as compulsively, persistently pursuing something despite unhealthy consequences.

31. PEOPLE WANT TO HELP.

If you don't ask, you don't get. –Mohandas Ghandi

When someone asks you for help, isn't your first inclination to try to help? Isn't it especially true if the person asks nicely and appreciatively? People tend to respond to your expectations and if you expect them to want to help, it is amazing how often they will. If you have difficulty asking for help, I would recommend the book or tape, *The Aladdin Factor* by Jack Canfield and Mark Victor Hansen.

32. I CAN GET EVERYTHING IN LIFE I WANT IF I JUST HELP ENOUGH OTHER PEOPLE GET WHAT THEY WANT.

This is motivational speaker Zig Ziglar's credo. It is a "win-win" philosophy. Note that he doesn't say that every time you help someone you will receive a one-to-one return. If the contingency were that direct, almost everyone would do it. It does say "what goes around, comes around." Einstein said the most fundamental question in life is, "Is the world a friendly place?" Zig Ziglar's philosophy says yes. The truth seems to lie with Henry Ford's maxim, "If you think you can or you think you can't, you are right." Thus if you believe and follow Ziglar's philosophy, it will be true for you and help you to be healthier and more successful. You might think of this belief as a proactive version of the Golden Rule (do onto others as you would have them do onto you).

33. IF I LOCK IN MY INTENT, THE UNIVERSE WILL PROVIDE.

What most people, or at least the unsuccessful ones, are unaware of is that life gives us exactly what we ask from it. The first thing to do, therefore, is to ask for exactly what you want. If your request is vague, whatever you get will be just as muddled. If you ask for the minimum, you'll get the minimum.
    –Mark Fisher, *The Instant Millionaire*, p. 44.

When we are clear about what we want, resources seem to appear miraculously. Our antennae are up and detecting things we didn't see before. It could be that our intentions send out energy fields that attract resources. Believing what we want is available opens our eyes to seeing it. To use Wayne Dyer's phrase and book title, *"You'll see it when you believe it."*

34. ANYTHING I NEED TO KNOW IS AVAILABLE TO ME–IN A BOOK, LIBRARY, THE INTERNET, OTHER PEOPLE, OR MYSELF.

It's amazing how often we assume that the information isn't there. We live in such a rich world. If we start with the assumption that the information is there for the finding and we decide it is worth tracking down, we'll find it.

35. MOST PROBLEMS ARE JUST INCONVENIENCES OR CHALLENGES.

In *Uh-oh*, Robert Fulghum[38] tells a delightful story about when he was a young man and had a 20-minute tantrum about being served wieners and sauerkraut every day for more than a week. His coworker listened patiently for 20 minutes and then told him the problem wasn't with the sauerkraut and wieners–but that he didn't realize the difference between an inconvenience and a problem. His coworker was a survivor of Auschwitz. When he was in Auschwitz, the sauerkraut alone would have been a dream come true. If we keep in perspective how blessed we are, we can easily see almost all of our problems as really just inconveniences. Will the belief take the passion out of our lives? Hardly. Rather it will make us more compassionate, cheerful, and resourceful. Often our inconveniences are begging, even screaming opportunities that we can use as springboards for being creative, helpful, or finding new solutions.

36. WE ARE FORTUNATE TO LIVE IN A LONGEVITY REVOLUTION.

As indicated in earlier chapters and Chapter 17, we live in extraordinary times. Life spans have increased as much in the last 100 years as they did in the preceding 5,000 years. Genetic engineering, tissue engineering, hormone therapies and other medical advances are likely to continue making dramatic innovations that enable us to look, feel, and function better. Advances in informational and educational resources are incredible and the technological advances show no signs of slowing. Changes in the marketplace and constant change are making it easier to work as long as we want and to be your own boss. There is an exciting longevity revolution going on and we are fortunate to be part of it.

Chapter 5

How to Change Beliefs

Progress is impossible without change,
and those who cannot change their minds
cannot change anything. –George Bernard Shaw

Life is exactly as you picture it. . . . if you want to change your
life, you must start by changing your thoughts.
–Mark Fisher, *The Instant Millionaire*, p. 50

Why is it that people can sincerely try to change a belief but the change doesn't stick? Sometimes there just wasn't enough power in the effort. Sometimes unconscious resistance put a priority on maintaining consistency with other beliefs and behaviors. Success is more likely when you use powerful strategies and address any subconscious "objections."

Principles for developing powerful strategies

- Make sure the belief is stated in the positive, e.g., I give lots of compliments.
- Make sure your words don't hedge, e.g., I'll *try*, I *can* (vs. I will).
- State or summarize the belief in a catch phrase that appeals to you, e.g., I'm spreading sunshine.
- Make up a song about the belief and sing it to yourself.
- Visualize the belief, hear the belief, and feel the belief.
- If you can, even taste and smell the belief, e.g., the sweet smell of success, I can taste victory.
- Inventory any beliefs or behaviors you have that conflict with the new belief, e.g., people might think I am patronizing or phony. Determine how you can reconcile the contradictions.
- Make sure you have an attitude of respect for your unconscious and any objections it might have. It has been working hard for many years to help you and protect you. Relax, close your eyes, "go inside" yourself, and ask whether there are any objections to the new belief. Listen for a quiet voice that has reservations or for unusual physical sensations. If there are physical sensations ask

what they are trying to tell you. If there are objections, determine the *intent* of the objections and how you can meet the needs of the intent.
• Develop an icon to represent the new belief.
• When talking about the belief, saying the catch phrase or affirmations, or visualizing the icon, use animated, enthusiastic, affirmative body language.

Exercise 5-1: Choose a belief you would like to change and map across the submodalities.[1]

People think in visual images, sounds, and kinesthetic feelings (modalities). If you change the way you represent a thought, it often changes what you feel and what you believe. Thus you can change the submodalities (qualities of the modality) to change your feelings and beliefs.

Think about something you strongly believe and picture a representation of the belief in your mind's eye. If you are not good at visualizing, sense the image in your mind's eye. Note the following qualities of the picture or image:
• How big is the picture?
• Is it in color or black and white?
• Is it still or moving?
• How far does the image seem to be from your face?
• Where does the image seem to be in space (e.g., up or down, right or left)?

Now think about the belief you want to have. Picture this belief in your mind's eye. Note how the qualities of this picture differ from the qualities of your strong belief picture. Change the qualities (submodalities) of the new belief to match the qualities in your strong belief picture. For many people, merely moving the picture to the location of the strong belief makes the new belief more credible.

Exercise 5-2: Physically installing a new belief [2]

This exercise is especially effective for installing a new belief. It is very helpful to have someone coach you through the exercise, but you can do it on your own. With each step of the exercise, it is important to remember exactly where in the room you did each step.

1. Think about the current belief you have that <u>you want to change</u> (e.g., I can't lose weight no matter how hard I try). Note your posture, mannerisms, and body sensations and make sure you fully experience them.

2. Move to another location in the room and think about the new belief <u>you want</u> to have (e.g., The real me is trim and healthy). Spend as much time as you need to find a phrase that really clicks for you and gets you excited. Amplify this belief so it generates great enthusiasm. Note your posture, mannerisms, and body sensations. (Do not proceed unless you are "salivating" to have this new belief.)

3. Move to another location and think of something that you are <u>unsure</u> about (e.g., Will the stock market go up or down tomorrow? or Will it rain next week?). Note your posture, mannerisms, and body sensations and make sure you fully experience them.

4. Move to another location and recall a belief that you once had but <u>no longer believe</u> (e.g., The Easter Bunny will bring me a basket of candy). Note your posture, mannerisms, and body sensations and make sure you fully experience them.

5. Move to another location and think about something that you used to believe but <u>now you believe the opposite</u> (e.g., a person that you once thought was wonderful but found out they were not, or vice versa). Note your posture, mannerisms, and body sensations and make sure you fully experience them.

6. If there is something in the room that represents <u>sacred and enduring values</u>, pick that location (e.g., a particular work or art, a collection of books, a Bible). Think of something that you feel very, very strongly about. This needs to be a sacred belief and a core value. It should be a belief that you would risk your life for, such as making sure children are not sexually molested. Note your

posture, mannerisms, and body sensations and make sure you fully experience them.

7. Go back to the location where you had the <u>unsure</u> belief (e.g., tomorrow's weather) and think about it again. While fully experiencing its posture, mannerisms, and body sensations, think about the old belief that <u>you want to change</u>.

8. Go back to the location for the belief that you <u>no longer believe</u> (e.g., the Easter Bunny). While fully experiencing its posture, mannerisms, and body sensations, think about the belief that <u>you want to change</u>.

9. Go back to the location for <u>now you believe the opposite</u>. While fully experiencing its posture, mannerisms, and body sensations, think about the old belief that <u>you want to change</u> and the <u>new belief</u>. Switch back and forth between the two beliefs, experiencing amazement at how strongly beliefs can change.

10. Go back to the location for <u>sacred or enduring values</u>. Note your posture, mannerisms, and body sensations. Keeping that posture and mannerisms, think about the <u>belief you want</u>. Switch back and forth between your <u>sacred belief</u> and you <u>new belief</u>. Amplify the feelings.

11. Go to the original location where you first thought about the old <u>belief you do not want,</u> taking with you your strong convictions about the belief <u>you want</u> and the posture and mannerisms that now go with it. Notice how the new belief <u>you want</u> has now replaced the old one and has many references in your mind and body to make it convincing and stable.

Exercise 5-3: Imagine what your life would be like if you change your beliefs–and if you don't. Feel the pain and joy.[3]

Remember Ebenezer Scrooge's dream in Charles Dickens' *A Christmas Carol*. He intensely experienced his past and present life and what his life would be like if he continued on the same path. You can use the same pattern. Imagine what your life will be like if you continue with your current belief. Imagine how painful it would be five, ten, twenty years from now. Don't just imagine it–feel it–feel the pain! Now imagine what your life will be like five, ten, twenty years from now following the new belief. Feel how much richer and more joyful your life will be.

Exercise 5-4: Put it to music

The movies *Jaws* or *Psycho* wouldn't have been nearly as scary without the soundtrack playing those ominous chords when the shark was near or the killer approached the shower. Movies count on soundtracks intensifying your emotions. If you want to change a belief or behavior, take a tip from Hollywood and add a soundtrack. So pair your new belief with Tina Turner singing *Simply The Best*, or Bette Midler singing *Wind Beneath My Wings*, or Bobby McFerrin singing *Don't Worry Be Happy*, or whatever works for you and the belief you want to permeate every cell in your body.

Exercise 5-5: Identify people you want to spend more time with because they are good role models for you.

For better or worse, people's beliefs and attitudes rub off on their friends and associates. Bonding comes from shared values and interests. If you primarily associate with people who are pessimistic, believe the conventional myths about aging, and don't take care of their mental and physical health, you are more likely to do the same. On the other hand, if you primarily associate with people who are optimistic, believe they can live a long life, and take good care of their mental and physical health, you are likely to do the same.

Exercise 5-6: Select and model healthy elderly people you greatly admire.

Imagine yourself developing their positive traits as you get older. Note what things you did to develop their positive qualities. Now pick some elderly people whose traits you dislike. Imagine yourself becoming more like them as you age and note what you need to do to make sure you don't develop those traits.

Exercise 5-7: Identify a belief you would like to change and how you will go about gathering supporting data.

I used to drink six or more diet colas a day. I was a caffeine addict. I tried a lot of behavior modification strategies, only to return to my previous caffeine habit. I read the medical literature and for the most part the literature indicated that caffeine wasn't all that harmful. That was all I needed to rationalize the habit. Intuitively, I knew that the caffeine was making me a little nervous and that so much caffeine was not healthy. But I enjoyed the lift and the ritual of drinking it. I kept asking questions. My doctor explained how caffeine disrupts body rhythms and the body's energy fields for several hours. From my knowledge of hypnosis and familiarity with polarity therapy, I believe body rhythms are important to good physical and mental functioning. My physician's information and my desire to live 150 years made it relatively easy to give up the caffeine habit and rarely drink caffeinated colas. I told my best friend about the accomplishment and he said, "Gee, body rhythms wouldn't convince me." You need to find the data that convinces you.

Here are some common examples of using data to counter limiting beliefs:

A man who is past 60 and doubts his ability to perform sexually could counter with data such as:

- Senator Strom Thurmond fathered three children in his seventies.
- Eighty percent of impotent men are smokers and I don't smoke.
- If testosterone levels, health, and blood circulation are good, there is no reason centenarian men cannot have firm erections.
- Exercise will help keep my cardiovascular system healthy and my testosterone level up and if that is not enough, I can take Viagra or testosterone supplements.

A person who worries about not remembering a name or information can counter with data such as:

- There is more and more information in my brain and it sometimes takes a little longer to do a mental search (a comparison with computer searches).

- I know from experience that if my conscious mind doesn't quickly come up with the information, I can relax and my unconscious will continue searching for the information and it will come to me.
- Is the problem that I am tired or stressed? Brains don't work as well when tired or stressed.
- Research on centenarians indicates that many centenarians have intact mental functioning (as indicated by neurological testing and by brain autopsies).

A person who has the thought, "I should grow older gracefully" can counter with:
- That means accepting what is average for my age group. I don't want to be average. I set a higher standard for myself than average and I take better care of myself mentally, physically, and spiritually than the average person does.
- Chronological age is only one measure of age. My spirit and health are much younger than my chronological age and I want to be with people who can keep up with me.
- The people I admire the most are not people who just go along with others' expectations. I admire and emulate people who blaze new trails and enjoy doing it.
- I suppose you believe that (fill in women, minorities, or whatever fits) should keep their place too. Bull!

A thought such as "I guess I'm getting old (and can't do what I used to do)" can be countered with:
- Skills are like muscles. If you use them, they keep working and working.
- As Deepak Chopra expresses it, "At this moment you are exhaling atoms of hydrogen, oxygen, carbon, and nitrogen that just an instant before were locked up in solid matter; your stomach, liver, heart, lungs, and brain are vanishing into thin air, being replaced as quickly and endlessly as they are being broken down. The skin replaces itself once a month, the stomach lining every five days, the liver every six weeks, and the skeleton every three months. To the naked eye, these organs look the same from moment to moment, but they are

always in flux. By the end of this year, 98 per cent of the atoms in your body will have been exchanged for new ones."[4]
- At my age I am free from worry about what others' think.
- The rule books for longevity are as out of date as 10-year-old books on computers.

When you buy a new car, you see that car everywhere. It's not that there are suddenly more of them on the road, it's that your "antennae are up" and you notice them now. Now that you are buying into living to 150, you want to notice information that supports the belief that you will live that long. Reading books like *Centenarians: The Bonus Years* can help. The author interviewed 150 centenarians and cites example after example of very vital centenarians. These centenarians fly airplanes, dance, conduct research, write books, and even run for Congress. It changes your conception of centenarians–which is exactly what you want. The critical question in reading such literature is whether it leaves you believing that centenarians are more vital than you thought. If you let your friends know you are looking for examples (role models) of vital centenarians, they might bring you news clippings or stories about them or even introduce you to some.

Exercise 5-8: Identify a belief that fits well with the "as if" approach and try it for a week.

Psychologist George Kelley called it fixed role therapy. You behave "as if" you had the belief, e.g., loving your spouse. Oftentimes the as if belief becomes natural and habitual. In *The King and I* Rogers and Hammerstein expressed it as "make believe you're brave, and the trick will take you far."

Exercise 5-9: Identify a belief or behavior you would like to have that is particularly appropriate for modeling.

Children learn sports by modeling great athletes. Adults also need role models. Models can be people you know, people you read about or see in the news, or even fictional characters from literature, movies, or television. They might be mentors or personal coaches.

Learn from others' experience and expertise rather than your own trial and error.

Exercise 5-10: Identify what change strategies have worked best for you in the past and apply the strategy to a current concern.

Ask yourself about beliefs you have changed and how that change came about. Formulas that worked for you in the past are likely to work for you now. The key might have been new information, finding a counter-example that contradicted your old belief, an inspiring role model, disciplined practice, a promise to someone, a bet, etc. Discover your best strategies and use the same formula to adopt beliefs that foster longevity.

Exercise 5-11: In addition to any prayers you already say, write a prayer that encompasses your goals, including your longevity goals, and chant it daily for a month.

Formal prayer is the repetition of words while in an altered state. Your unconscious mind is very receptive to words, especially when you are in an altered state. Rhythmically chanting or reciting formal prayers or affirmations can create an altered state and send a message directly to your soul, and possibly to God or your higher power. Informal prayer speaks from the heart. When you speak from your heart, your soul listens.

Metaphors and beliefs about aging

> *All perception of truth is the detection on an analogy.*
> –Henry David Thoreau

> *When imagination and logic are in conflict with each other,*
> *the imagination invariably takes over.*
> –Mark Fisher, *The Instant Millionaire*, p. 68

People often represent their beliefs metaphorically. In the movie, *From the Hip*, the head of the law firm says "The wounds pile up. After awhile you are afraid you are nothing but scar tissue." This is not a metaphor for living to be 150. Contrast her view of life with that of Deepak Chopra or Wayne Dyer, who see the spirit as eternal and our bodies as in a constant process of renewal. The difference between beliefs and metaphors is that beliefs state the idea directly and metaphors make abstract comparisons.

Many people in our culture devalue age. Old people are old geezers, grumpy old men, old hags, and over the hill. Some people have a reverence for age and believe age brings maturity and wisdom. Our pluralistic culture gives us choices from many metaphors. To live to be 150 you need to make sure you have positive metaphors for living a long productive life.

Metaphors and beliefs often pop up in our conversations. Here are some examples:

- It's a jungle out there. (This is likely to prompt an attitude of taking care of yourself, and possibly your family, and the hell with others.)
- Family is everything. (This is a companion to jungle out there and is seen in close families including the Cosa Nostra.)
- We are all children of God. (This is likely to prompt seeking opportunities to help others and do good deeds.)
- "All the world's a stage and all the men and women merely players; They have their exits and entrances, And one man in his time plays many parts." [Shakespeare's *As You Like It* 2.7.139] (This is likely to prompt an existential perspective, and possibly feelings of resignation and futility.)
- "Life's but a walking shadow, a poor player, That struts and frets its hour upon the stage, And then is heard of no more, it is a tale told by an idiot, full of sound and fury. Signifying nothing." [Shakespeare's *Macbeth* 5.5.19] (This is likely to prompt despair and nihilism.)
- Life's a game. (This is likely to prompt a competitive nature.)
- I'm a late bloomer. (This is a very positive metaphor for people whose careers get a late start.)
- What goes around comes around. (This fosters generosity and a sense of ultimate fairness.)
- Clement Stone's "reverse paranoia" in which he thinks of the world as conspiring to help. (This fosters optimism, gregariousness, and confidence.)

- We are all part of God's (or a great cosmic) plan. (This fosters a spiritual connection, sense of purpose, and a sense of fairness.)

We teach our children stories with metaphors to inspire them and to shape their character and behavior. For example:
- *The Little Red Hen* teaches that if you don't do the work, you are not entitled to the fruits of the labor.
- *Cinderella* teaches that virtue in the face of adversity is rewarded. (You might object, however, to the girl's dependence on a prince recognizing her virtue and rescuing her from her dire circumstances.)
- *Star Wars* suggests that life is a clash between good and evil and there is a hero hidden in each boy and girl if they will trust their unconscious wisdom (the Force).
- *The Little Engine that Could* teaches believing in one's self and persisting in the face of adversity.

Here are some examples of beliefs:
- Men are no damn good. (This belief, usually borne from painful experience, is likely to initially help protect a woman from further pain, but in the long-run sets up a self-fulfilling prophecy by pushing away men who contradict the belief, and feeling "comfortable" with men who validate the belief.)
- "The unexamined life is not worth living." [Socrates] (This belief fosters reading, philosophical discussion, and introspection.)
- Life is a gift. (This belief fosters an attitude of gratitude.)
- We are here to do God's work. (This belief fosters discerning God's will in decision making and obedience to what is perceived as God's will.)
- Life is awesome. (This belief fosters awe, amazement, and appreciation.)
- I will live to 150. (This belief creates a different sense of time, including a sense that careers don't end of 65 and it is OK to "be a tortoise" and make your mark in life well after 65.)

Exercise 5-12: *Identifying beliefs and metaphors*

Because metaphors and beliefs have a powerful influence on your thinking and behavior, it is important to periodically examine them, consider their implications, and consciously discern whether the metaphor or belief fits with who you want to be. If any do not fit, identify a metaphor or belief that is a better fit and determine how to adopt it. Identifying metaphors can be as simple as being vigilant for phrases you use and statements you make. Friends might be able to point out metaphors you use that are so ingrained that you might not notice them. Complete the following sentences and see what metaphors you come up with:

Life is like_____

My life is like_____

The world is like_____

People are like_____

The most important thing in life is_____

Men are like_____

Women are like_____

My favorite fairy tale as a kid was _____

Metaphors and beliefs about aging influence our thinking and behavior as well. Completing the following sentences can help identify some of your beliefs and metaphors about aging.

Growing old means_____

Sitting on an airplane next to a 20-year-old would be different than

sitting next to a centenarian because_____

Grumpy old men_____

Elderly people_____

The best thing about living past 100 is_____

Nursing homes_____

George Burns (comedian, actor) was_____

The idea of a centenarian flying an airplane_____

When someone calls a woman an "old hag,"_____

I would describe the oldest person I know as_____

Dick Clark (host of *American Bandstand* and *New Year's Rockin'*

*Eve)*_____

Supporting beliefs and metaphors are important ingredients for longevity. To put it concisely, "conceive, believe, and achieve."

Resources

There are many good resources on the relationships between mind, body, healing, and health. Bernie Siegel's books, *Love, Medicine & Miracles* and *Peace, Love & Miracles* give heartwarming case histories of how emotional healing has often cured cancer. Robert Dilts, Tim Hallbom, and Suzi Smith's *Beliefs: Pathways to Healing and Well-being* explains how to use Neurolinguistic Programming (NLP) strategies to promote health and healing. Caroline Myss' *Why People Don't Heal and How They Can* is a fascinating and useful explanation of how energy, chakras, and spirit affect healing.

The classic book on beliefs effecting success is Napoleon Hill's *Think and Grow Rich.* The best introduction to NLP is *Heart of the Mind* by Connirae Andreas and Steve Andreas. Tony (Anthony)

Robbins' tapes are particularly good at using NLP, passion, and enthusiasm to change beliefs and behaviors. His books, *Awaken the Giant Within* and *Unlimited Power* focus on beliefs. He and Joseph McClendon III also wrote *Unlimited Power: A Black Choice.* Zig Ziglar's tapes and books are excellent and are especially appreciated by committed Christians, e.g., *Goals* and *Top Performance.* Robbins and Ziglar are such great speakers they are best appreciated live or on tape or CD. Salespeople especially like Tom Hopkins' books and tapes, e.g., *How to Master the Art of Selling.*

The expert on optimism is Martin Seligman, who wrote *Learned Optimism* and *The Optimistic Child.* The definitive book on flow is Mihal Csikszentmihalyi's *Flow: The Psychology of Optimal Experience.*

People who say it can't be done
shouldn't interrupt those who are doing it.

Chapter 6

The Be-attitudes:
Optimism, Gratitude, Dealing with It,
and Embracing Lifelong Learning and Change

The Be-attitudes are outlooks that foster enjoying life and good mental and physical health. Here is why and how to cultivate be-attitudes.

Optimistic and pessimistic dogs

Optimism is pivotal to good health and longevity. Research has found that optimists are healthier, happier, live longer, and recover from illnesses better. And it costs nothing.

The scientific study of optimism began with a problem. Dogs were being trained for an experiment in which they heard a tone and then received a mild, brief shock. Each dog was then placed in a box with two compartments with a low wall separating the compartments. When the experimenter sounded the tone, the dog was supposed to expect a shock and escape by jumping into the other compart-ment—normally an easy task for a dog to learn. These dogs, however, responded to the tone and the shock by just laying there, whimpering.

Martin Seligman hypothesized that during their training the dogs had "learned to be helpless"—that is, no matter what they did, they could not avoid the shocks so they no longer even tried. Seligman devised an experiment with three groups of dogs:[1]

- The "escapable shock" dogs received shocks but could turn off the shock by pressing a button with their noses.
- The "no personal control" dogs were paired with the escapable shock dogs. They received the same shocks as the escapable shock dogs, but nothing they did affected when the shock ended.
- The "no shock" dogs did not receive any shocks.

Both the escapable shock dogs and the no shock dogs learned to jump to the other side of the box in seconds. The no personal control dogs, however, gave up and just laid down and received shocks. They never learned that the shock could be avoided by merely jumping to the other side. Dozens of variations of this experiment have now been conducted with dogs, rats, and even humans with comparable results.

There were interesting exceptions. In both animal and human research, one out of three no personal control subjects did not become helpless following a shock, noise, or other aversive stimulus. These were the optimists. One in ten of the animal and human subjects that were not shocked made no attempt to try to escape aversive stimuli when exposed to them. These were the extreme pessimists. Apparently their previous life experiences led them to believe they had little control over their lives.

At a time when B. F. Skinner and behaviorist psychologists were casting all behavior into stimulus-response terms, Seligman and his colleagues had demonstrated that even dogs and mice don't just respond to stimulus-response conditioning, but develop expectations about their ability to control what happens to them. This research helped to create the field of *cognitive* behavioral psychology.

What optimists do that is different

Many people think of optimism in terms of positive thinking and affirmations, e.g., Emile Coue's "Every day in every way I'm getting better and better," thinking of a glass as half full rather than half empty, or visualizing successful outcomes. Seligman described optimism as *how we think about the causes* of good things and bad things that happen to us, or our "explanatory style." Optimists bias their interpretations of events in a way that protects their egos and gives them hope to keep on trying. Pessimists have a neutral posture or a negative bias.

If an optimist does well on a math test, she is likely to say something like: "That just proves that I'm a good student." Note that she presumes her skills and success are ongoing traits, that she generalizes beyond math to being a good student in general, and that she attributes her success to her skills rather than external factors like being lucky or the test being easy. A pessimist who does well on a math test is more likely to say something like: "I guess I got some breaks on that math test." Note that her comments only apply to math, attribute her good scores to external, chance events, and do not suggest she will do well on the next math test. Thus optimists view favorable events as permanent, pervasive, and personal (i.e., internal or within their control). Pessimists tend to make the opposite attributions and see favorable events as temporary, specific, and external.

When it comes to bad events, the same principles apply but in reverse. An optimist who does poorly on a test is likely to say: "I'm a good student. I just had an off day and an unfair test." Thus she views her poor performance as a fluke, an exception to her usual performance, and not her fault. The pessimist is likely to say: "That proves I'm stupid and will never pass this course (or worse yet will never graduate)."

Seligman's three dimensions are summarized in the following table:

Explanatory Style of Optimists and Pessimists

	Good Events	Bad Events
Permanence (permanent or temporary)	Optimists: permanent Pessimists: temporary	Optimists: temporary Pessimists: permanent
Pervasive (universal or specific)	Optimists: universal Pessimists: specific	Optimists: specific Pessimists: universal
Personal (internal or external)	Optimists: internal Pessimists: external	Optimists: external Pessimists: internal

His book *Learned Optimism* includes a quiz that lets you rate yourself on these dimensions. He has a similar test for children in his book *The Optimistic Child.*

Seligman does not have a category for Importance (if sticking to his alliteration, we could call it Prominence). When good things happen, optimists tend to see them as important, for example, "Seeing that flower made my day." When bad things happen optimists tend to say, "It's really not very important anyway." Pessimists, on the other hand, discount the importance of positive events the way some people brush off a compliment about their clothes with an "Oh, this old thing," and amplify the importance of negative events with thoughts such as "But I know there is a spot on it even if no one else sees it." After all, many pessimists are also perfectionists.

Children are much more optimistic than adults and we enjoy their enthusiasm and resilience. They forget pain or anger in a few minutes and become intensely absorbed in playing again. Children's optimism protects them from an otherwise frustrating world of adult no's, sibling and peer squabbles, frustrations at learning to read, write, do math, play sports, and much more.

When my son was 5 years old and would spill milk or break something, he would say, "Oh well, that's OK," in a very credible manner. I would call this an example of discounting the *importance* of the undesirable event. Perhaps he was right, it was only spilled milk—not a reason to mentally beat himself up or get him off track from feeling good. As a parent it was tempting to challenge his attribution, lest he sluff off responsibility and not learn to be more careful. I restrained from challenging his attribution, as it would be just a matter of time before teachers and others would not go along with his minimizing the importance of breaking things or forgetting his homework. This is part of the process of how children learn to be less optimistic.

Another major factor in children becoming less optimistic is modeling parents, teachers, and other role models. Adults who manage to maintain a childlike quality, for example, opera singer Luciano Pavarotti and actress Ruth Gordon, are generally perceived as irresistibly charming.

One of the world's greatest optimists was Thomas Edison, who said:

> *Results? Why, man, I have gotten lot of results! If I find 10,000 ways something won't work, I haven't failed. I am not discouraged, because every wrong attempt discarded is another step forward. Just because something doesn't do what you planned it to do doesn't mean it's useless. . .There are no rules here, we're trying to accomplish something.*[2]

Note that while our society rewards optimism on an individual level, news and politics thrives on pessimism and fear.

Pessimists experience more depression

Depression is the "mental common cold" of our times. Depression has been increasing to epidemic proportions. A few decades ago most psychologists said that young children don't get depressed. In a study from 1985-1990, Seligman found that 35% of third and fourth grade boys were severely depressed at least once in these grades. The two major factors in their depression were a pessimistic explanatory style and bad life events (e.g., divorce, moving, death of a family member or pet). For preteens, boys are more likely to be depressed than girls and boys are more prone to acting out behaviors like fighting. After puberty, girls and women are much more vulnerable to depression.

Most people experience some mild depression at times in their lives. Seligman estimates that at any given time 25% of adults are experiencing some depression. Community studies indicate that at a given time 2-3% of men and 5-9% of women experience a "major depression." In one's lifetime, 5-12% of men and 10-25% of women experience a major depression.[3] (Men, however, are at greater risk for acting out behaviors such as alcoholism, drug addiction, and crime.)

Criteria for a major depression are the presence of several of these behaviors: depressed mood, markedly diminished interest or pleasure in most or all activities, increased or decreased appetite, increased or decreased sleep, agitation or slowing of physical movements, loss of energy, feeling worthless and/or excessively guilty, difficulty thinking, concentrating, and/or making decisions, and recurrent thoughts of dying or suicide. Thus, a major depression affects mood, thinking, and physiological functioning. There are between 20,000 and 50,000 suicides a year in the U.S. There were few optimists among them.

Like the dogs in Seligman's experiment, depressed people experience learned helplessness. They feel nothing they do can make much of a difference in solving their problems. There is a lot of overlap between depression, pessimism, and low self-esteem. Seligman's research suggests that pessimism tends to be the more causal element. For example, at the beginning of the semester, college students took tests for optimism/pessimism, a test for depression, and indicated what midterm grade they would consider a failure. Of the students whose midterm grades were at a level that they considered a failure, a much greater proportion of students who were pessimists at the beginning of the semester became depressed than those who were optimists at the beginning of the semester.

Pessimists have more health problems

When we are exposed to foreign entities such as viruses or bacteria, our T-cell and NK (Natural Killer) cell counts increase. T-cells recognize specific foreign substances and help kill them. NK cells kill anything identified as foreign. T-cells and NK cells in pessimistic or depressed people, however, are less likely to increase in numbers when exposed to foreign cells. Research with elderly individuals also shows that pessimists have lower T-cell and NK cell levels, whether they are depressed or not.

Thus, the effects of pessimism and depression filter down to the cellular level, rendering the immune system helpless. Pessimists have twice as many infectious diseases as optimists. Optimistic women with breast cancer have had better survival rates than pessimistic women with cancer. Women with a second bout of breast cancer (which currently has a poor prognosis) had better survival rates if they were optimists. A study of men who had a heart attack found that eight years later 24% of the optimists had died and 84% of the pessimists had died. Another study assessed optimism and pessimism and found that thirty years later, pessimists had higher mortality rates.[4]

In 1939-1944 two hundred very fit, intellectually gifted Harvard men from five freshmen classes were recruited for a research project to study the determinants of success and health over life spans. Studying people over a period of years is the ideal research methodology but is rarely done because of the enormous costs in time and money. The men in the study received physicals every five years, frequent interviews, and answered hundreds of questionnaires. Although they had "all the advantages in life," they had their share of divorces, bankruptcies, heart attacks, alcoholism, and other problems.

The current principal researcher, George Vaillant, found that before 45, psychological factors did not have much influence on physical health, i.e., the men's health at 45 was comparable to their health at 25. After 45, Vaillant found better health in men who had what he called "mature defenses"–humor, altruism, and sublimation. At 60 none of the men who used mature defenses in their twenties were chronically ill, while more than one-third of the men with immature defenses in their twenties had chronic illnesses at 60.

Seligman obtained access to this rich data source and analyzed essays that 96 of the men wrote in 1945-46 and rated the essays for optimism vs. pessimism. He found that starting at 45, those who had written pessimistic essays as college students had more health problems. By 60, the differences in health status had become more pronounced. When optimism was compared to Vaillant's mature defenses, optimism showed a stronger correlation with health. With the men in their mid-seventies now, mortality data soon will become available to determine whether the study's optimists live longer.

When pessimists become ill or face adversity, they are more likely than optimists to believe there is nothing they can do and thus do less than optimists do to help themselves. Since they are less likeable than optimists, they also tend to have smaller social support net-works–another factor that contributes to higher risk for illness and poorer prognosis for recovery from illnesses.

Optimists are better liked and more successful

Seligman's research found that depression is becoming an epidemic among school children. He went into elementary schools in Philadelphia's suburbs and taught the children a child version of the ABCDE model for coping (described in the next section). He taught ABCDE skills and skills for coping with social problems (e.g., teasing, divorce, rejection) in twelve two-hour group sessions. He was not only interested in whether the program resolved depression, but also if the benefits lasted over time.

He selected a group of 70 children who were depressed or at risk for depression. In pretesting 24% of these fifth and sixth grade children had moderate to severe symptoms of depression. Immedi-ately after the training, 13% of children in the training group and 23%

of children in the no training group had depressive symptoms. When retested two years later, 22% of the training group children and 44% of the no training group children were depressed. Thus, although rates of depression increased at puberty, children who had the benefit of the training program were only half as likely to become depressed as children who did not have the training. Seligman views this as "inoculating" children against depression and pessimism. His book, *The Optimistic Child*, describes how you can teach these skills to your children, grandchildren, great grandchildren, great great grandchildren, etc.

Seligman also measured optimism and pessimism for students entering Pennsylvania State University. As he expected, those who scored optimistic tended to achieve better grades than their SAT scores would suggest and those who were pessimistic tended to achieve worse grades than their SAT scores would have predicted.

In the workplace, optimists are more popular (and social skills are part of job success in most jobs). In jobs that require persistence, such as life insurance agents making cold calls, optimists are more likely to keep trying. Seilgman was invited to help Metropolitan Life Insurance Co. select its agents because despite Met Life's careful selection and screening, half of their new agents quit within the first year. Insurance agents are far more optimistic than the general population. Still, some are more optimistic than others. Seligman found that the agents who scored highest on optimism at hire were twice as likely to stay the first year. Met Life modified its selection process to include strong optimism and thereby increased retention of its agents. Optimistic agents also sold more insurance.

Seligman also worked with West Point to reduce their cadet dropout rates. At West Point more than eight percent of plebes (freshmen) quit within two months. Seligman assessed optimism vs. pessimism when plebes arrived at West Point. He found the plebes who quit had disproportionately scored more pessimistic than their classmates at arrival at West Point.

Seligman and his colleagues studied the speeches of presidential candidates and other politicians and found that those with the most optimistic speeches usually won the elections. They studied statements made by players and coaches on sports teams and found the most optimistic teams were more likely to exceed the point spreads than pessimistic teams, e.g., if a football team was expected to win by ten points and had optimistic rhetoric, odds were they would win the game by more than ten points.

Pessimists can become optimists

While identifying who is optimistic might help employers and coaches select the most successful employees and athletes, what is to become of the pessimists? Seligman believes optimism not only can be measured but can be learned and taught. His books, *Learned Optimism* and *The Optimistic Child,* describe how to learn optimism. Pennsylvania State University has taught optimism skills to thousands of its students. Seligman's organization, Foresight, Inc., gives workshops on optimism. A MacArthur Foundation grant is teaching cancer patients to be more optimistic. Optimistic skills are closely related to skills cognitive behavioral psychologists use with depression (e.g., David Burns' book *Feeling Good: The New Mood Therapy*).

The essence of learning to be an optimist uses Albert Ellis' ABC model to analyze and change self-talk. Seligman added a DE to improve the self-talk. When learning optimism, Seligman encourages people to keep a diary of events and analyze entries in the ABCDE format. The ABCDE acronym stands for:

- ANTECEDENT BEHAVIOR (OR ADVERSITY), e.g., My boss criticized my report.
- BELIEFS, e.g., I am in big trouble now. Nothing I do seems to please her.
- CONSEQUENCE, e.g., I'll cross my fingers and hope she forgets about it.

DISPUTATION, e.g., She usually likes my reports and one problem report isn't going to get me fired. She didn't criticize the whole report, just parts of it. I know how to rewrite it to meet her objections and she would probably be pleased with the changes and impressed that I listened well and cared enough to rewrite it. I also know more about what not to do next time.

- ENERGIZATION, e.g., I'll revise the report this afternoon.

To give another example:
- ANTECEDENT BEHAVIOR (OR ADVERSITY), e.g., My wife and I had a bad argument this morning.
- BELIEFS, e.g., I guess we don't have such a great marriage after all. I don't think there is any solution for this problem. It's going to be uncomfortable around here for a long time. What's the matter with us?
- CONSEQUENCE, e.g., I'll see if I can keep my distance for a few days and see if things cool down.
- DISPUTATION, e.g., All couples have arguments. I'm glad that we didn't let it deteriorate into name calling. I have a better understanding of how she sees things now. An argument doesn't mean we don't love each other. Even if I am not willing to do what she asks, I can let her know that I respect her wishes and would like to try to work out some kind of solution or compromise.
- ENERGIZATION, e.g., I'll give her a hug, tell her that I love her, and tell her that I'll give it some more thought and maybe we can discuss it again tomorrow to see if we can come up with a solution.

In disputing the beliefs and consequences, Seligman asks people to consider:
- What *evidence* supports the belief? e.g., What evidence is there that you are in "big trouble with the boss," that "nothing pleases her," much less that you might be fired.
- What *alternatives* are there to the consequence you choose? e.g., revising the report.
- What are the *implications* of the beliefs? e.g., While it's not a good day to ask for a raise, my good track record and good relationship with the boss makes any serious consequences unlikely.
- How *useful* is the belief? e.g., If I adopt the belief that nothing I do pleases the boss, I will feel bad about myself, avoid the boss, get depressed, and be less productive. This would set up a self-fulfilling prophecy. On the other hand, if I assume the boss cared enough about me and believed in my ability to improve enough that she took the time to give me constructive criticism, I will feel

better about myself, be more productive at work, and have a better relationship with my boss.

When you compare the consequences of the initial and more optimistic internal dialogues, the better results with the optimistic scenario should be very appealing (if not, something is probably wrong with the analysis).

Seligman's books use the term ADVERSITY and just discusses the system for dealing with unfavorable events. I prefer the more traditional term ANTECEDENT EVENTS and using the process to enhance good events as well. For example:

- ANTECEDENT BEHAVIOR, e.g., I was downright eloquent in my presentation today.
- CONSEQUENCE, e.g., That was really nice.
- DISPUTATION, e.g., You know, it's not necessarily limited to that presentation. My presentation skills have been getting better and better. I think I have developed a rhythm and style. I have gotten so good I am starting to pay attention to eye contact. This is becoming fun. Let me think about how I can make it even better next time.
- ENERGIZATION, e.g., I'm on a roll. I want to make sure I nurture this emerging skill so it gets better and better and becomes even more fun.

Seligman does not talk about specifically considering each ABCDE analysis from the perspective of permanence, pervasiveness, personalization, (and importance). Such an analysis can be very useful in fully understanding our thinking processes and how they might be enhanced.

Optimism research has focused on how people explain adverse events. Much still needs to be learned about how people explain positive events.[5] The two explanatory styles are certainly related but they appear to be somewhat independent of each other. Pessimism appears to be far more likely to effect anxiety, stress, and health problems than the lack of optimism. The emphasis on explaining aversive events probably reflects psychology's historical preoccupation with pathology as opposed to optimal functioning. Optimism has also been studied in terms of a general disposition of optimism vs. pessimism, and in terms of a global outlook toward life (e.g., our nation's future) vs. making specific decisions.

Exercise 6-1: Noticing optimism

Think of the most optimistic people you know. How do you feel when you are around them? Now think of the most pessimistic people you know. How do you feel when you are around them? Which would you rather emulate? Are there pessimistic areas of your life? If there are, try using the ABCDE process with these issues.

The ethical dilemmas with optimism

It's a disturbing idea that depressed people see reality correctly while nondepressed people distort reality in a self-serving way. As a therapist I was trained to believe that it was my job to help depressed patients both to feel happier and to see the world more clearly. I was supposed to be the agent of happiness and of truth. But maybe truth and happiness antagonize each other. Perhaps what we have considered good therapy for a depressed patient merely nurtures benign illusions, making the patient think his world is better than it actually is. –Martin Seligman[6]

I have always revered honesty and truth seeking. Learning that optimism is healthy, desirable, and a distortion of "truth" was quite a jolt. Perhaps it is analogous to good manners. Good manners do not endorse brutal honesty but call for saying an outfit we don't care for is "nice" and telling a white lie about "other plans" instead of just saying you don't want to go. The purpose of these distortions is to prevent the other party from experiencing pain unnecessarily.

Distorting the truth, however, does call for extra caution as one can stray too far from reality or distort too much when the risks of being wrong have serious consequences (e.g., being extremely optimistic about a poorly researched penny stock). While Mickey Mouse and Miss Piggy are healthy optimists, Wile E. Coyote is an extreme optimist who seems unlikely to ever catch the Road Runner and takes quite a beating in the chase. For some people, understanding the structure of optimism (permanence, pervasiveness, personalization, and importance) can help keep perspective on optimism rather than just doing what one normally does.

A second ethical dilemma is that the formula for optimism has optimists blaming others when unfavorable things happen. Our society has become overly litigious and quick to label people as victims. The last thing we need is to encourage more people to blame their problems on others instead of taking personal responsibility for their behavior and their lives. Consequently, I would not encourage people to blame their problems on others in order to be more optimistic. The other elements of optimism are sufficient to create a healthy optimism in most cases. Regarding unfavorable things as temporary and specific might reduce motivation to try to make sure something does not happen again. Externalizing the problem can greatly lower motivation to change and correct or prevent a problem. Although internal attributions can be brutal in someone who is severely depressed (e.g., it is my fault my spouse and children are unhappy), in many situations they can be important in effecting change (e.g., my drinking is negatively impacting my spouse and children).

When you shouldn't be an optimist

There are some jobs which are better suited for people who are mildly pessimistic. These are jobs in which the negative consequences of making a mistake are high and risk has to be minimized. Thus, we want nuclear power plant operators, airline pilots, utility company operators, bankers, auditors, safety inspectors, etc. to be worry warts who check, check again, and worry about all the things that might go wrong.

When people want to relate their troubles or concerns, an extremely optimistic response undermines rapport. Optimists need to be good listeners first and communicate that they heard, understand, and care. Then, with pacing, they can gradually introduce optimism.

Optimistic and pessimistic metaphors

Metaphors are the templates we use in interpreting what life means and what to do. Questioning, updating and choosing more optimistic metaphors can make wholesale changes in becoming more optimistic. Here are some illustrations·

Pessimistic and Optimistic Metaphors

Role	Pessimistic	Optimistic
Vocation	Another day at the salt mines.	I'm a lucky person to have a job that is so interesting.
Cartoons	*Garfield, Dilbert*	*Mickey Mouse*
Marriage	–Marriage is a three-ring ceremony–the engagement ring, the wedding ring, and the suffering. –My old lady/man...	Like a great wine, marriage improves with age as the companionship and shared experiences become richer and fuller.
Age	When you get to be my age...	Like wine I get better with age.
Memory	My memory ain't what it used to be.	Wisdom and good organization are more important than memorizing.
Sex	I'm too old for sex.	–Sex is to be savored like a fine meal, not like a starving teenager gobbling a burger and fries. –There is such a sense of freedom in not worrying about pregnancy.
View of life	Life is tough.	Life is sweet.

Things in life will not always run smoothly. Sometimes we will be rising toward the heights–then all will seem to reverse itself and start downward. The great fact to remember is that the trend of civilization itself is forever upward, that a line drawn through the middle of the peaks and the valleys of the centuries always has an upward trend.
–Endicott Peabody[7]

Progress is impossible without change,
and those who cannot change their minds
cannot change anything. –George Bernard Shaw

There are no such things as incurable,
there are only things for which man has not found a cure.
–Bernard Baruch[8]

Gratitude and perspective

Gratitude is about perspective. My children don't believe me when I tell them they are richer than 98% of the people in the world. Even Americans on welfare often have color televisions, telephones, central heating, shop at grocery stores, and perhaps even have air conditioning. The fact that you are reading this book suggests that you are probably in fairly good health and have a good intellect. If everyone in the world put their health, intellect, and finances into a lottery, would you really want to add yours and try your luck?

People fantasize about what it would be like to be a king or queen. Think about what it *really* would have been like to be a king or queen as recently as one hundred years ago. Queen Victoria reigned from 1837 to 1901 and her son, Edward VIII, was underemployed until he became king at 59 and reigned for nine years. In the winter you would live in a cold, dark castle with just fireplaces for heat. In the summer it would be hot and humid with no air-conditioning. While today you can choose to hear Pavarotti, Frank Sinatra, or the New York Philharmonic Orchestra at their best, any time of day or night, as a queen you would be limited to local musicians in live appearances or perhaps a relatively new invention, the gramophone. Radio, television, Internet, airplanes–forget it.

Dinner would be largely limited to local foods and England was not known for its cuisine. While you could get fresh meat all year, most fresh fruits and vegetables would only be available in the summer. Ice boxes provided refrigeration. Light at nighttime would be from candles, torches, or gas lamps. Instead of a heated/air-conditioned car with radio and CD or cassette player, you would travel by a horse-driven carriage at five miles an hour or by train or boat. There was the war in South Africa, international tensions, and contentious domestic politics. Would you want to trade places? Want to feel gratitude? Just compare yourself with a king or queen's life a hundred years ago (much less a peasant's life), instead of your neighbors.

I have counseled people who go into "road rage" when stuck in traffic or "slighted" by another driver. It is amazing how they let themselves become so upset over such trivial inconveniences and minor slights. When I'm stuck in traffic, it reminds me just how lucky I am–comfortable in an air-conditioned car with a collection of cassette tapes that makes the car a mobile university. If I'm not inclined to learn, I can get news at the touch of a button, or my favorite music at the touch of a button or insertion of a tape or CD. When I think about the other drivers, I figure: 10% are alcoholics, another 10% use street drugs, 20% have health problems, medications, colds, etc., 10% have just had an argument with their spouse, boss, child, etc., and are upset, 10% are distracted with cellular phone calls, putting on makeup, etc., 10% have serious emotional problems like depression, and 2% are feeling suicidal. Considering who is driving, I really don't feel any need to become upset and taunt them because they delayed my trip a few seconds or "invaded my space."

Other ways to feel gratitude

How do you wake up in the morning? Do you jump right out of bed brimming with enthusiasm and a song on your lips? Most people begin by arguing with their alarm clock for five more minutes. Just as the first impression can be critical in setting the tone for relationships and getting things off to a good start, our internal dialogue gets us out of the right side or "wrong side" of the bed. One way to get good start is to ask yourself what you are grateful for. But don't just rattle off a list. Associate into how you feel about each of these. If it is your daughter, see her in your mind's eye beaming with a big smile that says I love you, hear her voice, feel her hug. If you associate into several things you are grateful for, you can't help but feeling positive and hopeful, even if your life has been difficult lately.

Tony Robbins[9] recommends his "Morning Power Questions." Ask yourself, one at a time, questions about what makes you feel happy, proud, grateful, excited, passion, and enjoyment. Be sure to associate into your feelings. Also ask yourself whom you love and who loves you and associate into those feelings.

Richard Bandler,[10] a master at controlling mental states, describes how people can use the theater of their minds to wake up with enormous enthusiasm and motivation. Start by hearing (either in your mind or on a CD) a full symphony orchestra playing *Thus Spake Tharathusra* (the theme from the movie *2001: A Space Odyssey*). Then have some gospel singers singing to you about what a glorious day it will be for you and all the wonderful things you will do. If that isn't enough, imagine yourself leading a big brass band playing John Phillips Sousa music (perhaps like the scene in the musical, *The Music Man*). Or if you prefer you can have some great looking men or women beckoning you. What works for you will be different from what works for others, but you get the idea. Or you could settle for listening to whatever music gets you feeling positive and enthusiastic.

Religiously committed people find prayer gets them in a positive frame of mind. You could pray from the heart, thanking God for the things you appreciate. Most written prayers are directed at praising God, citing a metaphorical relationship to God (e.g., king, father, shepherd, savior) asking God for various blessings, or repenting. This is no accident as Jewish prayers were written from a perspective of a subject petitioning his or her king. Thus, the thrice daily Jewish Amidah prayer begins: O Lord, open Thou my lips and my mouth shall declare Thy praise. Praised are Thou, O Lord our God and God of our Fathers, God of Abraham, God of Isaac . . . . The Christian "Lord's Prayer" begins, "Our father who art in heaven hallowed will be thy name, thy kingdom come thy will be done . . . . " The 23rd Psalm begins by identifying your relationship with God, "The Lord is my Shepherd . . . . " Of course people who are smitten with love wake up preoccupied with how wonderful their beloved is. It is a great way to start the morning (though few can sustain that mental state for decades).

A lot of people's prayers focus on what they want. Even the Alcoholics Anonymous "Serenity Prayer" starts "God grant me the serenity . . . . "[11] This type of prayer helps in focusing on goals. Prayers emphasizing gratitude, however, strike me as a higher level of prayer. In Jewish worship, prayers are not allowed to ask God for anything on the Sabbath as it is a day of rest. Rather Sabbath prayers focus on gratitude and praise.

Prayers can become mechanical. This still can serve a relaxing hypnotic function. To receive the full benefit from prayer or expressions of gratitude, however, you must emotionally associate into the prayer or thought. Motivational thinkers emphasize that you will become what you focus on. As Proverbs 23-7 puts it, "for as he thinketh in his heart, so he is." Do you really want to focus on your problems?

The morning prayers in Judaism speak of the amazement at waking up, that one's eyes open. It goes on to view other "mundane" events as miraculous. Blessing daily events such as blessing food before eating, provides daily reminders for gratitude. Daily contributions to a charity box builds a daily gratitude and is a practice children can enthusiastically participate in, understand, and enjoy.

Rabbi Abraham Joshua Heshel spoke of radical amazement–an attitude of awe at how the mundane are miraculous. Judaism even has a blessing for toileting that expresses appreciation and amazement that one's "plumbing" worked. I am often struck at how electric lights, sewer systems, and other utilities work so reliably, much less things like television and computers. I especially loved a scene from the movie *Joe vs. the Volcano* in which Patricia (played by Meg Ryan) quotes her father as saying: "Almost the whole world is asleep–everybody you know–everybody you see–everybody you talk to. He says that only a few people are awake and they live in a state of constant, total amazement." Einstein put it simply, "There are only two ways to live your life. One is as though nothing is a miracle. The other is as though everything is a miracle." Feeling that sense of constant amazement and awe and wonder is the antithesis of aging.

Exercise 6-2: Feeling gratitude

What activities prompt you to feel gratitude? Is there a way that you can incorporate more of these activities in your life? Is there a way that you can use these activities or memories of them to start your day on a positive note?

Dealing with it

Poor Hamlet! He fretted, obsessed, tantrumed, and dallied. His ambivalence took a heavy toll–the deaths of Rosencrantz, Guildenstern, Ophelia, Polonius, the king, and even himself. Hamlet had several problems characteristic of people who have difficulty dealing with problems–obsessive ruminating, rigidity, procrastination, and lack of perspective. Centenarians rarely have these traits.

Obsessive ruminating Worry warts play the same mental "audio tapes" over and over. Their thinking is self-absorbed. Like Muzak, their tapes play on and on. They hear the tapes whenever something else isn't distracting their attention. Their audio tapes are in a constant loop and have no exit point. While progress with this problem is usually painstakingly slow with behavioral therapies, Neurolinguistic Programming (NLP) has some very effective strategies for dealing with worrying. One is to have some fun with the internal tapes by making them high pitched and squeaky (like Mickey Mouse), farther away (so they are less powerful), or moving them to your big toe where they seem downright silly. The effect is to scramble the pattern. Most of the time, your attention needs to be focused on other people or activities as opposed to self-absorbed ruminating.

Rigidity I once worked at a community mental health center that had an extensive program for domestic violence perpetrators and for recipients of domestic violence. We were perplexed at what diagnosis to give the men for insurance forms and records. Then it dawned on me that almost all of the men were rigid and fit the criteria for obsessive compulsive disorder. The world had to operate by their rules and if it didn't they blew up. If their wives didn't follow their rules and expectations, they hit them. Cognitive behavioral therapies challenge their rules and rigid thinking and have the best track record provided the men feel respected and buy into the process. Solution-focused therapies are especially effective as they encourage the men to take ownership of the problems and set their own goals. Longevity requires flexible thinking. Albert Ellis and Aaron Beck have both written readable and serviceable self-help books that help with rigidity.

Procrastinating Procrastinators focus on how they feel about doing something instead of the outcome they desire. In his mind's eye, the procrastinator sees himself struggling with writing a paper or filling out tax forms. He asks himself how he feels about doing it and gets a negative response. He then mentally sees an alternative, like a television program, and asks himself how that feels. It feels good so on goes the television. People who just get it done see the finished product and imagine the satisfaction and compliments. Then an internal voice says, "Let's do it."

Perspective Perspective includes realizing that one setback does not ruin your life. Often an adversity has an upside to it. Basketball great Michael Jordan was cut from the high school varsity basketball team his sophomore year because he wasn't giving it his all. Jordan said "It was the best thing that ever happened to me."[12] Planning on living to 150 makes perspective even easier. It's hard to believe that one setback is going to ruin the next hundred years of your life.

Baggage Baggage refers to unresolved issues and conflicts with parents, siblings, ex-spouses, children, etc. that interfere with current relationships. Barbara DeAngelis has an infomercial in which she talks about what sabotages marriages and wheels out a baggage cart with about a dozen suitcases. It gets the point across vividly. Dealing with it means no baggage. Seek professional help if you need it but clear up any baggage. Few centenarians tote baggage.

Forgiveness When we hold on to anger and resentments, we incarcerate ourselves and voluntarily serve guard duty. It takes a lot of energy and distracts us from more important matters. Forgiving doesn't mean condoning or asking for another punch. It does mean focusing on the positive and what is happening now.

Exercise 6-3: Dealing with it

Consider the issues of obsessive ruminating, rigidity, procrastinating, perspective, baggage, and forgiveness. Are any of these problem issues that are holding you back? If so what would be the best way for you to deal with it now?

Embracing lifelong learning and change

The illiterate of the future are not those who cannot read or write, but those who cannot learn, unlearn and relearn.
–Alan Toffler

In Cuba and the United States in the early part of the 20th century thousands of workers rolled cigars. It was boring, tedious work. The employers had professional readers read great literature and newspapers to the workers while they worked. The readers often had great voices that could make reading the phone book sound interesting. For four hours a day, the workers were treated to a classical education. They might not have gone to high school, but they were lifelong learners with great educations. Today's equivalent would be people who listen to informative programs on public radio. This is a roundabout way of saying that a person does not have to have a college education to be a lifelong learner. Indeed the libraries and the Internet have democratized access to information and learning.

Change is occurring at a logarithmic rate. In FY 96-97 the U.S. Library of Congress had 530 miles of bookshelves and was cataloguing over a quarter of a million books a year. The number of books published is almost doubling every decade. The content and usage of the Internet is currently doubling about every two years. Computer speeds and hard drive memories double about every two years. What does it mean? There are many kinds of change. There is the latest, fastest, newest syndrome–which is often a macho thing. That's OK if you can afford it. There are people who like to follow the fads. Are hemlines higher or lower this year? Fads are OK but have little to do with longevity. Longevity requires:

1. adapting to changes in the job market that affect or will affect you
2. learning technology well enough to access what it can do for you (For example, it's great to be able to program a computer but for most people it is sufficient to be able to access information from the Internet, use E-mail, and use a word processor and possibly a spreadsheet.)
3. sorting out what is valid and important enough for you to change your lifestyle and what is not (e.g., the latest recommendations on nutrition and health care)
4. understanding your personal finances and your investments well enough to prosper financially
5. striking a balance between preserving traditions and embracing change

Some people revere the music they "grew up on" and listen to that music almost exclusively (hence the popularity of "oldies" radio stations). People often cling to the food they grew up with as it is associated with family and revered memories. Religious and ethnic traditions encourage staying with traditional values and behaviors. An Orthodox Jew, for example, might embrace the latest in technology while keeping kosher, repeating daily prayers that haven't changed in thousands of years, and not answering the phone, driving, or even flicking a light switch on the Sabbath. In some ways Jews (whether Orthodox, Conservative, Reform, Reconstruction, or nondenominational) have an advantage in that their religion has given a lot of thought and debate to the tension between preserving tradition vs. embracing change.

Ask yourself the question, "What is the relationship between your work this year and last year? Roger Bailey[13] says your answer will show how much change you want in your life. If you said it was the same, you are in the 5% of people who desire little change and are on a 15- to-25- year change clock for major changes in life (e.g., choosing to change jobs, houses). People with this response gravitate to jobs that have minimal change over time, for example, farming, the gas utility company, or a tenured professorship in English literature. If you said the same but with some exceptions, you are in the 60%

who like change to evolve and are on a 5-to-7-year change clock. If you gave equal weight to same and different, you are in the 13% who are on a 2½-to-3½- year change clock. If you said it is different but cited some ways in which it is the same, you are in the 12% who are on a 1½-to-2½-year clock. If you only talk about how it is different, you are in the 10% who are on a 1-to-1½-year change clock and you probably have modern or hip furniture, a high-powered computer that is less than a year old, and lots of electronic gadgets. Bailey's theory illustrates that people have different paces for how much change they want in their lives. You don't have to be part of the 10% who see change as revolutionary. Centenarians can and do come from all of these change paces. What is important is to recognize your pace and be OK with it. As long as it meets the five functions cited in this section, it works for you. (Of course if your spouse is on a different change clock there might be a lot of conflict.)

There is no perfect path when it comes to dealing with change. What fits with your values, style, talents, and family and religious connections might not fit for someone else. Still, it helps to have a target. The target is to maintain enough ties with your past to give you a sense of roots and belonging while embracing enough change to meet your needs to adapt and make life interesting. Perhaps Bob Hope has an ideal solution when he said he doesn't consider himself old but a combination of all ages.[14]

Most of what I really needed to know about how to live life I learned in kindergarten . . . Share everything. Play fair. Don't hit people. Put things back where you found them. Clean up your own mess. Don't take things that aren't yours. Say you're sorry when you hurt someone. Wash your hands before you eat. Flush. Warm cookies and cold milk are good for you. Live a balanced life. Take a nap every afternoon. When you go out into the world, watch out for traffic, hold hands, and stick together. –Robert Fulghum[15]

Exercise 6-4: Embracing change and learning

What is your pace for change? Does it match those of your family members? How many books are you reading a year?

Exercise 6-5: What if you didn't know

How would you feel if you did not know how old you are? If the answer is freer, more energetic, or other positive traits, live a day as if you didn't know and see what happens.

Resources

Martin Seligman's *Learned Optimism* and *The Optimistic Child* are interesting reading and contain self-assessment quizzes. There are many books on cognitive behavioral therapy and the ABC or ABCDE models. Albert Ellis wrote *A New Guide to Rational Thinking* and many other books that have a colorful style and are easy to read.

The best sampler of how NLP (Neurolinguistic Programming) can help with common problems is in *Heart of the Mind* by Connirae Andreas and Steve Andreas. Its chapters include dealing with fears, traumas, allergies, criticism, assertiveness, grief, overeating, guilt, shame, decisions, and healing.

Chapter 7

A Lifetime of Mission and Purpose

*Some people sit on their butts [and buts], Got the dream–yeah,
but not the guts.* –song from the musical *Gypsy*

For too much rest itself becomes a pain.
–Homer's *The Odyssey*[1]

Get a life. –a mantra of the 1990s

Re-creating but not retiring

Retiring means coasting to most people–not learning or accomplishing much new, just enjoying yourself. Never, never, never retire. Living vibrantly to 150 means never retiring but always contributing and learning–always re-creating.

Let me share some of my favorite examples of re-creating rather than retiring:

- Lib Herndon "retired" from her state government job and turned her multistory old home into an art gallery. Every room was full of sculpture, paintings, photographs, and weavings. Artists visited frequently to talk about doing shows in her home/gallery. This is one of the most delightful lifestyles I could imagine.

- Mel Helitzer was a Madison Avenue advertising executive before "retiring" to rustic Athens, Ohio where he is a journalism professor and teaches a class in humor writing. It is no ordinary class. The final exam is to perform a stand-up routine in the Student Union. I know. I took his course and exam about fifteen years ago. I always got the impression that Mel couldn't believe he was being paid and called professor for something he enjoyed so much. After a few years of teaching the class, he wrote a book on humor writing.[2]

- Betty Rogers "retired" and became a professional speaker, speaking on retirement planning, successful aging, and humor. She loves stand-up comedy and persuaded retired people to perform at amateur night at the local Funnybones Comedy club. She also created a Comedy Club for Seniors.® She says the retirees initially tended to ramble and have difficulty developing discrete routines. With coaching, they became quite good comedians and their lives became much richer.

- When Colonel Harlan Sanders retired with little savings, he took one look at his Social Security check and started peddling his family recipe for Kentucky Fried Chicken.
- In his hundreds, Michael Heidelberger,[3] the "father of immuno-chemistry," still conducts research, publishes journal articles and lectures. When he turned 100, however, colleagues persuaded him, for safety reasons, to start taking taxis to work instead of two buses and walking several blocks in New York City. He also plays clarinet with amateur chamber music groups and friends.
- Centenarian and MIT professor Kirk Struik[4] still conducts research, lectures, and writes journal articles on ethnomathematics.
- When in her 70s Claire Willi[5] found her health and vitality were deteriorating. She enrolled in a dance and fitness class and it rejuvenated her life. Now a centenarian, she still dances.
- At 89 Selma Plaut[6] started auditing courses at the University of Toronto. She graduated with a bachelor's degree when she was 100. English wasn't even her native language as she was a Jewish refugee from Nazi Germany.
- Helen Langner[7] "retired" from her full-time psychiatry practice at 76. As a centenarian she still practices psychiatry on a part-time basis while pursuing many avocations.
- Dr. Henry Stenhouse[8] ran for Congress at 100 and is writing a book about his experiences in China before World War I.
- Centenarian theatrical producer/director George Abbott[9] is still consulting on Broadway productions.
- Louisa Groce[10] was a single parent who taught school in Philadelphia for thirty years, reared five daughters and, working a second job at night, put them all through college. After "retiring" she became a lay minister, attended a Lutheran seminary, and was ordained and assigned a congregation at 81.
- Centenarian Beatrice Wood[11] began making pottery when she was 40. She works several hours a day in her studio and her critically acclaimed work is in several museums. She wrote her autobiography, *I Shock Myself*, when she was 92.

- Grandma Moses began painting rural scenes for her own pleasure in her late 70s. Without formal art training, her work became internationally acclaimed and she was still painting at 100.
- Centenarian George Dawson, grandson of a slave, grew up in poverty in Texas and went to work on the farm at age eight to help support his family. He said "I got tired of writing my name with an X" and he enrolled in an adult education program when he was in his nineties. One result was co-writing his autobiography, *Life Is So Good.*
- The Energizer Bunny who just keeps going and going and going (and is playing the drum as well). You might say he marches to a different drummer.

I was at a conference on Medicare health services and there was a lot of discussion about patients taking more responsibility for their health, e.g., exercising, quitting smoking, eating healthy foods. During the break I was talking with a social worker from an intermediate care facility. She commented on how most of their patients have the belief that "I worked hard for forty-five years, I'm retired, and I want to be taken care of." Of course, not everyone has this attitude. It could partially be a generational attitude and future generations "won't be so retiring." I hope so because it is an attitude that is contrary to health and to long life. These people are coasting. It's like deciding that after a car is 10 years old, it's not worth keeping up so just use it until it dies.

The concept of retirement is only about a hundred years old. It was invented and used in some Western countries when employment and job mobility were far more limited than today. Its purpose was to remove older workers from the workforce so younger workers could get jobs or advance their careers. It was invented at a time when most people's bodies and minds were wearing out in their sixties. When Social Security was enacted in 1935 and the "retirement" age was set at 65, life expectancy was 60 for men and 64 for women. Thus, most people paying into the program were not expected to receive retirement benefits! It was intended as a safety net and brass ring. Today's longer life spans, better health, and abundance of employment opportunities make it time to retire retirement. Taking its place will be sabbaticals, respites, going back to school, long vacations, volunteering, part-time work, writing, speaking, grandparenting, mentoring, and community building. Universities are no longer just populated by students under 21. Some universities charge no fees for students over 65 to audit courses. There are between 50 and 75 retirement communities being built next to and linked with universities. The residents can mix with the students, take classes, attend artistic and athletic events, use university facilities, teach classes, and mentor students.[12] It can be especially appealing to people who feel strong ties to their alma maters.

While the stereotype of retirement is playing golf or shuffleboard, attitudes have been changing. An AARP (American Association of Retired Persons) nationwide survey[13] found that 61% of retirees and 70% of non retirees said retirement is "a time to begin a new chapter by being active and involved, starting new activities and setting new goals." Only 32% of retirees and 23% on non retirees said retirement is "a time to take it easy . . . [and] enjoy leisure activities." Note that younger respondents were more likely to see retirement as an active, goal-oriented time. A 1998 AARP survey found that 80% of Baby Boomers planned to work after retirement. Top role models were former President Jimmy Carter, retired General Colin Powell, and former Senator/astronaut John Glenn. Employment of older workers is likely to increase as employers discover their skills. Congress' repeal of the Social Security earnings penalty in March, 2000 will also encourage workers over 65 to continue working. (The earnings test penalized employment by reducing Social Security benefits by 33% for retirees 65-69 after an earned income floor of $15,500 a year. After age 70 there was no disincentive.)

Centenarians who work do so because it is their passion. Many do volunteer work. Some are taking university classes. Several have written autobiographies. Soon there will be so many centenarian autobiographies that their books will no longer be a novelty. It's just a matter of time before sporting events have a category for athletes over one hundred. A good example of athletic skills is centenarian Tom Spear.[14] He is an avid golfer who plays eighteen holes three times a week and scores below 90. His 3-wood shots travel 180 yards.

In *The Instant Millionaire,*[15] Mark Fisher asks what you would do if you knew that you would die tomorrow. He has found that unhappy people tell you they would be doing something totally different while happy people tell you they would do the same things they are doing now. If you don't like what you are doing, why continue doing it? If you like what you are doing, why wouldn't you want to continue it? As Fisher points out, Bach was writing music on his deathbed.

Your model of the world

Twenty years from now you will be more disappointed by the things that you didn't do than by the ones you did do. So throw off the bowlines. Sail away from the safe harbor. Catch the trade winds in your sails. Explore. Dream. Discover. –Mark Twain

There are a number of developmental theories about aging and stages of development. They all are laden with conventional thinking that suggests winding down. Consequently, they are all counterproductive in your quest for longevity. As hockey great Wayne Gretzky put it, "Most people skate to where the puck is. I skate to where it is going to be." Your model of the world needs to be based on the lifestyles of the mentally and physically healthiest people in the future, not on a description of people in past generations.

We don't know details about the lifestyles of people who will live healthy vital lives for 150 years (just as we don't know what transportation or communication will be like in twenty, fifty, or a hundred years). We do know a lot about their mental characteristics. They will be resilient, optimistic, independent thinkers who embrace change, learning, and self-renewal. They will have many of the 36 beliefs in Chapter 4. They will keep themselves fit, manage risks, and be knowledgeable about health. They will deal with problems, resentments, and disappointments and carry little "baggage." They won't be focused on "what's in it for me," but on how they can give to others, share with others, and help others. That is, they will be following a vision and a mission.

Remission

Robert Dilts[16] tells how he worked with his mother when she was given a diagnosis of "terminal" cancer. He went to medical libraries and asked for help in locating the literature on people who survive cancer. The librarians said they had numerous studies on mortality but couldn't come up with literature on survivors. Eventually, he asked what term they use for people who survive cancer and they replied remission. Remission is an interesting term as it suggests developing a new mission in life. Indeed Dilts' mother made a major career change and lifestyle change and went into remission. Bernie Siegel[17] reports a rich literature on how changes in beliefs, metaphors, and a sense of mission go with remission from cancer.

Choosing careers that enrich rather than erode

Some jobs use up the body. Some jobs use up the spirit. This is not to say that these jobs don't need to be done but that people who want to live to be 150 need to choose jobs that enrich rather than erode. What is eroding to one person is invigorating to another. One teacher at 70 might find the job exciting and feel she is lucky to be able to touch children's lives. Another teacher at 25 might talk about dreading those horrid kids. One customer service representative or nurse might feel good about helping people in need and another might feel the customers or patients are insufferable.

There are jobs, however, that seem to be especially eroding. Eroding elements include feeling unappreciated, unproductive, and feeling you are being treated unfairly. The most extreme examples are organizations with rigid bureaucratic rules and a negative esprit de corps. These organizations have no sense of mission or vision. Every year their regulations change and mount. It would be easy to feel like Mickey Mouse in the Sorcerer's Apprentice in *Fantasia* when the brooms kept coming with more and more buckets of water. I have worked with dozens of government employees who hate their jobs, have numerous psychosomatic complaints from job stress, but won't leave their jobs because the benefits are better than they can get in the private sector. They hang on until retirement. These employees have "tenured employee syndrome." That "gold watch" is much too costly.

Longevity calls for pursuing jobs that give you a sense of purpose and accomplishment. If your job isn't doing that, you need to either figure out how to make it meaningful or how to get a job that is. Meaning doesn't require a lofty goal. I can obtain a sense of meaning and purpose from washing dishes. When you feel like Dilbert, however, it is time to find another job. Some people find their career choice so fascinating and engaging that they choose to do it until they die. Scientists and musicians often fit this pattern. Some careers tend to foster burn out. Many attorneys get tired of law and choose new careers (some as psychologists). In *Future Shock*, Alvin Toffler predicted that, largely because of technological change, the average American will experience six or seven different careers. People who live to 150 will probably average even more careers.

One role model is actors. As dancer/choreographer Bella Lewitzky put it: "Artists do not retire because most artists do not have a job; they have a view of life which they practice and they continue that practice until they no longer draw breath."[18] Many entrepreneurs have the same view of life.

Finding your passion and mission

Some people know exactly what they are passionate about and maintain that passion their whole lives. Many people, however, have their passion wane and need to find a new passion or passions. Some people lose their passion when their circumstances change, for example, leaving college might include leaving behind certain sports, pastimes, and friends. A painful experience such as losing a job can take the joy out of a passion or career. Many physicians and psychologists found managed care so stifling they pursued other careers. Even achieving a goal can leave one without a passion or mission. Quite a few astronauts became depressed after they completed their missions. They worked single-mindedly on one goal and upon achieving it had no goal. Professional athletes often have this problem when they "retire" from the sport.

Mission Statements

I doubt if many current centenarians sat down and wrote a mission statement. Many, however, intuitively had one and probably could tell you what it was. They lived in a simpler time with fewer choices. Their sense of mission was often obvious to them from their religious or family traditions. There are two reasons that a mission statement can be extremely valuable to you. First, with so many changes and choices today, writing a mission statement helps you to be very clear and confident about who you are and where you are going. Second, if you are going to follow a different drummer, you need to be consciously aware of longevity aspects of your mission so you don't get sucked into conventional thinking.

Wait, I hear a cacophony of readers complaining that many organizations make a big show of mission and vision statements, put them on their annual reports, and forget them. Just because they drop the ball is no reason to discount the value of understanding and using a mission statement for your life.

Each author who writes about missions and goals uses the terminology differently and has a unique perspective on the issues. In trying to reconcile them, I found Robert Dilts' "logical levels"[19] provided the best framework for integrating differing view-points. I enhanced Dilts' system by integrating it with other theories, with an emphasis on Tony Robbins' and Laurie Beth Jones' ideas. Both Dilts' model and Robbins' ideas are based on NLP (Neurolinguistic Programming). Dilts' "logical levels" describes our minds and bodies as a network of systems which are organized in a hierarchy:

Adaption of Robert Dilts' Logical Levels
for Writing Mission Statements

Level	Question	Function	Written text
Spiritual	Who else	Trans-mission	Vision statement
Identity	Who am I	Mission	Mission statement
Beliefs/ Values	Why	Permission/ Motivation	List of beliefs & rules
Capabilities	How	Actions	Goals (+ purpose and action plan)
Environ-ment	Where When	Constraints	Schedules

The spiritual level addresses your connection and relationship with God, community, and family. The answers might come from your religious upbringing or from soul searching. Most adults have reached some conclusions on these issues. Profound life events often cause a reexamination of spiritual issues. Your vision statement includes your vision of how you can help make the world a better place. Martin Luther King, Jr. explained his in his "I have a dream" speech.

The identity level existentially addresses who you are and your purpose in life. Purpose isn't something you bestow upon yourself. It comes from connecting with something greater than yourself. It answers the question, "Why was I put on earth?" Or "What does God want of me?" Mission flows from inside and gives you a compelling sense of urgency in fulfilling your purpose. It uses whatever unique talents you have to make your contribution to the world. A mission has passion and makes you feel alive. If you hit on a mission statement that resonates with your purpose, your spine gets an electric jolt and your whole body says YES, YES. Martin Luther King Jr.'s mission was to preach the word of God and help people work together to achieve equal justice and racial harmony.

There isn't much consensus on what beliefs are. To keep it simple, they are your ideas about what is true and what is real. Values are a subset of beliefs that have positive or negative feelings about good/bad or right/wrong. Values are general, for example, it is important to be a good parent. Rules are criteria and strategies for how we implement values. The belief level is where we interpret reality and coordinate our interpretations with our identity, boundaries, values, and rules.

Capabilities are our talents and skills. Talents are abilities you were blessed with. They are genetic endowments like Mozart's musical talent or Einstein's abstract visualization talents. Skills are things you learn how to do. Your mission taps talents and seeks skill building. A person with low self-esteem underestimates his or her capabilities and a person with inflated self-esteem overestimates his or her capabilities.

Behaviors follow from your representation of your identity, beliefs, and capabilities. For example, a man who smokes cigarettes (behavior) might see smoking as manly (identity), think cancer won't really happen to him (belief), and think he is addicted and incapable of quitting anyway (capabilities).

Environment, the when and where of behavior, is the context in which our behavior takes place. Many people go to church because the environment helps them connect with God. Many smokers find they smoke more when they are with other smokers. Changes can take place at any level and reverberate to other levels. If you accomplish something you did not think you could, you might change your beliefs about your capabilities or you might conclude it was a fluke. When Tony Robbins has people walk on hot coals, some conclude "If I can do this I can do anything," while others only conclude "Wow, I can walk on hot coals."

Dilts' logical levels also have correlates in your nervous system:[20]

Logical Levels and Your Nervous System

Level	Nervous System
Spiritual	Your nervous system as a whole (holographic)
Identity	Immune system and endocrine system (deep life- sustaining functions)
Beliefs	Autonomic nervous system, e.g., heart rate, pupil dilation (unconscious responses)
Capabilities	Cortical systems, e.g., eye movements, posture (semiconscious actions)
Behaviors	Motor systems–pyramidal and cerebellar (conscious actions)
Environ- ment	Peripheral nervous system (sensations and reflex actions)

To illustrate, consider the difference in beliefs of a cancer patient who believes she will die vs. a cancer patient who believes she can conquer the disease.[21] Rational arguments about cancer not necessarily being a fatal disease are not likely to change the person's beliefs. Consciously making changes requires intervention at a higher level than the level at which you want the change. As Einstein put it, "Our thinking creates problems that the same type of thinking will not solve." A change in her conception of herself as a victim (identity level) or relationship with God (spiritual level), however, is likely to make her receptive to new beliefs about cancer.

Dilts' Logical Levels can also be used to contrast how victims and optimists think at each logical level.

Logical Levels: Victim vs. Optimist

Level	Victim/Pessimist	Optimist
Spiritual	God is punishing me.	God and prayer will help me.
Identity	I am a cancer victim.	I am basically a healthy person.
Beliefs	Cancer is a fatal disease.	This is a temporary problem.
Capability	I'm doomed.	Good health practices, prayer, and medicine will beat this.
Behaviors	I'll take my medicine but . . .	I'll work my program.
Environment	The cancer is attacking me.	My program is shrinking the cancer.

Dilts pointed out that when Jesus was asked which of the Ten Commandments was the greatest, he jumped to a higher logical level. Instead of talking about behaviors, he spoke to the spiritual level with the first Great Commandment: Love your God (spiritual level) with your heart (beliefs/values level), your mind (capabilities level), and your strength (behavior level). His second Great Commandment, To love your neighbor as yourself, was at the behavior level.

Writing your comprehensive mission statement

You will become as great as your dominant aspiration . . .
If you cherish a vision, a lofty ideal in your head,
you will realize it. –James Allen[22]

I've found that when you make a deep commitment,
unseen forces come to your aid. –Charles Lindbergh

Dreams come a size too big so that we can grow into them.
–actress Josie Bisset

Your comprehensive mission statement needs to include longevity. The process requires considerable time and soul searching. But if you are going on a journey you need a map. Here is the process from the top down:

1. Spiritual Level: Vision Statement

Martin Luther King, Jr. painted a picture of a better world. It was such a compelling vision that hundreds of thousands of black and white people risked their jobs and their safety to make the vision come true. Patch Adams looked over a hillside and had a vision of a free medical clinic that served people rather than patients. Jesus had a vision of a more caring world. Mother Teresa had a vision of people who were dying or hungry receiving loving care. Moses had a vision of leading his people out of slavery and into the promised land. They saw the end result and painted a vivid, compelling picture.

Vision is about your dream of a better world. It empowers you with a sense of connection, purpose, and passion. Your vision statement needs to include longevity but keep in mind that longevity is merely a means achieving other ends. You might need several vision statements to cover different areas of your life, e.g., work, family, spiritual, and health/longevity. Envisioning involves fantasizing about what you would really like. If you don't ask, for sure it won't happen. If you do ask, your mind starts figuring out how to do it. Vision statements:

- are stated in present tense
- describe the desired end state
- include vivid details to make it tangible
- inspire passion

If you are having difficulty identifying your vision, ask yourself:
- If I could create a perfect world, what would it be like?
- If I were to take a sabbatical and study one subject, what would I study?
- What talents and gifts has God given me?
- What epitaph would I like on my tombstone?
- What would I like my obituary to say?
- What legacy would I like to leave?

The vision statement can be short or lengthy. Visions need a headline to quickly communicate their essence. Martin Luther King, Jr. said "free at last, free at last, Lord God Almighty, free at last." Some of the best examples of headlines come from advertising, e.g.,
- Nike's "Just do it."
- The U.S. Army's "Be all that you can be."
- Federal Express' "When it absolutely positively has to be there."

Each of these crisply communicates a promise of a better you, a better world, or a problem solved.

2. Identity Level: Mission Statement

While vision paints your dream, your mission statement gives a general direction or strategy for achieving your dream. Vision is an end state; mission is a process. Martin Luther King, Jr.'s mission was to achieve equality with nonviolent protests and demonstrations. If you are having difficulty identifying your mission, ask yourself:
- If I were independently wealthy, what would I do to contribute to the world?
- What activities make me feel I am making a contribution?
- What do I enjoy so much I do it for free?
- When am I in a "flow" state in which I am absorbed in and captivated by what I am doing?

- What could I do all day long and not get tired?
- What fascinates me?
- What special talents do I have?
- What would I do if I knew I could not fail?

If you had more than one vision statement, you might need to write a mission statement for each. Most businesses mistakenly write lengthy mission statements to put on their brochures and reports and then forget them. Such a process is a waste of time. Laurie Beth Jones[23] has three excellent criteria for mission statements. They need to be:

- a sentence or less
- a process (not an outcome or goal)
- easily understood by a 12-year-old
- so memorable they could be recited at gunpoint

For work mission statements, the key to being successful (and to making lots of money) is "being very clear about what you love to do, what you are willing to do, and what you can do all day long without getting tired or it."[24] If you meet these criteria, you are likely to get very good at what you do, radiate your love of what you do, and attract clients and money.

Richard Leider asked people over 65 what they would do if they could live their lives over again.[25] They said they would be:

- more reflective
- more courageous
- clear earlier about purpose

3. Identity Level: Primary Question

Just as we use computers to try to answer questions, our minds continually ask us questions. For task-oriented activities, the questions are task oriented; for example, "What should I eat for dinner?" Our minds also ask us a primary question, for example, "How can I be helpful?" or, "Why does this always happen to me?" Whether your primary question is positive or negative, useful or not, your mind will try to give you an answer. Consequently, it is vital that your primary question is positive and generative for you. (The concept of primary questions comes from Tony Robbins.) To find your primary question, notice your internal dialogue and what question is the most central question. If it isn't positive and generative and supporting your vision and mission, change it.

4. Identity Level: Attributions, Injunctions, and Scripts[26]

It is natural that we model parents and other important people in our lives. Our role models give us messages about ourselves, the world, and our role in the world. These models were often formed when we were at an impressionable age and had limited intellectual abilities and knowledge for assessing the implications of the messages. Challenging the messages could have gotten us into trouble with our parents or teachers. Attributions can be positive; for example, "You're so smart." or "You have your mother's gift for music." Attributions may be negative, for example, "You're such a klutz." Injunctions are messages about what you are not supposed to do or be, for example, boys don't cry, girls should leave decisions to men, children should be seen and not heard. Scripts are roles that our parental figures suggest, for example, "You're going to be a doctor when you grow up." or "You're just like your old man." Naming someone Jr. suggests he will be like Sr. In many ways Martin Luther King, Jr. brought reform just as his namesake Martin Luther had done almost 500 years earlier. In school many children receive labels such as jock or nerd.

Consider what attributions, injunctions, and scripts your family and childhood transmitted and how these may still affect your life, positively and negatively. In what ways are you like your father, mother, and grandparents? Note the most important attributions, injunctions, and scripts and what you now choose to do about them. Do any of them have implications for longevity?

5. Beliefs Level: Longevity Values

The most important beliefs are the ones you feel strongly about–values. We begin with the list of 36 longevity beliefs from Chapter 4. Review the list and rate each value on a scale of 1-5 with 1= I don't believe this one yet or don't feel comfortable with it yet, and 5=Yes, I really believe this and believe it passionately. The 36 longevity beliefs are:

_____ 1. My mind is a muscle and I keep it strong and fit my whole life.
_____ 2. I can have a sexually fulfilling life my whole life.
_____ 3. I practice continuous quality improvement with my mental and physical health.
_____ 4. I listen to my body and proactively foster good health.
_____ 5. I always have a mission.
_____ 6. I search for the smart way to do things.
_____ 7. My mind, body, and spirit are constantly renewing themselves.
_____ 8. I cultivate my sense of humor.
_____ 9. I cultivate a positive vocabulary.
_____ 10. I cultivate fond memories and let bad memories wither.
_____ 11. Any suggestions of surgery prompt an intense search for alternative solutions.
_____ 12. I move like a 20-year-old.
_____ 13. I exercise my eyes to improve my vision.
_____ 14. I am a lifelong learner.
_____ 15. Every age has its benefits.
_____ 16. I expect to have an enjoyable, exciting life at 150.
_____ 17. I am a trailblazer who leaves behind conventional thinking about longevity.
_____ 18. I have a serenity about outliving most people I know.
_____ 19. I make new friends all my life.
_____ 20. I'm really younger than my chronological age.
_____ 21. I pace myself–I'm going to be around a long time.
_____ 22. I choose life enhancing risks and reduce risks with little benefit.
_____ 23. I use the serenity prayer to give me perspective.
_____ 24. I am cheerful.
_____ 24. I have a contingency fund.
_____ 25. I observe and follow what works for me rather than blindly following generic or expert advice.
_____ 26. The resources for living longer are improving every year.
_____ 27. There are no accidents in life.

_____28. I don't need many material things to make me happy and successful.

_____29. If I intelligently pursue what I love, the money will come.

_____30. People want to help.

_____31. I can get everything in life I want if I just help enough other people get what they want.

_____32. The universe will provide.

_____33. Anything I need to know is available to me–in a book, library, the Internet, other people, or myself.

_____34. Most problems are just inconveniences or challenges.

_____35. We live in a longevity revolution.

6. Belief Level: Your Other Values

Add to the 36 longevity values ten values that are most important for you. These may or may not involve longevity issues. After writing the list, review it and consider the implications of your values and how they limit or help you. You can state the values as statements or affirmations. Either can work, but only if you emotionally associate into the values and *feel* them. Divide the list into values involving things you want to do and values about things you don't want to do. Then rank order each list.

7. Belief Level: Toward Rules

Toward rules are rules that make it easy to follow your values and achieve your goals. Most people are quite hard on themselves. Self-criticism and trying to be perfect become demanding masters. It is easy to feel discouraged, feel you will never measure up, and give up. If your rules make it easy to achieve your values, you are more likely to follow your values. For example, one of your values is good health. If your rule is that you only eat healthy foods and exercise every day, it is easy to give up when you fall short of the rule. An example of a toward rule for health might be: Every time I exercise, engage in a physical activity, dance, stretch, drink a glass of water, or eat something healthy, I am following my values and life plan. Notice that it is easy to feel good about following your plan, and consequently easier to stick with the plan. From the 36 longevity values and your ten other values, take your top 12 toward values (more if you like) and write a rule that makes it easy to achieve the value.

8. Belief Level: Away Rules

Away rules are rules that make it difficult to follow values or engage in behaviors or emotional states that you want to avoid. Values you want to avoid often go with painful emotional states you wish to avoid. The strategy with away rules is the opposite of your strategy for toward rules. You want away rules to make the undesirable states or behaviors very unlikely. For example, if you find yourself becoming angry at people, you might want an away rule such as: If I start to become angry, I will consider all other alternatives and only if no other alternative will produce better long-term results than becoming angry will I choose anger instead of a more productive alternative.

9. Capabilities Level: Capabilities

Most adults with good self-esteem are familiar with their capabilities. Capabilities are talents and skills such as musical talents and skills, writing, public speaking, selling ideas, etc. If you are going through major life changes or career changes, inventorying your capabilities can be especially helpful. After you list your capabilities, ask yourself what compliments and feedback you receive from others to see if you might have missed some of your capabilities.

10. Behavior Level: Goals

State your goals as the outcomes you want (vs. what you plan to do). I suggest a list for one year, five years, ten years, your 100th birthday, and your 150th birthday. Most time management experts stress that goals need to be stated in measurable outcomes with time frames. Tony Robbins[27] added two very important elements–purpose and a "what it takes" action plan. They add the motivation and direction that get you excited about getting it done and focuses you on how to most efficiently and effectively do it. If reading the purpose doesn't get you excited about achieving the outcome and following the plan, you need a "juicier," more inspiring purpose statement. As Robbins puts it, "There is a major difference between simply having a dream and having enough reasons to push yourself through the inevitable obstacles and thereby achieve a worthwhile goal . . . You must know why you are going after it so that if your first plan or attempt fails, you have the necessary drive to follow through."[28] Examples of longevity-oriented goals might be:

Outcome: Be strong, look great, feel great, and have lots of energy as evidenced by:

1. doing Nordic Track for 40 minutes averaging at least 6 mph
2. bench pressing 150 pounds X 3 sets of ten reps
3. 60 uninterrupted pushups

Purpose: To be extraordinarily healthy and fit another 100 years

Action Plan:

1. Cardiovascular exercise three times a week
2. Lift weights three times a week

Time Frame: by July 1 or sooner

11. Environment Level: Environment

Walt Disney intentionally had three different frames of mind.[29] As the *dreamer* he free associated and used his imagination to come up with possibilities and ideas. As the *critic* he constructively pointed out the difficulties in carrying out the dreamer's ideas. As the *realist* he pragmatically determined how to do things. Disney had different postures, rhythms, mannerisms, and rooms for each of his three frames of mind. He appreciated the power of environmental cues.

You need to make a list of places and situations that bring out particularly resourceful states for you. For example, your resourceful list might include listening to Mozart centering you, exercising giving you energy, and dancing giving you a sense of freedom.

Review your comprehensive mission statement at least once a week. Pair it with something you do anyway so it will become a habit, for example, reading it while eating Sunday breakfast. As you read it, associate into the emotion that goes with your vision, mission, and goals. Then double the emotions and make them really intense. Pick areas you want to focus on and post the list of affirmations or beliefs somewhere so you will see it daily. Determine how to tie the system with whatever system you currently use for scheduling and goal setting. If you don't have a system, the two most prominent ones are Franklin Covey Planners and Day-Timers. Both have literature explaining how to get the most from the system. Tony Robbins has a system, Outcomes-Focused, Purpose-Driven, Action-Plan (OPA)[30] that promises to be even more effective. As of this writing, its complexity makes it difficult for most people to understand and effectively use.

Exercise 7-1: Write a comprehensive mission statement.

It should address your:
1.   Spiritual Level: Vision Statement(s)
2.   Identity Level: Mission Statement(s)
3.   Identity Level: Primary Question
4.   Identity Level: Attributions, Injunctions, and Scripts
5.   Beliefs Level: Longevity Values
6.   Belief Level: Your Other Values
7.   Belief Level: Toward Rules
8.   Belief Level: Away Rules
9.   Capabilities Level: Capabilities
10.   Behavior Level: Goals
11.   Environment Level: Environment

To give examples, I have outlined my current comprehensive vision statement in the Appendix.

Exercise 7-2: Write your obituary.

Writing your obituary helps you sort out what is important and what your legacy will be. Pick a target age, e.g., at least 150 years, and figure what year it would be then. You can indicate that your death was sometime after that year and imagine you gave or recorded the presentation a few years after you died. Decide whom you would be addressing, for example, those attending your funeral, just family members, your church, or an organization. (I chose my Toastmaster's group so I could actually deliver it.) Decide whether the format would be a formal speech, intimate living room presentation, or some other format. Then write away, keeping in mind that there will be enormous technological change. To give an example, my obituary is in the Appendix.

Resources

My favorite resource for writing vision and mission statements is Laurie Beth Jones' *The Path: Creating Your Mission Statement for Work and for Life*. Carol Adrienne's *The Purpose of Your Life* does an excellent job of helping people figure out the big picture in their lives. Barbara Sher's books, *I Could Do Anything If I Only Knew What It Was* and *Wishcraft* are also excellent. For a more businesslike approach to mission and goals, Steven Covey's books are excellent, particularly, *First Things First*.

Movies can be a rich source of inspiration. There are many movies about people seeking their vision and mission, e.g., *Jerry Maguire, Joe vs. the Volcano, Scrooge, Heaven Can Wait, It's a Wonderful Life, Oh God, Music Man, Sound of Music,* and many others. Martin Luther King, Jr.'s "I Have a Dream" speech can be helpful in getting into the flow of writing a vision statement. If you are Internet-oriented, you might think of your vision and mission statements as a web page, with each vision statement having its own page.

Chapter 8

Married for a Hundred Years?

*Keep your eyes wide open before marriage,
half shut afterward.* –Benjamin Franklin[1]

Did you ever see a homely looking couple that seemed madly in love with each other–always doting on each other, touching each other, and obviously very much in love? You might have thought to yourself, "Boy I couldn't imagine myself being in love with him/her, what is the attraction?" For that couple, both partners truly believe that their mate is the most wonderful person in the world. So why are they happier than most couples and perhaps yourself as well?

Let me make an analogy with optimism vs. pessimism (or feeling positive and cheerful vs. feeling depressed). Research has shown that mildly pessimistic people and mildly depressed people have more accurate perceptions of reality than optimistic and upbeat people. Yet optimistic and upbeat people are more successful and happier. People enjoy socializing and working with them and are more likely to want to do things with them and for them. Since they are more optimistic they initiate more activities. And because they are happier they have better physical health. Thus they experience a benevolent spiral of good fortune. Meanwhile, more "accurate" pessimistic and mildly depressed people have the opposite experience and a vicious circle punishing them.

The same thing happens in marriages. If a man believes and tells his wife that she is, like my wife, brilliant and gorgeous, good things happen. She feels better about herself, has a glow about her, dresses nicer, takes better care of herself, and is more pleasant. Again we have our benevolent spiral. If a husband is critical of his wife and focuses on her faults, the opposite happens. She might have some new gray hairs or new wrinkles, but pointing them out is not helpful. So our homely couple is brilliantly proficient at focusing on the positive and not worrying about conventional standards. If you love Barbra Streisand, her nose is beautiful. If you love a man, you will find a scar on his face a romantic sign of valor and virility. In effect we create our own realities. Creating a positive reality about your partner fosters a happier, longer marriage. To draw an analogy from another source, consider how Marva Collins drew national attention for teaching black Chicago ghetto elementary children to read and love Shakespeare and the classics. She tells her students, "You are the brightest children in the whole world . . . You know you are better than anyone else in this world."[2] The children aren't literally brighter or better than any other child in the world, but the belief helps them be better, brighter children.

> *Nothing makes a woman more beautiful*
> *than the belief that she is beautiful.* –Sophia Loren

There are times for being brutally objective; for example in deciding whether to purchase a stock. In much of life, however, putting a positive spin on your beliefs and thoughts yields better results than brutal honesty. Good manners place consideration of others' feelings above brutal honesty. Without manners our society would be quite brutal.

Exercise 8-1: Assessing Your Marriage

For each question, give yourself 2 points for usually, 1 point for about half the time or half true, and no points for rarely or never.

_____ 1. I have far more positive interactions with my spouse than negative interactions.

_____ 2. I remember what my spouse wore when I met him/her.

_____ 3. I know my spouse's favorite book.

_____ 4. I admire my spouse.

_____ 5. Each day I ask my spouse how his/her day was.

_____ 6. When I make decisions, I value my spouse's opinions.

_____ 7. I recognize when arguments are getting too intense or negative and do something to de-escalate the argument.

_____ 8. Arguments with my spouse are about one specific action or behavior (vs. global issues like being more considerate, more orderly, etc.)

_____ 9. There are a number of problems that we know we won't agree upon and we agree to disagree.

_____10. We practice good manners with each other.

_____11. We touch a lot.
_____12. My partner usually has good ideas.

Scoring:
17-24 – Your marriage is doing very well.
12-18 – Your marriage has a lot of room for improvement.
 0-11 – Your marriage needs CPR.

Exercise 8-2: *Assessing Your Priorities*

In the first column, rank the following values/activities in the order you feel are most important to you.

Importance		Time
_____	clubs/organizations	_____
_____	friends	_____
_____	marriage	_____
_____	parenting	_____
_____	personal fitness	_____
_____	recreation	_____
_____	religion	_____
_____	sports	_____
_____	television	_____
_____	work	_____

In the second column indicate the amount of time you actually spend at each activity each week. We will get back to this exercise later in the chapter.

What is marriage for?

In *Fiddler on the Roof*, Tevye's daughters wanted to marry men because they were "in love." They asked Tevye to go against the tradition of the papa and the matchmaker arranging marriages. A befuddled Tevye asks his wife Golda, "Do you love me?" She thinks it's a crazy question but concludes, "For twenty-five years I've washed your clothes, cooked your meals, cleaned your house, given you children, milked your cow, after twenty-five years why talk about love right now?. . . I'm your wife . . . For twenty-five years I've lived with him, fought with him, starved with him, twenty-five years my bed is his, if that's not love what is?" They conclude, "It (love) doesn't change a thing, but even so, after twenty-five years, it's nice to know."

Fiddler was set in Russia toward the end of the nineteenth century. Tevye not only was wrestling with the role of tradition in his life but with the purpose of marriage. In Western culture, love increasingly became the primary reason for marriage. People became more mobile. The 1960s brought hippies and free love. Movies and television made sex explicit and glamorized affairs. Feminism brought changes in male and female roles. The criteria for obtaining divorces were liberalized with no fault divorces and dissolutions. Divorce rates climbed. Prenuptial agreements became common. People divorced because they "were no longer in love" or had "grown apart." In our pluralistic society, a consensus on the purpose of marriage is unlikely.

Some celebrities, e.g., Mickey Rooney, Elizabeth Taylor, and Larry King have a pattern of serial marriages. Could this be the future of marriage if people live to 150? Yes, for some people. Not everyone has the commitment or qualities that will make a marriage last a lifetime. For people who marry serially, resilience in surviving divorces will be critical. That requires not interpreting divorce as failure. Just as a person might go through several jobs in a career and fondly regard each job, serial marriages call for viewing each marriage as a treasured experience. Rather than asking yourself, "How could I have been such a failure?" the questions are: What did I learn and gain? Can we continue a friendship? etc. This is not to advocate for serial marriage but to be realistic that it is likely to be common.

The current generation of centenarians formed their core values in the first two decades of the twentieth century–when values were not very different from Tevye's values. It was a time when divorce was rare and scandalous. People were less likely to marry because of romantic love and more likely to marry because a person was a suitable partner for rearing children and running the farm. Many of the current generation of centenarians had marriages that lasted several decades. Some outlasted their spouses and remarried.

Most people want their marriages to last a lifetime. What would make a marriage last for a hundred years or more? I reviewed a lot of books on marriage and found a disappointing collection of bromides and conventional wisdom. There is surprisingly little research on what makes marriages work or fail and much of the research is based on questionnaires rather than experiments.

There is, however, one shining star in marital research–the research by John Gottman, Ph.D. Gottman and his associates studied more than 2,000 married couples over two decades, videotaping their interactions, rating each verbal and nonverbal response, and studying their physiological responses during interactions. In three studies he was able to predict which marriages would stay together and which would end in divorce with 91% accuracy. He says he can often make such a prediction after hearing the couple interact for five minutes.[3] Gottman summarized his research in his best-selling books, *Why Marriages Succeed or Fail* [4] and *The Seven Principles for Making Marriage Work.*[5] Often psychological research ends up validating what seems obvious. Rather than dismissing such results, keep in mind that our culture's common sense advice is often contradictory, e.g., spare the rod, spoil the child vs. you catch more flies with honey than vinegar. The next three sections examine Gottman's findings–what works, what doesn't work, and widely held beliefs he discredited.

What works

A romantic night out really turns up the heat
only when a couple has kept the pilot light burning
by staying in touch in the little ways. –John Gottman[6]

1. Successful marriages have **five times as many positive interactions as negative interactions**. Despite enormous differences among the couples he studied, almost all of the couples who stay married had five positive interactions for every negative interaction. Marriages that eventually ended in divorce, however, had slightly more negative interactions than positive ones.

This finding can be seen as a validation of behaviorists like B. F. Skinner, who showed how our behavior is generally determined by the reinforcement and punishment we receive. Stephen Covey's concept of "emotional bank accounts"[7] also fits well with Gottman's 5:1 ratio. Covey relates that when you make more emotional "deposits" than "withdrawals" in a relationship, the relationship is healthy. When you make more withdrawals than deposits or are overdrawn, however, there is little *trust* or goodwill. It is not just the frequency of deposits or withdrawals, but how big they are. Covey is optimistic that there are unlimited ways to make deposits. It is interesting that some banks are called bank and *trust* companies. Our language has many metaphors equating relationships with banking, for example, investing time in a relationship.

It is noteworthy that happily married couples notice almost all of the positive things their partners do but unhappily married couples only notice 50% of their partner's positive actions.[8]

2. Successful couples have **fond memories**. Regardless of how romantic or crazy their courtship was, successful couples recall the events in detail and with great fondness. Unsuccessful couples either can't remember much about the events or view them negatively. We all selectively remember and color events. You can look for the fond memories, humor, and good times just as easily as you could look for the pain and bad times. The consequences of this choice are critical to a marriage. If you don't have fond memories, now is the time to construct them. You might start with making sure you have a positive spin and fond memories about how you met and courted.

Gottman found that the most predictive factor in whether a couple will divorce several years later is how they talk about the past. He asked 56 couples who had no intention of separating or divorcing about how they met, dated, wed, dealt with tough times, and experienced good times. When he reinterviewed the couples three years later, seven had divorced. In their initial interviews, all seven divorced couples had spoken negatively or could not remember much about their past. Of the 49 who stay married, 48 of them had spoken positively about their history in the initial interview.

Gottman relates: "Couples who later divorced tended to look back on their early days as a time of great confusion, uncertainty, and anxiety. Whatever the reality, they view their coming together as a stressful, almost haphazard occurrence, rather than one motivated by commitment and joy . . . Couples who recall their early days as chaotic often say that external events controlled their lives. For example, a couple might recall that they got married for financial reasons, or because of a pregnancy."[9] Couples who stay married, however, "look back at their earlier difficulties with pride that they were able to surmount the obstacles together."[10] Gottman also cited three factors for which the men's response was particularly important:

- Men who related their marital history as a joint undertaking and used *we* instead of *I* were more likely to remain married.
- Men who remembered their feelings and specifics about their courtship were more likely to remain married.
- Men who spoke fondly of their wives and took pride in their wives were more likely to remain married.

3. Successful couples **know a lot about each other**. Gottman's student, Alyson Shapiro,[11] found that 67% of newly wed couples reported a large drop in marital satisfaction the first time they became parents. What distinguished the 33% who reported no drop or an increase in satisfaction was that they already knew each other very well before parenthood. Knowing each other well strengthens a marriage against stressors in general. Couples who know each other well know their partner's friends, triumphs, tragedies, favorite foods and favorite colors. They know their partner's favorite brand of coffee, favorite movie, novel, actress, etc. If you don't know these kinds of things, ask. It will show your love. One option is to make a list of questions about favorite things and ask and teach each other the answers.

Exercise 8-3: How well do you know your partner?

Make a list of categories and see how well you know your partner, e.g., favorite movie, book, beverage, food, comedian, actress, actor. Have your partner do the same with you. If you find you don't know, the exercise will help you find out.

4. Successful couples have **fond thoughts and feelings and admiration for each other**. They routinely think of their partner as kind, wise, attractive, sexy, desirable, thoughtful, etc. They routinely think of their mate's admirable qualities. Sound like the homely love birds at the beginning of this chapter? That's how they do it. If you don't have these thoughts spontaneously, make a list of positive traits and keep adding to it. Read it several times a day until you spontaneously think of them.

Exercise 8-4: Write a eulogy

Imagine that your spouse or partner has died and you have been asked to deliver a eulogy. In preparation you focus exclusively on the positive qualities and events. Then read the eulogy to yourself daily for a month.

If two people agree on everything, then one of them is really not necessary in the relationship. –Ellen Kreidman[12]

5. They **share a lot of their thoughts, feelings, and activities**. Part of feeling lonely or misunderstood is feeling that your partner (or no one) knows, understands or cares. Sharing with your partner creates a powerful bond of feeling understood and loved. Thus, successful couples ask "How was your day?" and want to know the answer. They share the little things. They share their dreams.

6. They **let their partners influence them**. When partners act like they know better than their partners and don't take their ideas or feelings into consideration, it hurts and it is demeaning. Conversely, seeking and valuing a partner's views and feelings and making compromises shows respect and fondness. One-sided decision-making is more commonly a problem with husbands than with wives, though the gender difference has been diminishing in the last few decades.

7. They are **skilled at de-escalating arguments**. With some couples, one or both partners are skilled at recognizing when an argument is starting to get too intense or too negative. They de-escalate the argument by using humor, by suggesting they take a break, by pointing out what is happening, or with a calming voice and gestures. Gottman calls this "repairing." Thus, the spouse has the presence of mind to monitor and edit his or her comments, even in the heat of an argument. Even if one spouse attempts to de-escalate an argument, however, the other has to hear it and respond favorably. Often, when arguments become too intense or negative, one partner (usually the male) becomes overwhelmed and emotionally shuts down and withdraws. Gottman reports that de-escalating skills are critical to who gets divorced and who stays married.

Gottman found that during arguments, some partners experience an increase in pulse and blood pressure. Their muscles tense and their adrenal medulae secrete adrenalin. In short their bodies are preparing them for "fighting or fleeing." They feel anxious and distressed and have difficulty thinking clearly or staying in control. This is not a time when they can resolve conflicts effectively. Gottman calls this process flooding. His research found that in difficult marital discussions, men's pulse rates and blood pressures tend to rise higher and stay elevated longer than women's pulse rates and blood pressures.

Gottman believes that men's increase in pulse and blood pressure accounts for them being more likely to resort to stonewalling to maintain a sense of control. In stonewalling the partner withdraws emotionally. The term comes from the other partner feeling like she or he is talking to a stone wall. Gottman reports that 85% of partners who use stonewalling are men and stonewalling is usually more upsetting to women than to men (as indicated by an increase in women's pulses and heart rates when their partners stonewall them).

8. They **start arguments by focusing on specific behaviors** (vs. attacking character or making sweeping generalizations). Arguments that attack the partner usually end tensely and unproductively. Examples of attacking the partner include: "You are so stupid." "You're just like your no-good mother." "You are hopelessly insensitive." Attacking often includes blaming. Sweeping generalizations often include "you never" or "you always." Arguments that begin with a focus on specific behaviors and respect for the partner are far more likely to be productive and to foster marital stability.

Gottman reports that 96% of the time he can predict the fate of a conflict from the first three minutes. If a partner feels personally attacked, he or she is likely to feel defensive. Defensive responses include denying responsibility, feeling self-righteous, making excuses, yes but-ing, making counter charges, repeating one's view, whining, stonewalling, and body language such as a false smile or folding arms across the chest. The antidote for defensiveness is to reinterpret the partner's behavior as communication rather than an attack.

9. They **solve the problems they can solve and live with the unsolvable ones**. Like AA's serenity prayer, couples need to recognize what they can change and what they cannot. Almost all marriages have conflicts that appear to be unresolvable. For example, one partner might have a much higher sex drive, a stronger need for neatness and order, or want more children than the other. Gottman says 69% of marital conflicts are unsolvable ones (as indicated by the couple still arguing about the same issues when he studied them four years later).[13] I'm optimistic enough to never say never as I often see major personality changes. The point is well taken, however, that if arguing is not changing something, it is often best to live with it and get on with the marriage–that is, to develop an attitude of serenity. The things you can change, of course, are worth arguing about. Only 40% of marriages end because of frequent, devastating fights.[14] The more common reason is emotional detachment.

Without following the principles above, marriages often end with emotional detachment and disengagement. To paraphrase T. S. Eliot, "This is the way the *marriage* ends. Not with a bang but a whimper."

What does not work

I purposely cast the previous nine principles in positive terms. Each could be stated in the negative. Stating things in the negative should be avoided for two reasons:
1. It encourages negative thinking–and you tend to become what you dwell on mentally. People rarely fall down a flight of stairs, but if you think about not falling down the stairs, you are far more likely

to fall. Effective athletic trainers know this and focus on the performance they want instead of the performance they do not want. An athlete is much better served by watching films of his or her best performances than watching films of what he or she did wrong.

2. Our brains have difficulty processing negatives. Our brains have to make an image of the negative and then negate the negative image, e.g., make a picture and then cross it out. Not only is this complicated, but the image of what you don't want is still in the picture. Good hypnotists are careful not to talk about what they don't want. For example, in smoking cessation, the patter is about feeling free, clean, fresh, healthy, vigorous, and in control of your own life (vs. you will not want cigarettes).

Marital therapy myths

Gottman's research transformed many widely held beliefs into myths. These include:

Use active listening. Psychologists and marital therapists often encourage partners to use "I-messages;"[15] for example, "When you come home late without telling me you will be late, I feel you don't care about me or appreciate the work I put into fixing dinner. It would mean a lot to me if you would call if you are going to be late." Gottman's research, however, indicates that active listening "does not work" because even people who have been taught to use it rarely use it in real life.

Neuroses and personality problems doom marriages. Research has found only a weak correlation between neuroses or personality problems and marital instability. Often, a person with an emotional problem finds someone who complements his or her limitations.

A good marriage requires common interests. One couple might seem to share many common interests and complain they have little in common while another might objectively have very diverse interests and feel they have a lot in common. People in the same professions can get along splendidly or find themselves competing and clashing. The keys are your perceptions and how you interact when sharing common interests.

Affairs cause divorce. People with severe marital problems tend to seek emotional intimacy in affairs. Gigy and Kelly[16] found that only 20-27% of divorced men and women said an affair was even partially to blame.

Avoiding conflict ruins a marriage. Most marital therapists encourage couples to confront their conflicts in assertive discussions. Gottman found marriages tended to have one of three styles of dealing with conflict. All three styles can foster healthy, successful marriages. While there is no one right style of communication for dealing with conflict, mismatches of style are very hard on a marriage. With mismatched styles it is as if each partner were trying to follow a different script. Gottman's research suggests that couples with mismatched styles would be wise to try to develop a mutual style. His three styles are:

- **Validators** Validators fit well with the pattern generally advocated by marital therapists. They are excellent communicators and negotiators. They are effective at expressing their ideas and feelings and are good listeners as well. They let their partners know they respect and understand their ideas and feelings even if they don't agree. When necessary, they work out compromises. Validators often have separate spheres of influence and stereotyped sex roles. Usually, the men are more analytic and the women are more nurturant. Gottman notes the risk with validating marriages is they can be so polite and compromising as to be passionless.
- **Volatile** Volatile couples thrive on passionate, dramatic arguments at high decibels. As in Sophia Loren movies, they love to argue as much as they love sexual passion. Volatile couples usually see themselves as equal partners and value independence and individuality. The risk, of course, is that in the heat of passion they might cross the line and say or do things that will be difficult to forget or forgive.
- **Avoidant** Avoidant couples are uncomfortable with conflict and minimize conflict. They state their views and agree to disagree

rather than argue. They avoid discussions that they know will end in a deadlock. "They affirm what they love and value in the marriage, accentuate the positive and accept the rest."[17] They believe their common interests and values are far more important than getting into a conflict about a difference. They often leave problems unresolved, willing to disagree or let time take its course. Avoidant couples tend to lack psychological sophistication and introspection. The style can result in one or both partners feeling the other does not know or understand him or her very well. These marriage partners also are not skilled at resolving conflicts that demand resolution.

Gottman's research with older couples

Most couples research has been with young couples. Gottman, however, also studied "older" and "middle-aged" couples.[18] The study divided 156 couples into four groups: happy and unhappy older couples and happy and unhappy younger couples. Older couples had an average age of 63 and had been married at least 35 years; middle-aged couples had an average age of 44 and had been married at least 15 years. The study used Gottman's characteristic second-by-second ratings of each partner's behavior during discussions of events of the day, an area of continuing disagreement, and a pleasant topic. The older couples showed the same sex differences as the middle-aged couples (and younger couples in previous research). The women were more emotionally expressive, both positively and negatively, and the men were more likely to be defensive or even stonewall. Eighty-five percent of stonewalling was by husbands. Wives were more emotionally expressive listeners.

Older couples showed more affection and dealt with conflict with less negative emotion. They showed more affection even when dealing with negative emotions. They also showed less increase in pulse and blood pressure during conflicts. Even unhappy older couples, who expressed a lot of negative emotions, did not get stuck in these states. They seemed to have gained some control over these states and learned not to pursue subjects that were best left alone. The study suggests that age brings emotional maturity and happier marriages. It was consistent with a number of studies that indicate that after a decline in marital satisfaction in "mid-life," couples report increased marital satisfaction and less disagreement over a wide range of issues.

Summarizing Gottman's unique message

Gottman's writings contain the usual admonitions about communication but also contain some unique recommendations about what couples can do to enhance their chances of marital success. These are:

- make sure positive interactions exceed negative interactions by at least a 5:1 ratio
- develop a common style of arguing
- develop good skills at de-escalating arguments
- recognize when one of you becomes emotionally overwhelmed –avoid crossing that threshold and enhance your skills at not becoming overwhelmed
- cultivate positive memories

My own thoughts

I have a bias toward principles that are based on quality research as opposed to personal opinions–which is why I have emphasized Gottman's research. As a psychologist, I have some "rules" based on clinical experience that I would add to Gottman's recommendations for making marriages successful and lasting:

- **Partners need to commit to marriage as a permanent contract and/or holy sacrament.** Western laws used to regard marriage as permanent. Divorce required grounds such as adultery, abandonment, incarceration for a felony, or insanity. The Catholic Church refuses to sanction divorce without extraordinary justification. Just as there is a difference in commitment between most couples who live together vs. those who marry, there is a difference in commitment between those who are committed to their marriage as a lifelong contract vs. those who are committed for only as long as the marriage meets their needs. Couples who "keep score" on a short-term basis are the most likely, at some point, to conclude the marriage "isn't working" and they "want out." Couples who know they are in the marriage for the long term find it easier to manage a few bad years if their partner goes through a difficult period, wanes in commitment, or is preoccupied with other responsibilities (e.g., sick parent, child care, career commitments, college courses).

- **Partners need to commit to good manners.** Just as boxers have rules to keep from killing each other (e.g., not hitting below the belt or in a clinch), marriages benefit from rules to keep the partners from killing each other. Manners are about showing respect and consideration for other people's feelings and sensibilities. While volatile couples might find them too conventional or stifling, most couples would do well to commit themselves to not only practicing good manners with guests, but also with spouses and children. Good manners give the respect and positive spin to a marriage that Gottman found so critical.

- **Partners need to commit to not using the D word.** Threatening divorce violates marital promises and trust. It should be off limits in the heat of anger and should never be used as a threat. It raises the stakes to a dangerous level and undermines commitment to the marriage.

- **Partners need to commit to no verbal abuse or violence.** This needs to be a line that just isn't crossed.

- **Partners need to commit to fidelity.** While a partner might rationalize that he or she can handle it, it won't hurt anything, it didn't mean anything, or that it might even strengthen the marriage, it rarely turns out that way. Even if the unfaithful partner can deal with the deceit and guilt, the other partner usually finds it very difficult. Einstein's wife found he was cheating on her. If Einstein can't get away with it, what makes you think you can? There might be an exception for the few couples who mutually desire to "swing" as they are not promising fidelity to each other.

- **Partners need to set as few rules as possible.** While it is important for couples to follow sound principles for treating each other and the marriage with respect and reverence, the fewer rules a marriage has about expectations of the spouse, the stronger the marriage. Many people enter marriages with expectations about the spouse, e.g., he must never forget our anniversary, we must both have the same level of interest in sex, he has to like my mother, we must go to church together. The more rules and the more rigid the rules, the more justification there is for being disappointed and concluding the marriage is not working. (Making "toward rules" easy to achieve was discussed in the previous chapter.)

- **Partners need to express appreciation and give compliments.** We all need to feel good and to feel appreciated. How you feel about your marriage or relationship has a lot do with how you feel your partner treats you. Appreciation and compliments cost nothing and give rich rewards. The biggest reason people choose each other is how the partner makes them feel, e.g., intelligent, sexy, strong, appreciated, admired. They want to feel good. Why stop giving these messages just because you are married?

- **Partners need to touch a lot.** While couples often differ in how frequently partners want to have sexual relations, we all need touching and physical affection every day.

- **Partners need to look for common values and interests.** One of the most interesting contemporary marriages is James Carville and Mary Matalin's marriage. He was President Clinton's campaign manager and is a frequent television commentator. She was deputy campaign manager for George Bush and has her own television and radio program. They have coauthored a book and a baby. Do they have nothing in common because they are passionate spokespeople for opposing parties or do they have a lot in common because of their passion for politics? Whether couples have much in common has more to do with what they perceive than objective measures. Couples who stay together look for commonalities and respect and tolerate differences. (This is analogous to Gottman's research on couples recalling their marital history in positive terms.)

- **Partners need to end arguments when they reach a resolution.** There are quite a few partners who reach a resolution but don't have the presence of mind to end the argument. Sometimes both partners feel they have to have the last word. When a satisfactory outcome is reached, it is important to stop.

- **Partners need to recognize and minimize secondary agendas.** Sometimes arguments have secondary issues as well. Secondary agendas are tied to self-concept or control issues; for example, being right, being smarter, being "the man of the house." Routine tasks that generate an undue amount of conflict are red flags for secondary agendas; for example, a couple arguing about directions when driving.

- **Partners need to seek continuous quality improvement.** Just as our jobs require continually enhancing our skills and learning new skills, we need to continually work on improving our marriages. The continuous quality improvement can come from any number of sources, including identifying and studying role models, setting goals (e.g., to give three compliments a day), and reading literature on marital excellence.

  Like the Second Law of Thermodynamics, which says that in closed energy systems things tend to run down and get less orderly, the same seems to be true of closed relationships like marriages. My guess is that if you do nothing to make things get better in your marriage but do not do anything wrong, the marriage will still tend to get worse over time. To maintain a balanced emotional ecology you need to make an effort–you think about your spouse during the day, think about how to make a good thing even better, and act. –John Gottman[19]

- **Partners need a vision of what their marriage can be.** I developed the following scale to gauge the quality of marriages. It is not intended to predict whether couples will stay together. Many couples stay together in miserable marriages. To illustrate each level, I included some examples of movies or television programs with couples at this level.

Brickey Quality of Marriage Levels

Level 6   Partners are strikingly fond of each other, frequently touch, and obviously admire and adore each other. For example, *Hart to Hart, McMillan and Wife, The Thin Man, The Story of Vernon and Irene Castle,* Shelly Winter's character and the husband in *Poseidon Adventure*

Level 5   Partners love each other and are satisfied with their sex life. For example, *The Brady Bunch, Happy Days, Growing Pains, A New Leaf, Rocky, The World According to Garp, On Golden Pond*

Level 4   Partners get along pretty well and do the right things but there is little passion. For example, *Mr. and Mrs. Bridge, The Great Santini*

Level 3   One or both partners are emotionally detached and lacking in respect for the other, but usually civil. For example, *Ordinary People, A Doll's House*

Level 2   Partners are openly hostile and contemptuous of each other. For example, *Cat on a Hot Tin Roof*

Level 1   One or both partners engage in physical abuse and/or destroying the partner's self-esteem, or there is a serious problem such as alcoholism that is destroying the marriage. For example, *Who's Afraid of Virginia Woolf?, Days of Wine and Roses, The Little Foxes, War of the Roses, Poison Ivy*

Which level best describes your marriage? If you are not at Level 6, how would your life be different if you were at Level 6? Research suggests that people with the highest aspirations for their marriage usually wind up with the highest quality marriages.[20]

Growing up we had heroes and role models. Perhaps you have role models now. I tried to identify role models for Level 6 marriages. Boy was that a tough task. I started with movies. Most movies about couples are about the chase and falling in love. There are love stories in which love is tested as in *Love Story,* in which Ali McGraw's character died from cancer and *An Affair to Remember,* in which Deborah Kerr inspires Cary Grant to have a purpose in life but their reunion is postponed by an auto accident that cripples her. Married couples usually have big marital problems as in *Funny Lady* and *A Star is Born.* There are some films about historical figures that have healthy marriages. There are also some Level 6 adoring couples who provide comic relief in films, for example, Pappageno and Pappagena in *The Magic Flute* and the German refugee head waiter and his wife in *Casablanca.* The only good examples I found of Level 6 movie characters were movies about couples that worked together as detectives (*The Thin Man*) or dancers (*The Story of Vernon and Irene Castle*). I also came across two odd ones–*The Adams Family* and *The Munsters.*

Television has Level 6 couples in husband/wife detective teams–*Hart to Hart* and *McMillan and Wife.* In *Columbo,* we never meet "Mrs. Columbo" (or even know her first name) but Lieutenant Columbo (whose first name we don't know either) always speaks fondly of his wife. There are numerous situation comedies with Level 5 parents, for example, *Happy Days, The Brady Bunch,* and *Growing Pains.* There are a few situation comedies in which the main characters are Level 5 couples as in *Roseanne.*

I looked to famous people and found some loving marriages. I remembered a television interview with actress Ruth Gordon and her husband Garson Kanin (who incidently was eighteen years younger than his wife). They obviously adored each other. He said the difference between Ruth Gordon and other people is that most people would bite into an apple and say "This is a pretty good apple," but Ruth would bite into an apple and say "This is the best apple in the whole world." If her style intrigues you, she has written three autobiographies. My impression is that Paul Newman and Joanne Woodward have a very loving relationship despite the temptations and distractions of Hollywood. Jimmy and Rosalynn Carter appear to have a very loving relationship in which they love and admire each other and live their religious convictions.

Exercise 8-5: Identifying marital role models

See how many Level 6 marital role models you can identify from:
1. your friends and acquaintances
2. movies or television
3. literature

If you would like to be more like them, plan for how you can learn more about them, their beliefs, their habits, and their lifestyles. What would it take to take your marriage to a Level 6?

How to feel totally and completely loved

Richard Bandler, the principal developer of Neurolinguistic Programming (NLP), believes that people primarily think by using mental pictures, sounds, and feelings, and that most people are better in one of these modalities than in the others. Tony Robbins built on this theory by pointing out how people have very specific triggers for feeling loved.[21] Robbins reminds us that when we are first dating, we use all three modalities. We are always looking at our partners and doing nice things. We listen intently and tell of our love, and we are constantly touching. Thus, we are certain to use our partner's preferred triggers for feeling loved. With time, most people do not relate as intensely and slip into expressing their love in the ways that make them feel loved, assuming that what works for them works for others. At this point we get conversations like this:

She: You don't love me anymore.

He: What do you mean? Didn't I buy you a new car, take you to the country club, and even sit through that boring opera?

She: Yes, but you don't *tell* me that you love me.

For him, loving means *showing* love by giving her things, taking her places, and otherwise *showing* love. She, however, needs to *hear* him say "I love you" to feel loved.

Exercise 8-6: Finding what makes you feel completely and totally loved [22]

Follow these steps to learn what makes you feel totally and completely loved:
- Close your eyes.
- Think of a <u>specific</u> time when you felt totally, completely loved.
- Can you have these feelings of being totally loved if you experience these feelings without *seeing* anything?
- Can you have these feelings of being totally loved if you experience these feelings without *hearing* anything?
- Can you have these feelings of being totally loved if you experience these feelings without any *touching or physical sensation*?
- Note what was most powerful in eliciting the state. If it was hearing something, note the tone of voice and volume. If it was touch, note exactly where and how.

Now that you know what makes you feel totally loved, make sure your partner knows so he or she can do it often. Use the same procedure to learn what makes your partner feel totally and completely loved.

Romance vs. real love

Some authors, e.g., Barbara Sher,[23] make a convincing case that romance is all illusion and it is wonderful to outgrow it at "mid-life." She believes that romantic love's idealization of a partner is an unnatural state that cannot last and does more harm than good. With romantic love you want to possess your partner and bask in his or her idealized qualities. It's about meeting our narcissistic needs. Our music constantly reinforces that "You're nobody till somebody loves you." Our economy thrives on selling romance–flowers, cards, gifts, romantic trips and getaways, sexy clothes, and sexy undergarments. Sher believes that when the hormones cool down in mid-life (which will happen later with increased use of hormonal therapies) you see and appreciate your partner with your eyes wide open. She makes a good point. Many of John Gottman's recommendations are about an eyes-wide-open way of knowing what your partner really thinks and feels and how to communicate well.

To me real love is cake and romance is icing. Cake by itself can be pretty good and nourishing. Icing by itself soon becomes too sweet and is empty calories. Cake with icing is simply the best. The icing needs to be an enhancement to the cake and not the other way around. The icing meets many of our emotional needs to feel special. As with optimism, a little distortion in the positive direction can be very beneficial and healthy. So kiss passionately, exaggerate your partner's good traits, and downplay your partner's shortcomings. Do special little things to put icing on the cake. But don't confuse the icing with cake. Seduced by romance, many a person has left perfectly good cake to chase icing, only to have the icing lose its appeal and that cake they left behind look pretty good.

There is an alternative to the romance vs. real love controversy. Some people see wonder and awe in everything. Abraham Joshua Heschel[24] in particular encouraged people to learn to view the world with a sense of wonder and awe. These "lenses" not only help a relationship but your whole relationship with life. Many people experience wonder and awe when in nature. Some find it in religion or their spirituality. Wherever you find it, you can generalize it to your relationships with people and hopefully to all aspects of your life. As Einstein put it, "There are only two ways to live your life. One is as though nothing is a miracle. The other is as though everything is a miracle."

Can you spare ten seconds?

Ellen Kreidman[25] insists that if your kiss lasts ten seconds it changes the whole tone of the day. Time it—when kissing ten seconds is a lot longer than you would think. Kreidman recommends a ten-second kiss anytime you have not seen each other for an extended period of time (e.g., coming home from work). It is also very powerful when parting (e.g., leaving for work). Her books and tapes are excellent resources for finding ways to put icing on the cake.

If all else fails

Over the years I have had several couples who were "at each others' throats" constantly. I felt more like a referee than a psychologist. Out of desperation I suggested they take dance lessons. To my amazement three of these couples returned affectionate and cooing. My theory is that their arguing was at a verbal level. Dancing is romantic and is primarily at a nonverbal level. In marriages where there is jockeying for leadership, dancing makes it clear who leads. Obviously, dancing is not going to work with all marriages. It is, however, very powerful with some couples.

When you have somebody to share the problems and joys with,
the problems are cut in half and the joys are doubled.[26]
–Actor Hume Cronyn

Making marriage a priority

Consider the following marital statistics:
- Half of all marriages end in divorce within the first seven years.
- For first marriages, 67% of the couples divorce within forty years.
- Second marriages have slightly higher divorce rates.
- Marital conflict is associated with:[27]
  - shorter life spans
  - depression
  - 35% more illnesses
  - suppression of the immune system
  - increased rates of cancer, cardiac disease, and chronic pain
  - decreased endocrine system functioning
  - poorer mental health of children

Exercise 8-7: Imagining the costs and benefits

In Chapter 4 we introduced the "Scrooge" pattern[28] in which, like Ebenezer Scrooge in Dickens' *A Christmas Carol,* you are visited by ghosts. Take a few minutes to go through that process with your marriage:

1. The first ghost is of the early years of your marriage or marriages. Associate into the passions and feelings that go with those memories.
2. Next, think about your current marriage and experience your feelings about it.
3. Next, imagine what your marriage would be like thirty years from now if your marriage continues on the same course it is on. Fully experience your feelings about that future. Double your feelings, and then quadruple them.
4. Now imagine what your marriage could be like thirty years from now if your wildest hopes and dreams for the marriage come true. Double and quadruple those feelings. Feel how much richer and more joyful your life will be.
5. Now return to *Exercise 8-2: Assessing Your Priorities* earlier in this chapter. Do you want to reorder any of your priorities or change any of your time commitments?

Clergy report that few people on their deathbeds wish they had spent more time at the office. Rather, people who are dying usually wish they had put more time into family and relationships. Why live to 150 if the most important relationships in your life miscarry? The pain from failed relationships fosters depression and disillusionment. If you choose to marry, it should be in your top values/priorities in life.

Resources

Libraries and bookstores have several dozen books with opinions about what it takes to make a marriage work. If you find an author whose style and advice appeals to you, try the advice and see if it works. If you want principles that have the backing of research, the choice is clear–one of Gottman's books–*Why Marriages Succeed or Fail*[29] or *The Seven Principles for Making Marriage Work.*[30] Both are written for a lay audience and include quizzes and exercises. For inspiration on ways to make a marriage more lively and loving, I like Ellen Kreidman's *Light His Fire* and *Light Her Fire.*[31] A straightforward approach to changing what couples think and say is Aaron Beck's *Love is Never Enough.*

Research on consumer satisfaction for marital counseling indicates that marital counseling has a considerably lower satisfaction rating that other types of therapy.[32] Far too much marital counseling consists of listening to complaints. It might be briefly cathartic but is rarely helpful in the long run. Martial therapy needs to focus on solutions and how improving *your* beliefs and behaviors will result in a better marriage. (If you change, it is impossible for your spouse not to change as well.) For a step-by-step manual for saving a problematic marriage, my first choice is *Divorce Busting*[33] by Michele Weiner-Davis. She uses a solution-focused process that is positive, based on extensive research, and fits with common sense. Solution-focused therapy follows a formula of identifying goals, identifying what works (or could work) in achieving those goals, and figuring out how to do more of what works. Patricia O'Hanlon Hudson and William Hudson O'Hanlon's *Rewriting Love Stories* is an entertaining and helpful solution-focused approach to marital problems and marital enrichment. Another resource is John Gottman's weekend workshops for couples and workshops for clinicians in Seattle, Washington.[34]

Chapter 9

Sex

Men's three big fears

Men's first big fear is that as they age they will lose their ability to have erections and sexual intercourse. With age men's erections become less vigorous, less reliable, and require more emotional and physical stimulation. Nevertheless, at 70 only 15% of American men are completely impotent.[1] That 15% includes men who smoke, abuse alcohol or drugs, are obese, have medical problems, and take medications that interfere with having an erection. Men who are healthy and physically fit stand a good chance of being able to have adequate erections most of their lives. If a man does have difficulty, there are now a variety of medications that can help most men achieve erections. These are described in detail later in this chapter.

Men's second big fear is that they are losing their sexual drive. The decline is due primarily to testosterone levels decreasing with age. Men's testosterone levels vary considerably. On the average, at 50 men's testosterone levels average about 75% of their youthful levels. By 80 or 90 testosterone levels are only about 40% of their youthful levels. Even 40% is often within the wide "normal limits" for younger men. Testosterone supplements are available in pills, patches, and injections and can restore sexual urges to more youthful levels. The cost is about $50-$100 a month. Another option, Human Growth Hormone (HGH), prompts men's bodies to produce more testosterone. HGH requires several injections a week and costs about $1,000 a month. There are hundreds of products that claim to prompt the body to naturally produce HGH. Currently it is difficult to determine which ones actually do. Major pharmaceutical companies are in clinical trials for pills that will prompt the body to produce HGH. Data are accumulating on the effective and safe use of testosterone and HGH so men will be able to make the prudent decisions. Both testosterone and HGH require a prescription. Most of the products that claim to prompt HGH production are over-the-counter supplements.

Men's third big fear is that their partner will not be interested in sex. The primary consideration is whether the partner enjoys making love with the man. If he skips foreplay and romance, has missionary position sex, ejaculates, and rolls over and goes to sleep, he shouldn't expect his partner to maintain an interest in sex for decades. If he brings playfulness, romance, variety, love, and a genuine concern for his partner's enjoyment, there is a good chance she will maintain an interest in sex for a lifetime. Her interest will also depend in part on her health and vitality. Good health, estrogen replacement, lubricants, and an ongoing sexual relationship also help.

Getting erections

The best prescription for good sexual functioning is to cultivate good health by eating well, taking vitamins and minerals, exercising, and following the principles in *Defy Aging.* A healthy lifestyle lessens diseases, medications, stress, sleep problems, psychological problems, and enhances the body's production of testosterone and other hormones.

Getting an erection is a complex process and there are several steps where things can go awry. The process starts with the brain becoming aroused by sights, sounds and fantasies and the spinal cord becoming aroused by touch. Neurotransmitters activate the parasympathetic nervous system which prompts the release of nitrous oxide in the penis. The nitrous oxide triggers a series of chemical reactions that relax the smooth muscle in the penis, allowing the penis to engorge with blood (assuming the arteries and veins are healthy). The engorged penis pinches the veins of the penis so little blood is able to leave. After ejaculation, or if distracted, the parasympathetic nervous system stops prompting nitrous oxide. The blood gradually drains from the penis and when pressure on the vein is released, the blood rapidly drains from the penis. The process can get short circuited by a variety of factors which might affect thinking, brain functioning, nerves, or the circulatory system.

A good diagnosis is essential to knowing what to do about difficulty getting or keeping an erection. When a man's body is in good condition and every physical system is working well, he typically experiences two to five erections a night while dreaming (the dreams do not have to be sexual). Sleep laboratory technicians can tell when a man is dreaming by his rapid eye movements (REM).

If a man is having nighttime erections, a doctor can measure his *nocturnal penile tumescence* (*NPT*) response to measure the degree to which the penis engorges during sleep. A good NPT response usually indicates a psychological cause for erectile difficulty (about 20-30% of erectile dysfunctions). A poor NPT response usually indicates a physical cause. NPT can be measured with an overnight evaluation in a sleep lab (which is typically required when sleep apnea is suspected). In the sleep lab two stress gauges are placed around the man's penis and are wired to a computer. NPT can be measured less formally and less expensively with a velcro device known as a Snap Gauge. Even less expensive is a variation of the old "postage stamp test"–a band of paper placed around the penis at bedtime. If the paper is ripped (or the stamps separated at the perforations), the man experienced NPT and his problem probably is between the ears. A thorough diagnosis takes into consideration health, medications, how the problems developed (acute vs. gradual onset, associated with any events), nocturnal erections, masturbation, psychological factors (depression, stress, anxiety, bad experiences), and the partner's receptivity.

The most common reason for men to have difficulty obtaining erections is atherosclerosis and other medical conditions that affect circulation. Factors that can cause erectile dysfunctions include:

- Medical problems–the most common ones being:
    - diabetes–more than 50% of diabetic men have erectile dysfunction difficulties
    - atherosclerosis–plaque builds up and restricts blood circulation
    - thyroid problems (either too high or too low)
    - high blood pressure–can damage arteries and foster atherosclerosis
    - nerve damage in the prostate or pelvic organs or spine
    - multiple sclerosis
    - Parkinson's disease
    - heart disease
    - sickle cell anemia
    - kidney disease

- prostate problems or surgery (fortunately prostate surgeries are getting better at sparing the nerves necessary for erections)
- Smoking
- Alcohol abuse
- Drug abuse (street drugs, steroids)
- Medications–some of the most common culprits are for:
  - blood pressure
  - heart disease
  - cholesterol
  - anxiety, e.g., Valium, Xanax, Tranxene
  - depression
  - gastrointestinal problems, e.g., Tagament, Pepcid, Zantac (but not Alka-Seltzer or Tums)
  - antihistamines, e.g., Benadryl, Dramamine
  - muscle relaxers, e.g., Flexeril
  - diuretics
  - beta blockers, e.g., Inderal
  - cancer chemotherapy
  - epilepsy
- Psychological problems (20-30% of erectile dysfunctions)
  - depression–dulls the interest and has twice the rate of erectile disorder
  - anxiety–you must be relaxed to activate the parasympathetic nervous system, which prompts the smooth muscles in the penis to relax
  - stress
  - marital conflicts, hidden agendas, ambivalence
  - guilt
  - bad experiences
- Sleep apnea (42% of men with sleep apnea have erectile dysfunctions)
- Testosterone deficiency (about 5% of cases)
- Venous leak (with this condition, which is usually congenital, veins from the penis aren't sufficiently blocked during an erection and blood seeps out–it can often be solved by using a latex band around the base of the penis to constrict the veins)

Note that erectile dysfunctions are often caused by medications rather than their targeted medical problems. With depression, some SSRI[2] antidepressants (e.g., Prozac) often delay orgasm. Men usually regard this as a desirable effect. (Some physicians even prescribe a low dose of an SSRI antidepressant as a treatment for premature ejaculation. The success rate is modest as there are often psychological or other factors contributing to the problem). Women, of course, have no need to delay their orgasms and medication delaying orgasms is an undesirable effect.

The most common psychological cause of erectile dysfunction is performance anxiety. Performance anxiety activates the sympathetic ("fight or flight") nervous system instead of parasympathetic nervous system that sends nitrous oxide to the penis so it will fill with blood. Not getting an erection increases the anxiety next time and sets up a vicious cycle. Almost every man occasionally experiences a problem getting an erection, e.g., due to stress, preoccupation with problems, anxiety, illness, medication, inebriation, or just being tired or exhausted. Often men assume the cause is aging and assume or fear they have lost their ability to get an erection. Keeping perspective and not catastrophizing can help keep a temporary difficulty from becoming a permanent one. Another thing that helps is not trying too hard. If you adopt a mind set that you can have a wonderful sexual experience without an erection and do so, you find that sex can be exciting and fulfilling without an erection. It takes your mind out of achievement mode and an erection often happens anyway. Sex researchers Masters and Johnson[3] found that performance anxiety often includes "spectatoring" in which men focus on their sexual performance instead of being mentally and emotionally absorbed in making love.

There are many ways to get an erection

Even if you have a medical problem or medication that is causing an erectile dysfunction, chances are very good that you can still have erections. Resources include:

Viagra Pfizer researchers in England were trying to develop a medication that increased blood flow and reduced chest pain (angina).

They gave up on the experiments but an odd thing happened–the experimental subjects wanted more of the medication. Many of the patients had vascular problems that caused erectile dysfunctions and the medication was prompting erections. Thus Viagra (sildenafil) was developed by serendipity.

Seven million American men are taking sixty million pills a year to help them obtain erections.[4] Viagra works by causing the nerves in the penis to release nitrous oxide, which leads to the smooth muscles in the penis relaxing and allowing the penis to engorge with blood.

Here are some key facts on Viagra:

- works with 70-80% of men (including those with medical conditions and medications)
- does not increase desire–if the desire is not there, nothing happens
- does not enhance sexual performance if performance is already normal
- peak effect is about 60 minutes after taking it
- half of the medication dissipates in four hours
- works best on empty stomach (large or fatty meals slow its absorption)
- costs about $10 a pill
- available in 25, 50, and 100 mg doses
- recommended frequency of use is no more than once per 24 hours (though clinical trials included doses as high as 800 mg)
- side effects are more likely with higher doses
- possible side effects include:
  - can be fatal if taken with nitrate-based heart medications or the nitrate-based street drug ("poppers")
  - headaches (16%)
  - facial flushing (10%)
  - upset stomach (7%)
  - nasal congestion (4%)
  - urinary tract infection (3%)
  - color vision distortion (3%)
  - diarrhea (3%)
  - dizziness (2%)
  - rash (2%)
  - priapism (rare)–this condition involves an erection that lasts six hours or longer–the condition is painful and four hours is

considered an emergency as the penis can be permanently damaged
- is least likely to be effective with:
  - lack of desire
  - radical prostate surgery
  - long-term insulin dependent diabetes
- other possible medication interactions include: Tagament and certain antibiotics including erythromycin
- caution is needed if you have sickle cell anemia, leukemia, Peronie's syndrome (a bent penis), a peptic ulcer, or any history of priapism (erection that won't subside)
- if you have a heart condition and need emergency attention, it is important to tell emergency medical personnel if you have taken Viagra as they might administer nitroglycerin or other nitrate-base medications
- the penis may remain erect after ejaculation and further intercourse may be possible
- Viagra researchers are looking into a nose spray version that would cut the response time to 5 to 15 minutes (and help people who have difficulty swallowing pills)

Viagra has had some interesting social consequences. It can upset the status quo and require readjustments in attitudes and roles. Some wives don't welcome their husband's sudden increased interest in intercourse. Men need to be sure they don't leave the love and romance out of their increased interest in sex. Some wives or lovers complain or fear that their partner isn't interested in them, just their erections. The term Viagra divorces refers to divorces that result from men trying their new-gained potency outside their marriages. The Pentagon drew a lot of criticism over its plan to spend $50 million for Viagra for soldiers with erectile dysfunctions. Finally, who would have guessed that straight-laced World War II veteran and former presidential contender, Senator Robert Dole would be promoting Viagra?

Vasomax Vasomax (phentolamine) also works by improving blood flow to the penis. Its big advantage over Viagra is that it does not interact with nitrates. This makes it medication of choice for men on heart medications with nitrates. It works by dilating blood vessels and blocking the effects of adrenaline. Data indicate a 25-60% effectiveness rate and a 15-to 30-minute response time. Some users have reported having a second erection after ejaculation. Side effects appear to be even less than for Viagra, with nasal congestion the most common complaint. Other complaints are headaches and flushing. Vasomax was approved for use in Mexico in 1998 and is likely to be approved in the U.S. On the average it does not appear to be quite as effective as Viagra but individuals vary in their response to medications and it may be more effective with some men.

Spontane   Spontane (apomorphine) stimulates brain cells to overcome anxiety. This allows desire to win out over anxiety. Data indicate a 46-60% success rate in men who did not have any physical basis for an erectile dysfunction. The most common side effect is nausea. It was submitted for FDA (Food and Drug Administration) approval in 1999.

Herbs   There are many herbs that purportedly help with erectile dysfunctions. Yohimbe is the only herb that has FDA approval as a treatment for erectile dysfunctions. Research has not supported its alleged aphrodisiac effects. It has been shown, however, to increase blood flow to the penis. Studies report success rates ranging from 14% to 85%. Yohimbe can be overstimulating, raise blood pressure and pulse, and cause flushed skin, dizziness, headaches, and hallucinations. The prescription form of yohimbe is preferable to over-the-counter yohimbe as there is more assurance of a quality product. There are many other herbs that are touted as helping with erectile dysfunctions but data specific to erectile dysfunctions benefits are scarce.

Ginkgo biloba has shown some efficacy in enhancing blood circulation in general. Many herbs are supposed to offer numerous benefits or be aphrodisiacs, but it is difficult to find good research support for their effectiveness with erectile dysfunctions. Some may help contributing problems such as depression or anxiety. Saw Palmetto has good research support for helping to prevent prostate cancer.

Testosterone By 50 testosterone levels average about 75% of youthful levels. By age 80 or 90 testosterone levels are only about 40% of youthful levels. Testosterone has a big effect on desire but only 5% of erectile dysfunctions are caused by low testosterone levels. If you are one of those 5%, however, it is an important 5%. Testing needs to not only look at testosterone levels but also free (unbound) testosterone levels.

Injections Two prostaglandin medications have a 90% success rate in producing erections by causing the penis arteries to swell and penis veins to contract. The catch is they have to be self-injected into the penis. The generic name alprostadil has two brand names–Caverject and Edex. They cost about $20 an injection. Erections occur in 10 to 15 minutes and last up to an hour (if they last longer the dosage needs to be decreased). The penis often remains erect after ejaculation and further intercourse may be possible. The procedure requires instruction in a physician's office and a prescription.

Mild to moderate pain was reported by 37% of users. Other side effects include: prolonged erection (4%), penile fibrosis (3%), and bleeding (3%). A long-term study indicates a risk of bruising (17%), prolonged erection (13%), pain (13%), hardening of tissue (10%), curvature of the penis (10%), superficial infection (3%), and dizziness (1%). There is some risk (less than 1%) of priapism (painful erection lasting six hours or longer).

Some men use a low dose of medication in combination with a vacuum pump to keep the medication dose minimal. While Viagra requires desire to work, injections work even if there is no desire, problems with anxiety, or other psychological issues. The medication should not be used more than once in 24 hours or three times a week. Diabetics who administer insulin by injection are already used to the idea of self-injections. Other less commonly used injections are papaverine or a combination of papaverine and phentolamine. They act by relaxing muscles so blood can be drawn into the penis.

MUSE The MUSE (Medicated Urethral System for Erection) system uses an applicator to insert a grain-of-rice-sized alprostadil pellet one inch into the urethra. (This is the same medication used with Calverject and Edex.) The medication is absorbed through the urethra, producing an erection in about ten minutes. Erections last 30-60 minutes. Success rates are 60-70%. The most common side effects are discomfort or pain. The cost is about $20 a treatment.

Vacuum devices A vacuum device has a plastic cylinder that fits over the penis. A hand or battery operated pump draws the air out of the tube, creating a vacuum that causes the penis to fill with blood. The process takes a minute or two. A rubber retaining band slides off the cylinder and onto the base of the penis to trap the blood in the penis. It must be tight to work. Usually, when the ejaculation reaches the retaining band, it is forced back through the prostrate and into the bladder (*retrograde ejaculation*). This is not physically harmful or uncomfortable. The erection remains, even after ejaculation, until the constriction band is removed. The band must be removed within thirty minutes (so it is important not to fall asleep before removing it).

In the U.S. physicians prescribe 150,000 vacuum devices a year at a price of $200-$500. In the long run they are cheaper than Viagra. Nonprescription vacuum devices of varying quality are sold in magazines, the Internet, and sex stores starting at $40. While a vacuum device might distract from romantic ambiance, it is the safest option and is usually effective in producing erections.

Penile implants This should not be considered lightly as it involves surgery and permanently changes the structure and appearance of the penis. If the other options are not applicable, however, implants can give satisfactory results. The simplest type of implant consists of a silicone-coated rod or rods, making the penis always erect. Since the penis does not fill with blood, there isn't the satisfaction of the penis enlarging and the sensation is different. The other disadvantage, of course, is the full-time bulge in your pants. Surgery is on an outpatient basis and complications are rare.

A more sophisticated device uses a spring and cable system that allows the penis to hang naturally when disengaged and be erect when the device is activated. Even more high tech is a system with two cylinders. Squeezing the head of the penis pumps fluid into the cylinders and causes an erection. Bending the penis near the glans releases the fluid back to the storage area. The surgery requires inpatient hospitalization and six weeks of healing before using. Five percent of patients need further surgery within five years. The Cadillac of implants has balloon-like cylinders that cause the penis to enlarge, as it would if engorged with blood. The fluid reservoir is in the lower abdomen. Squeezing one part of the scrotum activates the pump and squeezing another part of the scrotum returns the fluid to the reservoir. It also requires inpatient surgery.

The rule of thumb is that more complex systems have more things that can go wrong (e.g., a mechanical malfunction or leaking fluid) and require further surgery. In the U.S. there are 21,000 penile implants a year. A Taiwanese ten-year follow-up study[5] with 331 implant recipients found an 87% satisfaction rate.

Creams A cream version of Alprostadil (which is used in Caverject and Edex injections) has had successful clinical trials in Argentina.

The future Caverject was introduced in 1996, MUSE in 1997, and Viagra in1998. Pharmaceutical treatments for erectile dysfunctions are in their infancy. Pharmaceutical companies are likely to develop combination medications for men who do not obtain good results from current medications. Topical creams are also likely to be approved.

Currently, physicians do what can be done for any medical conditions, consider possible side effects from any medications, and use the following decision tree:
- first choice–Viagra
- second choice–injections or MUSE
- third choice–implants
- (vacuum device a choice at any point)

In the future first choices are likely to include pills, creams, and patches. Eventually, gene therapy may offer options as well.

Enhancing sex for women

The older woman has seen more, heard more,
and knows more than the demure young girl . . .
I'll take the older woman every time. –Clark Gable[6]

Women don't have to get an erection to have intercourse but an estimated 65% of women don't have an orgasm during intercourse. Many factors contribute to this statistic. Inadequate foreplay can lead to inadequate lubrication and uncomfortable intercourse. Most women need a lot more time than men need to become sexually aroused and many men don't take the time to help their partners become aroused. Some men ejaculate within a few minutes and intercourse doesn't last long enough for the woman to reach an orgasm. Most sexual positions, especially missionary position, don't provide enough clitoral stimulation. Because of mixed messages about sex, or bad experiences with sex, or their personality styles, some women have difficulty "letting go." Fear of pregnancy can cause anxiety. Health problems or medications can interfere with blood circulation to the clitoris and vagina. Not having an orgasm during intercourse is not considered a dysfunction as a majority of women do not have orgasms during intercourse.

What can a woman do? If your partner doesn't understand what you need, you need to explain it. It may be difficult but it sure beats decades of an unsatisfactory sexual relationship. He needs to know what helps you get in a romantic mood, what arouses you sexually, how much arousal you need, how to notice when you have enough lubrication, what sexual positions give you the most stimulation and what positions give you the least stimulation or are uncomfortable, and what helps you have an orgasm if intercourse is insufficient. For most women the "missionary position" (man on top thrusting and woman relatively inactive) is the least stimulating. Women often get far more stimulation from the "female superior" position with the woman sitting on top of her partner and sliding forward and back and rubbing against his pubic bone.

It is important to make sure vaginal tissues do not become dry or thin. Estrogen replacement can help. Water-based and water-soluble gels like K-Y Jelly or Astroglide can help. As with physical fitness, sex is a "use it or lose" it proposition. If you have a period of time when you are not sexually active, masturbation can help you stay physically and mentally sexually responsive. Vibrators can be especially helpful. A psychologist/sex therapist told me he advised one of his clients to get a vibrator and she was delighted, saying she had her first orgasm since her husband "lost interest" twenty years ago. For women who have difficulty experiencing orgasms, "directed masturbation while employing erotic fantasy" has the best record of success.[7]

While men's hormones and sexual drive peak between 18 and 25, women's hormones and sexual drive don't peak until around 40. With menopause women's ovaries stop producing estrogen. Estrogen replacement has a number of health benefits including reducing the risk of heart disease, osteoporosis, Alzheimer's disease, colon cancer, tooth loss, and skin aging. It can also prevent mood swings, hot flashes, problems with memory, and feeling like you are going crazy. All of these contribute to maintaining a healthy sexual drive and sexual functioning.

Whether women take estrogen supplements or not, many women in their fifties find they are losing their interest in sex and attribute it to aging. Women's bodies produce testosterone (the principle male sex hormone) as well as estrogen. At menopause, however, women's bodies stop producing testosterone. The result can be weight gain, doldrums, and loss of sexual drive. Often a small amount of testosterone can reverse weight gain, slow aging, and rekindle the sex drive.

What happens if women start taking Viagra? They already are. During sexual stimulation and orgasm women's clitorises and vaginas become engorged with blood. Viagra has been shown to increase blood flow to the clitoris and vagina, which presumably increases a woman's sexual response. Strong placebo effects are likely since women's orgasms are very subjective. Eventually, women might consume more Viagra than men. Currently, physicians have to prescribe it "off label," meaning is not for the purpose approved in the application to the FDA. Pfizer's research department is busy generating research data to justify an expansion of Viagra's indications to women and looking into a spray or cream versions of Viagra.

Vivus pharmaceutical company has been doing clinical trials in Argentina on a cream version of alprostadil (used in Calverject and Edex, and MUSE). It has obtained a patent on an alprostadil cream for women to rub on their clitorises. In 1999 they applied to the FDA for permission to conduct clinical trials.

Unfortunately most men still tend to judge women's sexual desirability by their youth and appearance. The good news is that with medical advances, hormone replacement, and skin care products, women can look a lot younger and healthier and more vibrant than then women did even a decade ago. In the next few decades gene therapy and further hormone replacement (e.g., HGH or IFG-1, or testosterone or related hormones) will help women and men look even younger. Also, a sizable number of men are becoming more receptive to relationships with older women. By the time people are 70, a partner's chronological age becomes less important than the partner's vitality.

Sex is a lot more than intercourse

Sex is a smorgasbord of choices. Lifelong sexuality calls for keeping your thoughts about sexuality multifaceted. Facets of sexuality include:
* Romance–consider the millions of women who read dozens of romance novels a year and Hollywood's thousands of romantic movies.
* Touching (caressing, cuddling, massaging, fondling, etc.)–Many women say touching is more important to them then sexual intercourse. Many people receive touching from massage, playing with children, playing with pets, and cosmetologists and beauticians.
* Fantasy–Women tend to read romance novels and watch romantic movies while men tend to view pornography and watch adventure/hero movies.
* Orgasm–While most people think of sex as intercourse, it is just one aspect of it and there are many variations of intercourse including manual, oral, anal intercourse, and masturbation.

- Connection and emotional intimacy–This is the end state that many seek from sex.
- Presence or charisma–Clark Gable had it, Cleopatra had it, Marilyn Monroe had it–some people have a magnetism.
- Repartee–consider the repartee between Cybill Shepherd and Bruce Willis in the TV series *Moonlighting* or Humphrey Bogart and Lauren Bacall or Katharine Hepburn and Spencer Tracy. Sex sometimes has a repartee like a dance or tennis match.
- Inexplicable attraction–a certain smile, a breathy voice, a swagger
- Love–those positive feelings toward a partner or lover.
- Making a partner feel good emotionally–compliments, admiring looks, etc.

If a man equates sex only with having a stiff erection that lasts long enough to have mutual simultaneous orgasms, every time he becomes physically intimate, he is putting his self-esteem on the line. Ironically, the pressure can undermine his "sexual performance" and set up a negative spiral of impotency. A man who regards orgasms as just icing on the cake, however, can enjoy the cake even if it doesn't have icing. If he regards sex as multifaceted, he has many ways to be sexual without having mutual, simultaneous, earth shaking orgasms.

Joan Crawford said Clark Gable had an animal attractiveness and any woman who worked with him felt "twinges of sexual urge beyond belief."[8] His wife, Carol Lombard, agreed but added "I adore Clark but he's a lousy lay."[9] A writer and mistress for over a decade said of Gable, "It never amounted to much and was never very good. But then I would open my eyes and realize this was the Clark Gable–Gable himself–and only then would I truly feel excited."[10] Many men could quickly become heartthrobs merely by listening, being romantic, cuddling, and complimenting.

Think about the best sexual experiences you have ever had. Did you remember how great the orgasm was? Most likely, you primarily remembered what was especially romantic and what made you feel very special and very loved. Most women will cite romance, tenderness, caring, caressing, leisurely enjoying the experience, and possibly the fantasy aspect of being swept away by a bold man. They may even experience more enjoyment from oral or manual stimulation than intercourse as many women don't experience orgasms from intercourse. While macho bull sessions may focus on sexual performance, privately many men say they derive even more pleasure from pleasing their partner than from their own orgasm.

Resources

Many primary care physicians are knowledgeable about erectile dysfunctions. Urologists usually have the most medical expertise regarding erectile dysfunctions. Helpful books on erectile dysfunctions include *The Unofficial Guide to Conquering Impotence, The Virility Solution, Viagra and You,* and *The Viagra Alternative: The Complete Guide to Overcoming Erectile Dysfunction Naturally.* Since new medications are coming on the market, however, check to see if there are more recent books. The Food and Drug Administration's web site, www.fda.gov/cder/, lets you look up the latest technical information on medications, though you have to use the generic name (e.g., sildenafil for Viagra). Internet searches can yield a lot of data on medications and treatments.

Gail Sheehy's books such as *Further Passages* are very helpful to men and women in understanding sexuality issues in the context of generations and aging. Her *The Silent Passage* gives a very helpful big picture of menopause as does chapter 9 in *Further Passages. Becoming Orgasmic* by Julia Heiman and Joseph Lopiccolo and *For Yourself: The Fulfillment of Female Sexuality* by Lonnie Barbach have helped many women more fully experience a more satisfying sexual life.

For psychological problems affecting sexuality, I recommend a psychologist who has expertise in sexual issues.

Chapter 10

Outliving Friends and Family

Death is not a failure.
Not choosing to take on the challenge of life is.
–Bernie Siegel[1]

Without death, life would be boring: everything would be
indifferent, alike, repeatable, and susceptible to deferral.
–Harald Wagner[2]

Death ends a life, not a relationship.
–Tuesdays with Morrie[3]

If you are going to live a very long time, you are going to outlive your parents, most of your friends, and possibly your children. Unless you learn to cope with their deaths positively and effectively, your longevity will be cut short. Effectively coping with outliving friends and family is a critical skill for longevity.

The loss of a child is one of the most difficult challenges in life. Consider how King David coped with the loss of his son. David was a poet, a warrior, a king, and a very religious man. His one sin that we know of was sending Bathsheba's husband to the front lines so her husband would likely be killed in battle and he could marry Bathsheba. David and Bathsheba had a son, who became very ill. David fasted, prayed, and slept on the ground to try to reverse God's punishment. When the child died, David arose from the ground, bathed, anointed himself, changed his clothes, and ate. His courtiers asked him, "Why have you acted in this manner? While the child was alive, you fasted and wept; but now that the child is dead, you rise and take food!" He replied, "While the child was still alive, I fasted and wept because I thought: 'who knows? The Lord may have pity on me, and the child may live.' But now that he is dead, why should I fast? Can I bring him back again?"[4] David went to Bathsheba and consoled her and they had another son, Solomon. Solomon was one of the wisest and greatest of Israel's kings. Apparently God was pleased with how David handled his first son's death.

Too many people who lose others–mothers, fathers, children, friends–become people who see grief as a tent pole for their life. They cherish it almost, they clutch it to them, they never let it go, and that grief becomes the impelling force for a negative, bitter, unhappy, vengeful unforgiving life. Other people, like myself, use it as a springboard for being a better person and for enjoying life more and for appreciating all the good things in it as a counter to the other things that are going to happen . . . I'm convinced that the most important single thing that affects people–whether they're young or old–is their attitude.[5] –Art Linkletter, whose daughter committed suicide at 19 and son died in an automobile accident at 32.

Dealing with death has become more difficult for Americans in the last fifty years. Death now occurs in hospitals or nursing homes rather than at home. Hospitals, however, are dedicated to preserving life and see death as an enemy and failure. They use euphemisms for death and hospital staff are often uncomfortable dealing with death. (A positive antidote has been the hospice movement.) Television and movie violence have distorted our thoughts and feelings about death. Our youth-centered society does not want to deal with aging or death (though this will change as people over fifty become a larger and larger proportion of the population). There are religious traditions for grieving but fewer people know or follow their traditions. Consequently, people are unsure about what to do or what is "right." Family members are often scattered across the country. Most of us live in urban cultures and easily lose a connection with the rhythms and wonder of nature. In view of these challenges, it is especially important to have good skills at dealing with outliving friends and family.

As a psychologist I have worked with many clients who were stuck in grief. They will speak about losing someone with poignant emotion–as if it happened yesterday. But it happened years ago, sometimes decades ago. Some people, however, deal with loss very effectively and come to terms with a loss within a few months. What accounts for the difference? The effective group has better mental "strategies" for dealing with loss.

Resourceful visual images

People who get stuck often form unresourceful visual images in their mind's eye. Perhaps it is everyone gathered around the table for Christmas dinner–but there is the empty chair where momma is supposed to be. This image freezes the loss in time. It compares a picture of the way Christmas "is supposed to be" with the absence of momma and concludes that Christmas will never be the same again. Other people who get stuck see mom (or whomever they lost) in a hospital bed, wasting away with tubes and machines droning on. This image of mom is sure to elicit sad feelings. The empty chair or hospital bed scenes, however, are only two of billions of possible images. They do not represent the essence of who mom was. More resourceful images would have her with the family, or in a favorite activity, or a symbol that embodies her fine qualities.

Let me make an analogy with computers. When you turn on your computer, you get a default image on the screen. You can click options to have the computer change the default image to a more useful image. The first image is still in the computer if you need it, but the more useful image is now the default. If you have an unresourceful default image, change it to a resourceful image that honors the person who lived.

Neurolinguistic Programming (NLP) offers a number of strategies for making a memory more or less intense. The idea is to make resourceful images intense and unresourceful images seem to be a distant, far away memory. Moving a visual image away from your head, making the image smaller, making it black and white, and making it dimmer, all make the image less intense. Conversely, making an image closer to your head, bigger, colorful, and bright usually makes an image more intense. Thus, people who experience losses can make unresourceful images less intense and resourceful images more intense by changing the qualities of their visual imagery.

Exercise 10-1: Developing more resourceful visual images

Imagine someone you love. Picture that person in your mind's eye.
1. Note how close the image is to your face and how you feel when you look at it.

2. Move the image across the room and note how you feel when you look at it.
3. Move it close to your face and note how you feel when you look at it.
4. Note whether the picture is in color or black and white and how you feel when you look at it.
5. If it is in color, make it black and white (or if it's black and white make it color) and note if it feels different.
6. Note how big the picture is and how you feel when you look at it.
7. Make the picture much bigger and note how you feel when you look at it.
8. Make the picture smaller than the original picture and note how you feel when you look at it.
9. Note how bright the picture is and how you feel when you look at it.
10. Make it brighter and note how you feel when you look at it.
11. Make it dimmer than the original picture and note how you feel when you look at it.
12. Now choose someone who you care about who is no longer living and go through the same process.

The process is not just for developing resourceful feelings for someone who has died. You can use it to feel more positively about people who are living. You can also use it to feel less intensely about someone you broke up with or an overbearing boss, etc.

Attaching positive meaning

While not everyone consciously visualizes images, everyone attaches meaning to a loss. Let me give some examples:

• A single parent lost her only son, a teenager, in an auto accident. She was understandably overwhelmed with grief months after the accident when I saw her for psychotherapy. As she told me her story, she described how she had been a very withdrawn, bitter person before her son was born. He was a remarkable kid who had a zest for life and was very close to her. He drew her out and taught her to laugh, to love, and to connect with people. Had he never been born, she probably never would have come out of her shell. When she focuses on how he touched her life and the lives of many others, the loss is easier to bear, and she feels a sense of mission to pass on the love he gave to her and others.

- A young husband and his shy wife had an extraordinarily close marriage for ten years. He developed a serious illness and died after several operations. He had been her husband, best friend, and social partner in almost all of her non work activities. Not only did she not feel like socializing with others, she felt she did not fit in with single people or married people. Drawing on her strong Christian faith, she too was able to focus on how rich her life had become from being with him, how his presence can always be with her, and how she can now experience life more fully and help people because of their relationship.

- The dynamics are not limited to loss of a loved one. I have seen many people who experienced trauma, e.g., physical abuse, sexual abuse, growing up in an alcoholic family; center their identity on being a victim. They are so focused on what happened to them that they keep re-experiencing the trauma again and again instead of living in the present and getting on with their lives. They remain scared, angry, hurt, unhappy, and vulnerable. Fortunately, there are a number of resources for them. Some get beyond the impasse by participating in self-help groups. A number of newer therapies[6] have achieved remarkable results in resolving past traumas in a surprisingly short period of time.

- Captain Gerald Coffee describes how he felt his imprisonment in a Vietnamese Prisoner of War (POW) camp actually enriched his life[7]. He even says the experience was so valuable that if he had the choice, he would do it all over again.

- Art Berg,[8] who was rendered quadriplegic from an auto accident when being driven to his wedding, echos Captain Coffee's sentiments–if he had to do it over again, he would. Berg is now a successful author and motivational speaker.

- Perhaps the most dramatic example of how the meaning you attribute is critical comes from Victor Frankel's[9] account of his imprisonment in a Nazi concentration camp. He describes how those who survived were prisoners who were able to create meaning from the madness. Sometimes the meaning was as simple as surviving to tell the world what happened.

Exercise 10-2: Attaching meaning

Think of someone who died who was important to you. What meaning do you attach to his or her life? What additional meaning might you attach? What are some things you could do to honor his/her memory and pass on his/her qualities?

It is true that grief is a teacher. For awhile it may be our master and a hard one as we learn each lesson. Grief teaches us to find options and to reach within to depths we probably did not want to explore. Grief teaches us compassion so that we may become the guide for others who will follow, for others who need our help to make choices in life, to accept challenge and change as part of living.
                                                     –Dr. Sandra Graves[10]

Much of the literature on grieving emphasizes beliefs that are contrary to effective grieving. One, for example, said: "Losing a parent . . . is different from any other loss for several reasons: . . . your parents are irreplaceable . . . your relationship with your parents is one in which all others are based . . . you believe in your parents' unconditional love . . . a parent's death is an encounter with mortality . . . Often people refer to the death of a parent as splitting their lives into two: "There was the BDD–Before Dad Died–and the ADD–After Dad Died . . . I saw everything through that prism."[11] These beliefs are good for developing a therapy practice but not good for effectively coping with a parent's death. The beliefs intensify the anguish as opposed to a belief system that parents dying is a natural event in the natural order of things and one that you are mature enough to handle. Another author referred to her husband dying as "amputation without anesthesia."[12] This is a vivid metaphor, that fosters self-pity rather than healing.

Believing that death is followed by something positive helps. Such beliefs won't be credible unless they fit with your other beliefs. Seeing death as a positive thing can come from religious beliefs about an afterlife. They might be based on beliefs about our souls being eternal. This idea is at least as old as the ancient Egyptians and is common to many religions. Socrates took a little more intellectual approach that thought and souls are eternal. He chose death over keeping his mouth shut. Many eastern religions speak of our essence being energy which merely transforms at death. Deepak Chopra and others speak of the paradoxes of life and death (i.e., at any moment parts of our bodies are alive and parts are dead in a constant process of renewal).[13] Many religions believe in reincarnation with people returning to another life until we learned what we need to learn. For the skeptic, the tens of thousands of reports of near-death experiences raise the possibility of an afterlife experience. These are cases in which someone was apparently dead but revived. The reports have a remarkable similarity in describing out-of-body experiences, light, a tunnel of light, and a very reassuring, comforting feeling.[14] [15] Supporters of the veracity of near-death experiences include the world's most prominent thanatologist, Elizabeth Kübler-Ross, M.D. The medical advances in emergency rooms have made such experiences much more common. Reports of these experiences are remarkably similar to out-of-body experiences reported by people who have become very skilled at meditation. This would seem to support the Judaic, Christian, Islamic, and Eastern views of the soul as immortal.

An ongoing presence

People who deal effectively with loss often see the deceased as an ongoing presence in their lives. My model is Fred Sanford from the television show *Sanford and Son*. When Fred (played by Red Foxx) was having a hard time he would feign "having the big one" (a heart attack). He would then look up and talk with his deceased wife Elizabeth. He wasn't crazy. He just knew her so well that he could sense her presence, imagine a conversation with her, and gain comfort and guidance from the experience. Actually, he probably got along better with her after her death than in real life as he was a cantankerous character. Many religious people find it easy to think of the person who lived as an ongoing presence. New agers also believe in an ongoing presence. But even if you don't believe in powers or forces beyond known natural laws, your memory of the person who lived and what he or she meant to you can live on in your heart and in your mind and be a source of inspiration and guidance. At the end of the movie, *The Story of Vernon and Irene Castle,* Irene Castle is told that her husband has died in a plane accident. She is tempted to become morose but instead makes mental pictures of them dancing together. While grieving is more complicated than the movie went into, it is a good example of an ongoing presence helping with grieving.

Exercise 10-3: Sensing an ongoing presence

Think of someone who died who was important to you. Look up and carry on a dialogue with him or her. Note how you feel after the discussion.

Happened for a reason

When someone believes that what happened was God's will, I respect their view. They might believe that God punishes and rewards people. As in the Biblical story of Job, they might believe that the reason God made it happen is beyond human understanding and they should trust in God. Sometimes people tell me that God gave them a mentally retarded child because He knew that the child would need extra love and care. To this I say Amen (even though my personal view differs). Other people are overwhelmed by the senselessness and ask, "Why me?"

Harold Kushner[16] was a successful rabbi who had a huge challenge to his faith when his son was born with progeria, a condition that causes a child to age rapidly and die within a few decades. After much soul searching, Rabbi Kushner's conclusion was that God created a wonderful world with incredible laws of nature. After creating the world, God did not interfere with these laws. If He did, it would be a crazy world indeed. Imagine a bus about to hit a child and the child or the bus levitating to avoid the accident. There is predictability in the world and there is random chance. We all experience some unfortunate events and some people experience a lot more unfortunate events than others. Bad things sometimes happen because of the choices we make (e.g., smoking leading to lung cancer) and sometimes because we happened to be in the wrong place at the wrong time (e.g., being hit by a drunk driver while waiting at a traffic light). Kushner's philosophy can give some sanity, perspective, and meaning back to a person whose world has been turned upside down by tragedy.

Particularly when a death was unexpected, it is easier to deal with if you can ascribe meaning. If meaning doesn't come naturally, you can choose to give the person's death meaning. Often the most obvious meaning is to carry on what the person stood for. Another way of making meaning is to work to prevent the disease or cause of death from happening to others. For example, after her teenage daughter was killed by a drunk driver, Candy Lightner founded Mother Against Drunk Driving (MADD), which has saved tens of thousands of lives.

Dealing with "what should have been"

If Bill Clinton can hold his head high after Monica,
you can hold your head high too.

Often what gets a person stuck are beliefs about what should have been. Unlike Robin Williams' character in the movie, *The Best of Times,* you don't have to recreate the high school football game in which you dropped the winning pass. If you are stuck with the thought that "I didn't get to say goodbye," or "I never told her that I love her," it is important to honor the importance and intent of the belief but to get unstuck from the idea that it can't be done now. Begin by asking, "Where do you think she is now?" Few people stuck with these beliefs will say they are an atheist, or she is dead, and that is that. Otherwise they would not be upset about something that is over and done. Thus, they believe she is in heaven or transformed in some cosmic way into a continuing presence. Consequently, there is no reason not to say goodbye or "I love you" now. This can be done informally in one's heart, by imagining a conversation, by writing a letter, or performing a ritual. Photo albums or a visit to the grave can facilitate the process. Another alternative is to develop ways to honor the person. If the person had exceptional qualities, these can be passed on through the generations in stories, quoting things she said, and espousing her values. Holidays can be an especially good time for traditions honoring family and friends.

Often people try to forget losses, hurts, or disappointments. The attempt at amnesia doesn't work. The feelings go underground and brew and stew in your unconscious thoughts and feelings and in your dreams. The solution is to forgive. It frees your emotions and energy and lets you embrace life fully. As Bernie Siegel put it, "God has no unforgivable sins, only people do."[17] Forgiving is about forgiving yourself and letting go of what you are convinced should have been. Certainly you want to make sure you learned whatever there was to learn and are not a patsy for people taking advantage of you. Beyond that, you are the person who is punished when you do not forgive.

A resourceful interpretation of what dying means

The key factor, however, in dealing with outliving friends and family is having a philosophy of life that gives a healthy perspective on what dying means. Western culture is very oriented to controlling and mastering our environment. Death, however, requires a spiritual perspective and attunement to the cycles of nature.

There are several perspectives for viewing what happens. *First person perspective* is about what I think, feel, and want. It is an important perspective for getting things done, e.g., a physician taking charge in a hospital. *Second person perspective* is about what others want, e.g., a nurse discerning what the patient wants and what the doctors want. *Third person perspective* is about being objective, e.g., the research scientist dispassionately conducting experiments. *Meta position perspective* is "above" the other three perspectives and appreciates all three perspectives and how they are part of a system. Love can be about what you want from your lover (first position), what you can do for your lover (second position), or intellectually understanding how your love can make the world a better place (third position). Love can also be a transcendent experience in which you are tuned into the larger harmony of life (meta position). This can be triggered by hearing music, experiencing works of art, meditation, prayer, or many other ways. Meta position is a spiritual position.

You can experience death from all four of these perceptual positions. In first position you are focused on how you miss and want to be with the person. In second position you are focused on how you can carry on what he or she wanted to accomplish or share his or her qualities. In third position you dispassionately realize that he or she had lived a full life and was in a lot of physical pain. In meta position you might sing "Amazing Grace" and become caught up in a spiritual feeling, sensing a oneness with the universe and a sense of harmony and awe.

Having a meta perspective on life and death can come from many sources but it needs a wellspring. For some, religious traditions fit. Some feel connected with new age beliefs about mother earth, vibrations, synchronicity, oneness and connectedness. For some it might be a simple homespun philosophy; for example, Robert Fulghum's observations and stories, such as *Everything I Ever Needed to Know I Learned in Kindergarten.* Perhaps Deepak Chopra's interweaving of quantum physics, mind/body medicine, and Ayvurdic traditions speaks to you, as in *Ageless Body, Timeless Mind: The Quantum Alternative to Growing Old.* Perhaps it comes from meditation, the arts, or communing with nature. It can come from anywhere but it needs to come from somewhere. It is stronger if you can identify a role model who follows the philosophy and/or a written source that explains the philosophy.

Teachers and professors are particularly good role models for letting go. They have their students for only a year or a few years and then must focus on inspiring a new cadre of students. Do they complain that they can't bear to let their babies go? No, they realize that it is time for the students to leave the nest and fly. While they could become sad at the students leaving, they instead are joyful to see them move on to new challenges. They feel enriched and invigorated from having worked with them. They have a vision of helping to change the world.

Proactively dealing with it

You also need to decide what actions you are going to take. Do you want to follow certain customs and rituals for mourning? Probably the best developed Western mourning customs are Jewish customs. Jewish custom requires full mourning for parents, children, spouses, and siblings. These immediate family members are to be at bedside if it is known the family member is dying. This encourages closure between family members and makes the death real (contrast this with the difficulty accepting death for mourners when a body is not recovered, e.g., in war, airplane crashes). The body is lovingly cleaned and wrapped in a plain white shroud by men or women who have volunteered for this duty. Burial is soon after the death. The service includes prayers and eulogies (reminding everyone of what has been lost). The service is simple. There is no viewing of the body or embalming (which is regarded as denying death by trying to make the person look alive). The casket is a simple wooden box put into the earth. This suggests that everyone is equal in death and that the body is meant to decay (vs. denying death with an impenetrable casket and vault). At the funeral, immediate family members tear a piece of clothing and wear it for seven days to symbolize their loss. After the funeral, community members serve a "meal of recuperation," which continues the caring for mourners and implies that life goes on. The meal starts the seven-day period in which the family stays at home together and other members of the family and community visit, prepare meals, and do light housekeeping. There is no music, radio, or television. Mirrors are covered and people sit on low benches or on the floor. Visitors join in prayers. Mourners wear slippers to signify they are not going anywhere. They do not engage in vanities such as shaving. Having the family together solidifies family unity and sharing. The constant parade of visitors keeps mourners from brooding and self-blame and gives mourners people who will listen and care. After seven days immediate family members may return to work but are to refrain from recreational and entertainment activities until thirty days after the burial. Remarriage is permitted after ninety days (the primary intent is for children to be able to have two parents). Daily prayers with at least ten other Jews continue for eleven months after the burial.

The rituals are brilliant in providing a "formula" for grieving, helping people know what is expected and when enough is enough, reintegrating mourners back into everyday life at a respectful pace, and emphasizing life. The mourner's Kaddish (prayer) that is said three times a day for eleven months says nothing about death. It focuses solely on affirming life and faith in God. It strengthens the connections between generations and history. Kaddish also is said when attending services and at special services four times a year. On each anniversary of the death, immediate family members pray, fast, and make charitable contributions. Even if you are not Jewish, you might want to use some of these time lines for mourning immediate family members. Thinking out what customs, time line, and restrictions you want to follow facilitates and paces mourning. Mourning is the process of dealing with the loss. Grieving is experiencing the feelings.

The meaning of each death is different. Our charge is to glean inspiration from the good in their lives, incorporate that goodness in ourselves and share it and pass it on to others. For some this will come naturally, while others might consciously wrestle with what was special about the person and how to derive inspiration from those qualities. Charitable contributions can be one way to create a legacy. If you have mixed feelings or unexpressed feelings toward the person, "writing" the deceased a letter can help you sort out your feelings as can talking with others.

Levels of coping with loss

The following is a scale I developed to indicate how effective your skills are for dealing with outliving friends and family. To illustrate each level, I have included some examples from movies or literature.

Brickey's Outliving Friends and Family Levels

Level 6   You have a sense of awe and wonder about life and the big picture, you have a sense of being fortunate to participate in life's grand plan, you feel that knowing each person is a gift that was entrusted to you, not an entitlement, you feel a sense of rhythms and cycles in life, you don't take yourself too seriously, you are OK with all the deaths you have experienced and sense an ongoing presence in your life of several people who have lived before. For example, the movies: *Joe vs. the Volcano, Little Big Man, Harold and Maude*

Level 5   You believe something positive happens after death and that death isn't necessarily a bad thing. You have good strategies for dealing with death and putting it in perspective. For example, *Goodbye Mr. Chips*

Level 4   You have spiritual beliefs that support you in dealing with death and traditions and the support of family and/or friends help you cope fairly well with someone's death. For example, *Love Story*

Level 3   When someone close to you dies, you feel a big hole in your life. With time the pain fades but there is little healing and you still view the person's death as a loss. For example, *The World According to Garp*

Level 2   The death of a close friend or family member brings on depression and despair and it takes years before you enjoy life again. For example, *Used People, Ordinary People*

Level 1   You have a rigid script about the way life is supposed to be and have never gotten over major losses in your life. You feel you are a victim. For example, *Hamlet, Sophie's Choice*

Exercise 10-4: Which level best describes your coping strategies? If you are not at Level 6, how would your life be different if you were at Level 6?

Resources

The first step in choosing resources is to determine your spiritual beliefs and traditions. Almost any book I would suggest would mismatch most people's spiritual beliefs and not be very helpful. Harold Kushner's book, *When Bad Things Happen to Good People,* can be especially helpful in addressing the "why" question. Deepak Chopra has enormous integrity and his *Ageless Body, Timeless Mind* is a good resource for those who appreciate a Vedic philosophy.

Bernie Siegel's *Prescriptions for Living* is very helpful with dealing with love, loss, and forgiveness. When someone dies it is often unclear what to do, e.g., arrangements, legal matters, manners and customs. An excellent guide on the subject is *What to Do When a Loved One Dies* by Eva Shaw. It covers everything from military funerals to how to handle the media if the death draws media attention.

The library and bookstore shelves are full of books in which people share their experience with death. There are books for all types of deaths including: stillbirths, children dying, suicide, widowhood, a parent dying, a sister dying, and even a pet dying. If it is helpful to you to read about what others have experienced and know that you are not the only one who has had these feelings, by all means use these resources. Many of these books, however, were written by people who had a particularly difficult time in dealing with the loss and might not be the best role models for effective grieving. Some wallow in their misery and spend a lot of time being victims. It is better to spend most of your time on literature that affirms life. A good book for relating with children is *Telling a Child about Death* by Edgar N. Jackson. If you like New Age or Eastern religions, Anya Goos-Graber's *Deathing* has a well-thought-out case for viewing death and dying positively or helping someone who is dying have a positive, emotionally "prepared" death. It is based on wisdom from Tibetan Buddhism and yoga.

> *Resentment is warmed-over anger.*
> *Anxiety is warmed-over fear.*
> *Self-pity is nothing more than warmed-over grief.*
> *Warmed-over feelings happen when*
> *there isn't anything better to do.*
> –Robert Jean Bryant[18]

> *It is important to go to other people's funerals*
> *because if you don't go to theirs, they won't go to yours.*
> –Yogi Berra

Chapter 11

Time and Change

Ah but I was so much older then, I'm younger than that now.
–lyrics from *My Back Page* by Bob Dylan

It's hard for old age to hit a moving target. –Joan Rivers[1]

I'm in love with the past,
but I'm having a love affair with the future.
–Ruth Gordon[2]

Time isn't money, it's everything. Spend it on who and what you love.
–Bernie Siegel[3]

Self-concept and self-esteem

I worked with a successful businessman who had some business setbacks and was very depressed. Normally it would take several months to pull out of his level of depression. I probed for what mental process he went through to feel depressed. He said he would just look up and see (a big picture) of someone saying they didn't want to hire him. When I asked him how he used to know to feel good, his demeanor shifted and he described looking at a large "spreadsheet" with ten years of data on several life areas–family, business financials, customer feedback, peer feedback, spiritual, etc. About 90% of the "cells" were positive and bright and 10% were not. This was a superb structure for self-concept. It was realistic, represented his self-image through time, and specified key areas of his life. It gave him specific information on strengths and weaknesses. I encouraged him to reinstate his previous strategy for accessing his self-concept (and determining his self-esteem). Within days he was his old self again and had a job within a few weeks.

Our self-concept is the system of generalizations we make about ourselves. Everyone's self-concept is uniquely organized and some work better than others. The ideal self-concept:
• is accurate
• is optimistic

- is resilient
- represents traits and abilities through time
- operates in the background most of the time
- involves all three major senses–seeing, hearing, and feeling

An accurate self-concept enables you to make good judgments about yourself and what you can do and currently are not able to do. When self-concept isn't accurate, you get people who think they are bright when they aren't or think they are stupid when they have good intellectual abilities, etc. We saw from Seligman's research how and why optimism is important. When our businessman's "spreadsheet" was only based on his assessment on one piece of data (e.g., current unemployment), his self-concept was unstable and reacted to the mental image of the moment. When he based his self-concept on ten years of detailed data, his self-concept was stable and resilient. If you ask yourself if you are lovable and base your conclusion on just one person's opinion, your assessment is unstable. If it is based on feedback from many people, it is stable and resilient.

Our businessman's spreadsheet strategy gave his self-concept continuity through time. When he saw just one image (e.g., current unemployment) he was often consciously aware of his self-concept and self-esteem. When he used the spreadsheet strategy, he usually was not consciously aware of his self-concept or self-esteem as they did not change very often. We can only consciously track 7 ± 2 things at once so it is best that our self-concept does not occupy our conscious thinking unless we need to consciously think about it. People who frequently concentrate on their self-concept become distracted. A football player who is focused on whether he will fumble is more likely to fumble than if he just played and allowed himself to slip into a "flow" state. (It's like saying, don't think of a pink elephant.) People sometimes experience difficulty if some of their self-concept is in one representational system and other parts of it are in another. A person might see symbols of her accomplishments (e.g., education, jobs) but still hear an internal voice saying "you'll never amount to anything."

Self-concept also operates at multiple levels. Our self-concept operates at all of these levels. Some traits might be represented at all levels and some not. Contradictions can occur when different levels have different representations. For example, when a person marries, the capabilities level might remember and want to use premarital flirting skills while the values level might emphasize marital fidelity.

Robert Dilts' Logical Levels gives a good framework for appreciating the multiple and sometimes contradictory levels of our thinking, feelings, and behaviors.

Robert Dilts' Logical Levels[4]

Level	Question	Function	Written text
Spiritual	Who else	Trans-mission	Vision statement
Identity	Who am I	Mission	Mission statement
Beliefs/ Values	Why	Permission/ Motivation	List of beliefs & rules
Capabilities	How	Actions	Goals (+ purpose and action plan)
Environ-ment	Where When	Constraints	Schedules

It is complicated but the complexity also gives many opportunities to make changes in self-concept. Some of the easiest changes can come from:
- enriching the system with more details and examples
- enriching the system by including seeing, hearing, and feeling
- mapping across from parts of the system that work well to parts that do not work well yet
- reconciling contradictions in the system
- changing the structure of your time line

Exercise 11-1: Determining the structure of your self-concept

Think of a trait that you believe is true about yourself, e.g., I am honest. How do you know the trait is true? Did you see a visual image in your mind's eye? Did you hear a voice in your head say you are honest? Did you hear someone else's voice say you are honest? Did you have a physical sensation in some part of your body that signaled yes? Was it a combination of these ways of knowing? To what extent does your strategy meet the criteria at the beginning of this chapter? Now go for the bigger picture by asking yourself how you think of yourself. What structure emerges?

Self-esteem

Many self-help books and programs have focused on trying to improve self-esteem. Self-esteem, however, needs to follow naturally from a healthy self-concept. There are lots of street gang members who have good self-esteem. They think they are cool, powerful, and have the answers. Their self-concept, however, is unhealthy. The emphasis on self-esteem in our school systems has often yielded children who feel good about themselves and their academic skills but don't have the academic skills they should have. The point is illustrated by a *Calvin and Hobbes* cartoon in which Calvin decides to quit doing homework because it is bad for his self-esteem. Instead of trying to learn, he decides to concentrate on liking himself the way he is. Hobbs questions whether self-esteem is enhanced by being an ignoramus, but Calvin calls it merely informationally impaired.

Exercise 11-2: Fit with mission

Turn back to your comprehensive mission statement in Chapter 6. Does your self-concept fit well with your mission statement? If not, what can you do to reconcile the two?

Time lines

Exercise 11-3: Your time line

Imagine yourself brushing your teeth now. Visualize it in your mind's eye if you can. If not, sense it. Note where the image is located in space (e.g., forehead height, twelve inches in front of me). Now think about when you brushed your teeth when you were a child. Picture it in your mind's eye. Note where the image is located in space. Now imagine yourself at 100 brushing your teeth. Note where the image is in space. These three images give you reference points for how you mentally represent your present, past, and future.

In addition to a self-concept, we have an internal representation of time. The most typical representation is left to right (perhaps because we read left to right and graphs display time from left to right).[5] The ideal time line will:
- allow you to easily "see" past, present, and future
- either extend to at least 150 years or allow for the possibility of extending that long (e.g., it fades into the horizon but presumably continues)

There are many variations of time lines and each has its advantages. Western timelines usually run left to right in front of a person. Some Eastern time lines run through the person with the past behind the person, the present in the person, and the future ahead. This makes for a strong connection with time and intensely feeling the present. People who cannot see their past often have pasts they find painful and do not want to see. So their minds cooperate and make the information difficult to access. Some people have their present in front of them and their past and future wrapping around behind them. This makes the present intense and the past and future "out of sight, out of mind." This strategy contributes to being impulsive or self-indulgent as the consequences are "out of sight." I worked with one woman whose past was to her left, her present in front of her and her future straight up. It made the future very intimidating. I had her try moving her future to the right and she immediately relaxed and liked the change. Some people have their past, present, and future all straight ahead of them. This makes it difficult to see all three unless they are at different heights or transparent. I suspect that with Picture in Picture functions in TV sets (in which the screen has an inset showing another channel) and computer "windows," some people will develop time lines that use these formats.

As with other visual images, you will be drawn to images that are close, big, bright, clear, colorful, and moving. Associated pictures are also more intense (in an associated picture of skiing you would see a ski slope in front of you; in a dissociated picture you would see a picture of yourself skiing). People who dwell in the past have intense pictures (e.g., large, close, colorful, associated) of the past and have less intense or compelling pictures in their present or future pictures. They are great storytellers and historians. People whose present outshines their past and future are very focused on now and enjoying the present. This is especially helpful for a task such as skiing down a slope. People whose future pictures are more appealing than past and present focus on tomorrow and have difficulty being here now or enjoying the past. Be sure to put them on your planning committee.

For people who want to live a long time, the most effective time line is usually left to right with the present right in front of you. It is OK for the future to stretch as far as you can see. It's not OK for the future to seem to end at any time that would correspond to before 150. (By the time you get close to 150, you can always adjust the time line or renegotiate.) It can be difficult to represent the future since much of it is unknown. Often people's minds use symbols or streams of light to represent unspecified good things.

If you find you have difficulty with time, you can experiment with your time line. Begin by reassuring yourself that you are only experimenting and that you can always go back to your current time line. Then try changing the location, height, size, color, brightness, etc. of various aspects of your time line and see what difference it makes. If you like a change, take a few minutes to imagine what it would be like using the change and the consequences of the change. It is not unusual for changes in your time line, which can be made in a matter of minutes, to effect profound changes in your life. Certainly, if your time line doesn't extend to 150, adjust it so it does.

Time lines are primarily an NLP (Neurolinguistic Programming) concept. Mind/body physicians Bernie Siegel[6] and Herbert Benson[7] describe numerous examples of how people who are told they are dying have short time lines in their drawings and dreams. Typically they fulfill the script in their time line. The dynamics of a doctor saying you have two months to live can be similar to voodoo prompting death.

Religious and cultural representations of time

Many cultures and religions conceptualize time as cyclical, e.g., Indian, American Indian, Hindu, Buddhist, Chinese, and ancient Greek. Circular time concepts include mandalas, reincarnation, and life repeating itself endlessly in cycles. Judaism and Christianity broke with the Egyptian cyclical concept of time and structured time as primarily linear. In doing so Western time became less tied to nature and its cycles. Jews view time as: God created the world, made a covenant with Noah, made a covenant with Abraham, led Moses out of Egypt, established a homeland in Israel, helped the Jews survive exile and the Holocaust, helped the Jews reclaim their homeland, and expects Jews to continue to work to make a more perfect world. The Bible, genealogy, prayers for those who have died, and holidays like Passover emphasize ties to a linear history. Christians view history as: Christ was born (in the year 0), fulfilled the prophecies of the Old Testament, died for our sins, was resurrected, and offers redemption to all who follow his teaching. Many Christians add an end to time with a fiery apocalypse. Both Jews and Christians view their Bibles as canonized and not subject to change. Both Judaism and Christianity also have holidays that give a cyclical feeling to the year, but the stories in the holidays are linear.

Long life time lines

People who will live to 150 will have time lines that:

Extend 150 years or longer. Our unconscious minds are very suggestible. There are numerous instances of school children, workers, subway riders, and soldiers who were near but not exposed to environmental hazards developing the symptoms of the toxins.[8] Bernie Siegel is a big believer that patients' unconscious minds often hear and respond to what physicians say during surgery. He tells a fascinating story of a man whose heart stopped after abdominal surgery and the anesthesiologist left the room. Siegel said, "Harry, it's not your time. Come on back." The patient's heartbeat returned and he made a full recovery.[9] Hospital death rates ironically dropped substantially in several instances of physician strikes.[10] In a medication study, patients who were on placebo medications but did not take them consistently died at twice the rate as patients who took the placebo regularly.[11] In the same experiment, patients who did not take their beta blocker medication consistently also had death rates twice as high as patients who took their medication consistently. (Overall, the beta blocker patients had lower death rates than the placebo patients.) Women are more likely to die the week after their birthday. Men are more likely to die the week before their birthday.[12] The researchers speculated that birthdays are a celebration and social event for women but a deadline for life achievements for men.

Put things in perspective. If you have a setback in life, knowing that you are going to be around for another hundred years or so makes the setback seem smaller. If this effect does not happen spontaneously, you can mentally prompt it by imagining yourself fifty years in the future looking back on the current setback and considering what it meant. People say, "Someday you will laugh about this." Why wait?

Stages of life

Beautiful young people are accidents of nature,
But beautiful old people are works of art.

The literature on stages of life can give us helpful guidance on how to navigate our lives. A major premise of this book is to seek role models rather than learning by trial and error.

Freud was the first modern stage theorist with his theory that children go through oral, anal, and genital stages and compete with their like sex parent (Oedipal conflict for boys and Electra complex for girls). Jung extended Freud's theory to adulthood and emphasized individuation and becoming more uniquely individual.

Erik Erikson proposed eight stages of development with each stage highlighting an existential struggle. For adults the themes are: identity vs. role confusion (in adolescence), intimacy vs. isolation (in early adulthood), generativity vs. stagnation (in middle ages), and ego integrity vs. despair (in "retirement" years). Erikson studied individuals over time and also wrote about the development of famous people such as Ghandi and Martin Luther. Building on Erikson's work, Daniel Levinson also emphasized cultural influences for generations, e.g., wars, the spurt in birth rates, and the computer revolution. Thus, we have generational cohorts, e.g., Baby Boomers, Generation X. His book titles, *Seasons of a Man's Life* and *Seasons of a Woman's Life* illustrate his metaphor for aging.

Gail Sheehy popularized this type of research with *Passages* and *New Passages*. Her metaphor of passages is more optimistic than Levinson's seasons. Her catch words for ages are: the tryout twenties, turbulent thirties, flourishing forties, flaming fifties, serene sixties, sage seventies, uninhibited eighties, nobility of the nineties, and celebratory centenarians. She is particularly adept at addressing how men and women cope with the "marker events" of menopause and andropause (male menopause). Sheehy found that most women in their fifties reported that 47 was the nadir of their life and their fifties are one of the best times of their lives. Among professional women she interviewed, 90% described their fifties as "an optimistic, can-do stage in life." More than half of the working class women agreed. She and other researchers who interviewed people in their sixties, seventies, and eighties often heard that their age was the best age and the best of times. Men typically have particular difficulty with retirement, especially if it was not their choice. Women are more inclined to keep working (partly because their careers were interrupted with babies and child rearing and partly because they had fewer retirement benefits). Women over 50 seem to do well without men, but single older men have considerably higher rates of depression, suicide, and death. Presumably this is due to more women than men being skilled at social networking and supportive friendships. Sheehy found that women in families with incomes less than $30,000 a year (in early 1990s dollars) lacked the security to try new things and flourish in their later years.

Erikson, Levinson, and Sheehy's data were primarily from interviews. George Vaillant had some of the most comprehensive data. He headed a research project that mentally and physically tested 204 white male Harvard sophomores every few years to 65. While this was certainly an elite population, it had its share of problems, setbacks, and deaths. Factors during the sophomore year that correlated with mental health at 65 were: good psychological adjustment, practical organizational skills, and a low resting pulse rate (probably reflecting a relatively calm person). With age, the student's lower socioeconomic status, being an orphan, and being an introvert lost their correlation with poorer mental health. The only major correlate of later physical health in Vaillant's data was family longevity. (As noted in earlier chapters this effect could be due to inheritance of diseases, inheritance of longevity potential, lifestyle issues, and/or role model issues.) (Also, as discussed in Chapter 5 Seligman accessed this research data and found optimism when a Harvard sophomore correlated with physical health beginning at 45.) Avoiding problems with alcoholism or depression in midlife was associated with good mental health at 65. At 65, good relations with siblings emerged as a correlate of good mental health.

Some stage theories (e.g., Freud's psychosexual stages and Piaget's cognitive stages in children) describe stages that must be completed in sequence and that higher stages are superior to earlier stages. Erikson, Levinson, and Sheehy are much more flexible. As Levinson puts it: "Entry into a new period reactivates the unresolved problems and deficits of previous periods. These problems form the 'baggage from the past' that makes it harder to deal with current tasks."[13] Sheehy's metaphor for growth and stages is: "The lobster grows by developing and shedding a series of hard, protective shells. Each time it expands within, the confining shell must be sloughed off. It is left exposed and vulnerable until, in time, a new covering grows to replace the old. With each passage from one stage to the next we, too, must shed a protective structure. We are left exposed and vulnerable–but also yeasty and embryonic again, capable of stretching in ways we hadn't known before."[14]

Some stage theorists posit that you must let go of something to mature at the next stage. I question whether this is true and think it is a limiting belief. Except for Peter Pan, children progress from one stage to another without a sense that they are giving something up. They can't wait to be older and more mature. While some people who marry perceive they are giving up something, some would find the idea foreign. There are several factors that distinguish people who handle life transitions well:

- They have learned what to expect and how to do it well from reading, observing, and/or role models (vs. trial and error).
- They are working on the next issues before they are imminent and have already developed some of the skills and perspective before the transition is upon them (c.f. procrastinators vs. planners).
- They have positive attitudes and beliefs about change.

Lest this sound too idealistic, consider a few concrete examples. Some people get married rather impulsively and are rudely awakened when marriage isn't effortless bliss. Others have given marriage a lot of thought for years and have ideas and plans about what it takes to make a marriage work. Consider the impact of losing a job due to downsizing. For one person it is a shock that brings on depression. Another person might have anticipated that sooner or later the job would end and has been learning skills and networking for the next job long before the old one ended.

Erickson and Levinson stop at about 65. Sheehy dabbles a little farther but most of her interviews are with people in their fifties and sixties or younger. Their studies also are based on where people have been (or what I call rear view mirror vision). One of the most astute observers of aging is Betty Friedan. Her book, *The Feminine Mystique*, helped launch the feminist movement and she was the founder of the National Organization of Women (NOW). Her *The Fountain of Age* echoes many of Sheehy's findings. In a scholarly manner she examines the politics of aging, e.g., media images, mandatory retirement, the medical professions, pharmaceutical companies, retirement centers, and the hospice movement. She presents a positive view of how being an elder can be a great time of life and good for society. Like Sheehy, she notes that around 50 men become more like women and vice versa. Part of this might be maturity. Part of the coming together is hormone driven as men's testosterone levels decrease and women's estrogen levels decrease. (By 60, most men's bodies have more estrogen than women's bodies if the women are not taking hormonal supplements.)

Friedan asks the question, why do women live longer than men? While estrogen and social networking are likely factors, Friedan also suggests that women have more experience in dealing with change. Women's bodies and careers are more impacted by childbirth. Menopause is a more dramatic change than male menopause and women's roles in society have been changing more dramatically than men's roles. Women are much more likely than men to seek counseling or coaching on how to cope with change. If men's longevity is to catch up with women's longevity, men need to become more comfortable with learning social change skills and developing friendships that emphasize emotional support as well as sharing activities. Friedan calls for an end to the battle of the sexes and sees elders as participating, contributing, and passing wisdom and experience on to future generations. Friedan is attempting to start a much needed dialogue on the contribution, vitality, and quality of life that can go with living a very long time.

We need to develop positive images of what it is like to be an elder. As researcher Cecilia Hurwich found in her interviews, "Old age is the best time in life."[15] Erickson, Levinson, Sheehy, and Friedan are all helping to get the message out. Television and the movies have few positive roles for older people. This is especially true for women. Notable television exceptions are Angela Lansbury in *Murder She Wrote* and the situation comedy, *Golden Girls*. It is just a matter of time before television networks wake up to how their potential viewers are increasingly older and not interested in *Baywatch*. If they don't wake up, their market share will continue to shrink as viewers choose other networks on cable or other interests. Stereotypes of elders are full of amusing contradictions. Elders are supposedly childlike and sexless, yet rigid and crotchety. If older men think about sex, they are dirty old men and if older women think about sex they are silly and oversexed and should act their age. I once did some consults at a nursing home and was aghast to discover that every man in the nursing home was on salt peter (which inhibits erections). What were they afraid of? Pregnancies?

The American Association of Retired Persons (AARP) is careful about political endorsements to protect its nonprofit status and because 40% of its members are Democrats and 40% are Republicans. There is nothing, however, to prevent AARP from public relations and lobbying campaigns to promote public images of seniors as vital, healthy, wise contributing members of society. It shouldn't be difficult to feed the news-hungry print and TV media stories of elders who are creating and contributing. The media should be giving as much coverage to elder activists like Maggie Kuhn (the late founder of the Gray Panthers) as they do to Jessie Jackson. On the less flamboyant side, Hugh Downs and Art Linkletter are doing excellent work in highlighting positive role models. If the public doesn't develop more positive beliefs about elders, the pessimists will persuade the public that old geezers are a burden on society, draining the country's financial resources, and something needs to be done. The extreme case was in Nazi Germany where millions of elderly and disabled people were murdered because they were "a drain on the German economy and society." Already, numerous articles are appearing in the media about how few workers will be "paying for" the Social Security benefits of the Baby Boomers. Younger generations allegedly will be "taxed to death" and there will be no funds left for them when they retire. What will actually happen is that many people over 65 will still be working and paying taxes, including Social Security taxes. Many of those who are not competitively employed will be contributing to the economy by performing volunteer work.

The stage theories have all been based on a rear view mirror of life–studying what people have experienced or are currently experiencing. Your model of your life, however, needs to be built on what can be but hasn't happened yet. If some of the current stage theories fit for you, it is OK to glean help from them. I would not adopt any of them as a model for your life, however, as you are charting a different course. Your course says my mid-life is 75 and I will be active and vital for 150 years (or more). Rather than a usual career path, I will have a career all my life, though I might change my career path many times and some of my careers might be performing volunteer work. My parenting isn't just with my children and grandchildren, but eventually with great grandchildren and great great grandchildren. My health and sexuality aren't going to decline at 50 but will be vital long after I become a centenarian.

How change occurs

In considering behavioral change, Prochaska's[16] research is outstanding. It provides a useful explanation of how and why people change, or don't change. It also cuts across theories and explains how so many different approaches could all report a moderate level of effectiveness. Prochaska studied people who were successful at changing–both those who changed on their own and those who had therapy. He has been particularly interested in smoking, alcoholism, and weight loss. He found that with habits and lifestyle changes, people go through stages of change–precontemplation, contemplation, preparation, action, maintenance of the change, and termination. Successful changers are skilled at navigating all six stages.

In **precontemplation** people tend to deny there is a problem, e.g., I just drink beer, I don't have a drinking problem. They also often use minimization, rationalization and intellectualization. Precontemplation is the Scarlett O'Hara stage when you say "I'll worry about that tomorrow." In **contemplation**, people are ambivalent–they want to change, but. . . . Contemplation is the Woody Allen stage in which you are racked with guilt but have difficulty getting going. People transition to the preparation stage when they begin to focus on the solution rather than the problem and when they focus on the future rather than the past. In the **preparation** stage people develop and plan and increase their motivation and commitment. Preparation is the Columbo stage when you carefully gather information and lay out your strategy. In the action stage people put their plans into action. The **action** stage is the Arnold Schwarzenegger (or Xena Warrior Princess) stage when you take charge and take action. The **maintenance** stage is to ensure that the changes stick (e.g., the difference between losing weight and keeping it off). Maintenance is the Rocky stage when you have great heart and keep slugging it out. Ideally, the change eventually becomes so habitual that it is no longer necessary to consciously think about it. Sometimes maintenance needs to continue without end, for example, some ex-smokers still want to smoke years after they quit and most alcoholics are unsuccessful at returning to social drinking.

Prochaska's model has many interesting implications. In changing, it is important to know which stage you are in and what works in that stage. A lot of treatment programs and therapy fail because they are just oriented to the action stage while the person is in an earlier stage of change. (A good therapist or coach is skilled at recognizing the client's stage and pacing therapy or coaching to the client's stage.) The model also notes that on the average people usually require three or four attempts before succeeding at changes such as permanently losing weight, quitting smoking, or beating alcoholism. Not succeeding or relapsing should be viewed as a learning experience and you should focus on what you learned from the attempt. Some people move through the stages quickly and some take years or never make it through the stages. Prochaska found that addressing multiple problems is often as or more successful than addressing problems one at a time (consider how smoking, drinking, and eating can cue each other). His research has studied more than 30,000 people and his principles have been adopted by several national health organizations.

Rapid changes

I have been privileged to help many people make profound changes in their lives in a matter of minutes. How? Remember Dilts' logical levels–spiritual, identity, beliefs/values, capabilities, behaviors, and environment? Rapid change can take place at any of these levels. Here are some illustrations from movies:

Identity Level: In *It's a Wonderful Life*, George is 30, faces bankruptcy, identifies himself a failure, and considers suicide. After re-examining his life (with the help of an angel), he realizes that he has touched many lives and is successful. At that point the events had not changed; just his interpretation of them. We have a similar scenario in *Scrooge.*

Belief/Values Level: In *A New Leaf,* aristocratic, penniless Walter Matthau marries rich, inept, and dowdy Elaine May. On the verge of killing her, he has a change of heart and values and decides instead to help her and take care of her. In *Magnificent Obsession*, playboy Robert Taylor (1937) or Rock Hudson (1954) causes a woman's blindness in an automobile accident and then, in a change of values, devotes his life to becoming a surgeon and curing her blindness. Often a reinterpretation of facts causes a change in belief. In *An Affair to Remember*, Cary Grant believes Deborah Kerr does not love him when she doesn't show up for their rendezvous on top of the Empire State Building. Later his belief changes again when he learns she did not go because she was crippled by an automobile accident. In *Casablanca* both Humphrey Bogart and Claude Rains decided in a moment at the airport to be patriots.

Capabilities Level: *Dumbo* believed he was capable of flying when he had the red feather. He quickly learned he could fly without it as well. In *The Miracle Worker,* after weeks of frustration, Helen Keller's teacher finger spells water into her hand and Helen gets the concept and becomes exuberant with the realization of her new capability. In movies like *North by Northwest*, the hero has no idea that he is capable of scaling Mount Rushmore until he is pursued by criminals.

Behavioral Level: In *The King and I*, we learn that the behavior of whistling a happy tune makes you feel brave. While not instant, we find massive changes at all levels prompted by learning new behaviors in *The Karate Kid* and in *My Fair Lady*.

Environmental Level: In *Oklahoma* fickle Annie just can't resist loving whatever man she is with and sings, "I'm Just a Girl Who Can't Say No." The dilemma is echoed in *Finian's Rainbow* in the song, "When I'm not near the one I love, I love the one I'm near." In *Lord of the Flies* we see how easily culture can unravel when British school boys are stranded on an island and become savages.

So what distinguishes rapid change from slower change? Rapid change is effected by one or more of the following conditions:

- a new definition or conceptualization of what happened or what things mean, e.g., *Scrooge, It's a Wonderful Life, An Affair to Remember, Heaven Can Wait*
- leverage, e.g., when a spouse says, "Quit drinking or I'm leaving," when a parent's dying words are a request, when the boss gives an ultimatum
- highly emotionally charged situations, e.g., losing your job or lover
- choices that are thrust upon us, e.g., illnesses, accidents, opportunities, *North by Northwest,* the airport scene in *Casablanca*
- markedly changed circumstances, e.g., moving to another home or city, changing jobs, *Lord of the Flies*
- mental reprogramming, e.g., the Neurolinguistic Programming (NLP) strategies mentioned in this and previous chapters

Ultimately, it is people's interpretations that determine whether there will be a rapid change. One person can walk barefoot across forty feet of hot coals and conclude, "If I can do this I can do anything." Another will only conclude, "Wow, I can walk across hot coals."

Sometimes we make changes and have no idea of what the long range consequences might be, for example, when Rosa Parks refused to sit in the back of the bus. Woody Allen, on the other hand, has been in psychoanalytic therapy for decades and his personal life is still a mess. What's the problem? Ambivalence–he is successful and becoming mentally healthier might affect his artistic productivity or acceptance, much less his comfort level with his neuroses. Like Hamlet, he's stuck in that ambivalent, indecisive contemplation stage.

You are a paradigm pioneer

Paradigms are rules and boundaries about what we believe and how we do things. A paradigm shift occurs when the conventional thinking is successfully challenged with a paradigm that works better. "Paradigm shifters," like Jack LaLanne and Betty Freidan, conceptualize and begin the change. "Paradigm pioneers" are the early supporters of the change. Your interest in the mental maps for longevity makes you a paradigm pioneer. Knowing that you are a pioneer can help you keep a sense of confidence about thinking differently and charting a different course than most people. Consequently, it is worth looking at some examples of paradigm shifters and pioneers to appreciate how paradigm shifts work.

The Swiss were the world's greatest watch makers and dominated the market. They continually improved watches by making them waterproof and introducing self-winding watches. The electronic quartz movement was invented in Neuchâtel, Switzerland. The Swiss, however, were too entrenched in gears and movements to appreciate the implications. The Japanese appreciated the implications and took over domination of the watch industry in less than ten years.[17]

The Swiss watch story is hardly a unique one. American engineer Edwards Deming developed the concept of continuous quality improvement. The American automobile and other industries dominated world markets and were content with the way they did things. Shortly after World War II, when the Japanese economy was in shambles and Japanese products were synonymous with cheap goods and poor quality, the Japanese embraced Deming. Within a few decades Japan became a world leader in quality products including automobiles, electronics, and computers. In Japan Deming is a national hero and the Deming award for continuous quality improvement is coveted.

Resistance to new paradigms is illustrated in the following comments on computers:

I think there is a world market for about five computers. –Thomas Watson, Chairman of the Board of IBM (1943)[18]

There is no reason for any individual to have a computer in their home. –Ken Olson, President of Digital Equipment Co. (1977)[19]

640k ought to be enough memory for anybody. –Bill Gates, Founder and CEO of Microsoft (1981)[20]

Before the 20th century, paradigm shifters usually were not appreciated in their lifetime. With our era of rapid change, paradigm shifters are becoming appreciated within a few decades, e.g., Einstein, Picasso, and Steve Jobs, developer of the Apple personal computer. Paradigm pioneers might need a tough skin or a lot of confidence.

Initially, people react to paradigm shifters with "that's absurd." Later, they often reap great benefits.

Resources

Gail Sheehy's *New Passages* is very helpful in providing role models and knowing what to expect as we travel through time. Interviews with celebrities make it even more interesting. Betty Friedan's *The Fountain of Age* is a lengthy book and not easy reading. It does, however, contain seminal thinking about the future. Time lines are covered in Connirae Andreas and Steve Andreas' *Heart of the Mind* and in their *Change Your Mind and Keep the Change.* The best introduction to NLP (Neurolinguistic Programming) is Connirae Andreas and Steve Andreas' *Heart of the Mind.* There are also at least a couple dozen organizations in the U.S. and other countries offering NLP training. The largest and best known is NLP Comprehensive (www.nlpcomprehensive.com), 800-233-1657. *Changing for Good* by James Prochaska, John Norcross, and Carlo DiClemente is easy to read and does an excellent job of walking you through the change process. An excellent and easy-to-read book on paradigm shifts is Joel Barker's *Paradigms.*

People with complicated emotional problems or problems that don't respond to self-help efforts should consider psychotherapy. Overall psychologists have the most training in psychotherapy. Therapists vary greatly in their approach and competence and it is important to choose a therapist carefully. People who are emotionally healthy but want help in being even more effective at achieving their goals might consider a coach. Coaching became popular in the latter part of the 1990s. Much of coaching is done by telephone. More information on coaching is available at www.drbrickey.com, www.coachfederation.org, or the International Coaching Federation's toll free Referral Service at 1-888-236-9262.

Do not go gentle into that good night,
Old age should burn and rage at the close of day;
Rage, rage, against the dying of the light.
–Dylan Thomas in a poem addressed to his dying father

Chapter 12

Eating and Drinking and Common Sense

The Chinese do not draw any distinction
between food and medicine. –Lin Yutang[1]

Eat to live and not live to eat. –Proverb

Nutrition is a young subject: It has been kicked around like a
puppy that cannot take care of itself. Food faddists and crackpots
have kicked it pretty cruelly . . . They seem to believe that unless food
tastes like Socratic hemlock, it cannot build health. Frankly, I often
wonder what such a person plans to do with good health when they
acquire it.[2] –Adelle Davis, 1954

You probably think I am going to lecture you on eating only
healthy foods, shopping at health food stores, and becoming a health
fanatic. Not so. Ewell Gibbons, famous for eating wild berries and
nuts and advertising Grape Nuts cereal, did not live long enough to
collect a Social Security check. This chapter advocates not making
nutrition an ordeal but making sure your eating is healthy and
balanced. Manners used to dictate not talking about politics or
religion at social events because people often become livid and upset
about these topics. Perhaps the advice should be updated to include
diet. It is amazing how many people have a religious zeal that they
have discovered the one true diet.

Nutrition information–A tower of Babel

Many alleged nutrition experts are more interested in selling
products or promoting a viewpoint than using scientific research and
common sense. Large pharmaceutical companies and agribusinesses
often are more interested in profit than in health. There is more profit
in selling pills and packaged foods than in selling fresh produce. The
media fuel the fires as they thrive on fear, "breakthroughs," and
victims. For example, there is currently a "war on heart disease" that
focuses on lowering cholesterol levels. First it was total cholesterol,

then LDL (low density lipids or "bad") cholesterol, then the ratio of LDL to HDL (high density lipids or "good cholesterol").

I have not been able to find any research that clearly indicates that higher cholesterol levels lead to higher mortality. To the contrary, in some of the major studies, mortality was higher for people who took cholesterol lowering drugs than people in the placebo group. Although 80% of our cholesterol is produced by our livers, we are admonished to decrease our consumption of food containing cholesterol. There is a good reason that your body produces cholesterol–it needs it. Cholesterol is essential to building all of our steroidal hormones (testosterone, estrogen, DHEA, cortisol, etc.) and is a structural component in every cell in our bodies.

Certainly extremely high cholesterol levels (e.g., over 300) scream that something is terribly wrong. It is not clear, however, that trying to lower cholesterol levels does more good than harm. In 1991 the *Journal of the American Medical Association (JAMA)* reported that there was "no direct evidence that a nationwide cholesterol screening program for the elderly would lessen overall morbidity and would be worth the cost."[3] In 1994 *JAMA* reported on a study of 997 people with an average age of 78. Neither high cholesterol nor low HDL was a risk factor for coronary heart disease mortality, hospitalization for myocardial infarction, or overall mortality.[4] A 1998 *JAMA*[5] study found no relationship between high or low density cholesterol in almost 6,000 participants 65 and older. An editorial in *JAMA* said, "The most important harm is that cholesterol lowering interventions could actually increase, rather than decrease, the overall death rate."[6] The editorial also noted that cholesterol lowering programs with middle-age men led to increased rates of cancer.

Despite the lack of research support, the pharmaceutical companies have made millions from medications to lower cholesterol (never mind the side effects that accompany the medications). Meanwhile, agribusinesses have made a lot of money charging premium prices for packaged foods that are low in cholesterol. And your doctor fusses over your cholesterol levels in your annual physicals.

To give another example, there is currently a crusade to get fat out of our diets. The media admonishe us that fat is making us fat. Our supermarkets are full of no-fat and low-fat foods (at premium prices) to make us feel OK about eating potato chips, cakes, and junk food. Many consumers believe that as long as they buy no-fat or low-fat products they will lose weight or at least not gain weight. The irony is that research shows that most people on low-fat or no-fat diets eat more food because the fat was not there to curb cravings.

Without fat, our bodies could not absorb fat soluble vitamins, build new cells, or build hormones and neurotransmitters. Women who reduce the fat in their diets reduce the amount of estrogen their bodies produce. That lowers the risk of breast cancer but increases the risk of heart disease. Fat reduces the likelihood of depression and reduces the risk of dementia (particularly dementia following a stroke).

Most Americans' fat consumption is well over 30% of the calories in their diets. Research projections on the benefits of reducing fat to 30% of our calories concluded that the change would increase life spans by three months for women and four months for men.[7] Another study projected what our life expectancy would be if saturated fats were reduced to 10%. The increased longevity was 3½ days to 2 months for women and 11 days to 5 months for men.[8] As if this were not confusing enough, it seems that saturated fat (that is the "evil" fat) reduces the risk of a stroke. One study found that each 3% increase in total fat was accompanied by a 15% decrease in the risk of strokes.[9] Dr. Ronald Krauss of the American Heart Association concluded, "We know that individual responses to food cannot be predicted reliably on the basis of studies of large populations of people."[10] He concluded that because of genetic differences in how people metabolize fat, dropping fat below 30% would benefit one-third of the population, harm one-third, and have little effect on the other third. Unfortunately, there is no simple test or classification system for these kinds of individual differences.

Antioxidants are the rage in health supplements. Antioxidants conquer "evil" free radicals, reducing the risk of cancer and slowing the aging process by preventing DNA and cellular damage. While there certainly is sound research support for the benefits of antioxidants, there is research that indicates beta carotene, one of the big three antioxidant heros, actually increases the risk of cancer for people who drink heavily or smoke.[11] Free radicals do a lot of damage. But they are also essential to fighting bacterial invaders and to producing eicosanoid hormones, our bodies' master hormones.[12] They also are essential to producing ATP (adenosine triphosphate), which is essential for your body to produce energy.[13] Thus, if we take too many antioxidant supplements, we might run into unintended consequences. It is a matter of balance.

Placebos, like Dumbo's magic feather, help people get better because they believe in the intervention. One theory is that placebos work by causing your body to produce endorphins (your body's natural painkillers and mood elevators). The power of suggestion gets improvement 33% of the time.[14] The opposite of placebos is nocebos. Did you ever read through a medical text or dictionary or pill book and start worrying that maybe you had those diseases? If you believe something is going to cause you harm, the power of suggestion might make it so. Thus, if you spend a lot of time worrying about whether electrical fields, microwave ovens, or eating the wrong foods are going to make you ill, there is a 33% chance that they will. An extreme version of nocebos is voodoo. Yes, you should periodically study up on health issues. A steady diet of alarmist news, however, can literally make you sick.

Because placebos are such an important issue, let me cite two examples. In one study,[15] 13 Japanese students were touched on one arm with a poison ivy-like Japanese tree leaf they believed to be poisonous. All 13 students had skin reactions to the leaf even though in reality the leaf was harmless. Their other arm was brushed with a leaf that they were told was harmless but was really poisonous. Only two had skin reactions to the poisonous leaf. In a meta analysis (a study analyzing many well-designed studies on a subject), researchers studied the effectiveness of the antidepressant Prozac.[16] The conclusion was that 50% of improvement was due to expectancy (placebo effect), 25% was attributable to untreated depressions getting better with time, and only 25% of improvement was attributable to Prozac. Two other independently conducted analyses found essentially the same result.[17]

In trying to make sense of the tower of Babel, my commentary:
- favors research that supports living a healthy vital life to 150
- favors research that contributes to an integrated big picture (as opposed to considering isolated single research studies)
- favors studies that indicate large differences

- gives consideration to the source's biases and motivations
- presupposes that different people have different needs and different desired outcomes (e.g., an athlete's needs and outcomes are different from a mystic's needs and outcomes)

Conclusions

So what can you do about this tower of Babel?
- Appreciate that what we do for one system affects your body's other systems. A news headline that we should eat more tomatoes or take beta carotene supplements means little out of context. You need the big picture. Americans use a lot of war metaphors. We have wars on crime, drugs, heart disease, poverty–almost any problem–we will declare war on it. We talk about medicine in military language with killer T-cells, antioxidants, beta blockers, etc. Our bodies, however, are exquisitely complicated systems that need balance and harmony. If we "nuke" one symptom, we could be declaring a civil war on another system in our bodies.
- Recognize that there are enormous biological individual differences. The question is what works for you.
- Avoid extremes. Any health practice taken to an extreme runs the risk of being problematic.
- In most cases, don't be the first to try new products or theories. Wait several years for research to give a clearer idea on whether there were unforseen side effects and whether the benefits were overrated by initial studies.
- Question sources and motives behind news stories and health care products.
- Ask yourself if it makes sense for you.

Current centenarians' nutritional habits

Here is what we know about the nutritional habits of today's centenarians:
- Few if any have gone on weight loss diets. Rather, they maintain a fairly constant weight all of their adult lives.
- They have a wide variety of nutritional habits and most eat a wide variety of foods.

- Many drink alcohol but in moderation (supporting Aristotle's philosophy of all things in moderation). Belle Boone Beard's study[18] of centenarians found that slightly over half consumed alcohol but almost all of them in modest quantities.
- Belle Boone Beard's study[19] of centenarians found that fewer than 3% reported ever smoking cigarettes.
- When they were young, many of the foods they ate were salted, smoked, or pickled and fresh fruits and vegetables were often scarce. Electric refrigeration was not commonly available until the 1920s. Thus, they did not have ideal diets by today's standards.
- While it is possible that some took vitamin/mineral supplements, printed interviews and books on centenarians do not mention them taking supplements or emphasizing their importance. Thus, it is probable that most of their lives most of today's centenarians did not take vitamin pills, calcium supplements, etc. They might live or have lived even longer if they had. (Daily multiple vitamins didn't become commonplace until the last two or three decades. Pregnant women used to take "special" vitamins because most were not taking daily vitamins.)
- When in their hundreds, many centenarians lose their robust appetites and their diets often beccome deficient in important nutrients.[20] (Taking a daily vitamin/mineral pill could help a lot.)

Our current understanding of nutrition and the resources available to us today (not to mention the future) enables us to eat more healthily than current centenarians did. To date the oldest person (with good documentation of age) was Jeanne Calment who lived in Arles, France. She died in 1997 at 122. She was always a physically active woman who wasn't overly concerned about others' expectations. She had a good appetite–not just for food but for everything. She never had fluctuations in her weight. She smoked a few cigarettes a day until she was 117 when she quit on her own initiative with no explanation. She enjoyed port wine and chocolates. She still rode a bicycle at 100. Part of her "secret" was that "I never get bored." At 109, largely because of visual limitations, she moved into a retirement home where her diet was unappealingly institutional. Her quality of life was compromised by failing vision and hearing. She declined eye surgery for the severe cataracts in both of her eyes. Her biographer reports that she never adjusted to the facility's routines nor they to hers. She would wake herself at 6:45 a.m. and begin her day with prayer and exercise. Her days were very (self)-structured. Although virtually blind, she got around the facility faster than most of the other residents. How long might she have lived if:

- She had taken a multiple vitamin and calcium supplements most of her life?
- She had opted for the eye surgery her doctors recommended to improve her vision? This would have enhanced her quality of life and allowed her the physically active lifestyle she so enjoyed. Being more physical and seeing better would have made her spirits even higher, strengthened her bones, increased her balance, and lessened the likelihood of her falling and injuring her hip.
- A future medical advance that would allow her to hear better had been available to enhance her quality of life?
- She had not smoked?

Individual differences

Different people's bodies react differently to foods. What is good or inconsequential for one person can make another ill. Consider some of these individual differences:

- **Metabolism** Some people have a high metabolism and can eat and eat and not gain weight while some people gain weight on 2,000 calories a day. People who fidget a lot burn off hundreds of calories a day from fidgeting (though purposely becoming a fidgeter is not recommended). If you tend to gain weight even though you routinely consume a low number of calories, have your physician rule out thyroid or other problems. It would probably be worth experimenting with some specialty diets to see what results you obtain.

- **Salt sensitive** Some people's blood pressure shoots up with just a little salt while some people can consume large quantities of salt with little effect on their blood pressure.

- **"Food allergies"** Food intolerances are very common and require diet modifications. The five most common food intolerances or hypersensitivities are: wheat and corn cereals, dairy products, caffeine, yeast, and citrus fruits. The complete list is very long. Common intolerant responses include: headaches, migraine headaches, hives, asthma, eczema, arthritis, rashes, depression, sluggishness, increased heart rate, gastrointestinal difficulties, anaphylactic shock, and even seizures. Food intolerances make life complicated as it is often difficult to know what is in processed or restaurant food. People who have not consumed dairy products for several years can lose their ability to digest them and develop a lactose intolerance.

  If you are having health problems and cannot find a cause, consider the possibility of food allergies. Begin by identifying a possible problem food and making sure you know what foods contain or might contain that ingredient. This requires reading labels and being cautious when eating out. Then eliminate the food from your diet for two to four weeks and note the effect. Chart the effects, rating target symptoms in morning, afternoon, and evening.

- **Constipation** Some people can eat junk food diets with no fiber and never become constipated while some people eat lots of fruits, vegetables, and higher fiber foods and have chronic problems with constipation. Chronic constipation is a cry for help. It calls for ruling out medical causes and finding a diet that gets along with your gastrointestinal system. Exercise also helps reduce constipation. People with chronic constipation might want to see if symptoms improve with a series of colonics (treatments that cleanse the colon by spraying purified water in the colon).

- **Blood sugar levels** Some people have fairly stable blood sugar levels even when they eat simple carbohydrates with no protein or fat. Most people's blood sugar levels go a little too high when they eat meals or snacks with just carbohydrates. Hypoglycemics' blood sugar levels skyrocket in response to carbohydrates and then plunge an hour later, leaving them feeling tired and irritable. They crave carbohydrates and the cycle continues.

- **Sex differences**   Different hormones, different reproductive organs, different ratios of muscle to body fat, and menstruation all contribute to different nutritional needs for men and women.

- **Ethnic differences**   It is plausible that over the years, natural selection led to ethnic groups that lived in a geographic region faring better with foods that were indigenous to that region.

Weight loss diets only help their promoters

A third of the food we eat keeps us alive.
The other two-thirds keeps the doctors alive.
–Orson Welles

Weight loss diets cause a lot of harm and guilt and don't work. Is it just coincidence that the first three letters of diet are die? In the last fifteen years of the twentieth century, the average body weight for Americans increased by 7.6 pounds.[21] At any given time 40% of women and 25% of men in the U.S. report trying to lose weight.[22] Long-term success rates are very poor. By weight loss diets I mean choosing to give up certain foods for a period of time in order to lose weight.

Part of the problem is that your body adapts to a decrease in food intake by lowering your metabolism. Thus, the lower food intake does not result in as much weight loss as expected. When you "go off the diet," your body is still metabolizing food at the lower rate until it readjusts (if it does). The resulting weight and metabolism fluctuations or "yo-yo dieting" is worse than staying at that same weight (not to mention the diet's possible nutritional deficiencies). If you subscribe to Barry Sears' views (described in the next section), the proliferation of no-fat foods makes it more difficult to lose weight as our bodies need some fat to maintain stable blood sugar levels and prevent carbohydrate cravings.

Quitting drugs, alcohol, or cigarettes is a snap compared to taking weight off and keeping it off. With these addictions there is a 20% success rate after one year. So on the average people have to make five serious efforts to overcome these addictions. Every year 80 to

100 million Americans go on a weight loss diet. Two-thirds are women. Ninety-five percent do not reach or maintain their goal. Many end up depressed, terribly frustrated, and heavier than when they started. Weight loss diets are not the answer.

There are three ways you can beat the odds on losing weight and keeping it off–and without starving yourself:

1. Changing eating habits involves permanent changes that are comfortable because they are consistent with your values and self-image. If you believe that white bread is neither as healthy nor as tasty as brown bread, it is no sacrifice to choose brown bread over white. If you believe that a diet soft drink is more sensible and healthy than a sugary one, before long the diet soft drink will taste better than the sugary one, which will taste too sweet. Many people stopped eating red meat either for humanitarian reasons or because they have a mental image of globs of fat clogging their arteries. People might choose to raise their spiritual awareness by not eating foods that are contrary to their religious tradition (e.g., pork, meat). Learning the ingredients of some of our favorite foods sometimes is enough to reduce our interest in them. Changing eating habits might also involve finding a belief system about healthy eating that works for you (discussed in the next section).

Most of us are more likely to make changes by "ratcheting" our way into a healthier style of eating. This involves asking yourself if there is one small, relatively painless change that would make your eating habits healthier. You implement the change and when it is firmly established as a habit, you ask yourself if there is another small, relatively painless change that would make your eating habits healthier. Round one might involve switching from whole milk to 2% or skim milk. Round two might have snacks starting with vegetables like celery or baby carrots until that new behavior is established. In twelve months the accumulated benefit from several small new changes can make a huge difference. Behavioral approaches such as eating more slowly, putting your utensil down after each bite, using a smaller plate can also be helpful. If you make large reductions in calories to lose weight, caloric cycling might trick your body into not lowering its metabolism in response to lower calories. With caloric cycling you consume less than your maintenance level of calories for two or three days and then consume your maintenance level of calories for two or three days. Caloric cycling also is more enjoyable and less discouraging than diets that require sacrifice day after day.

2. Exercising aids weight loss in several ways. It:
- consumes calories
- raises metabolism for several hours
- builds muscle (and muscle consumes more calories per pound than body fat consumes)
- improves your energy level so you are more active and thus consume more calories
- tones muscles so you look and feel better and are likely to be more active

3. Zone eating habits   Barry Sears makes a powerful argument for why and how our meals and snacks need to balance carbohydrates, proteins, and fats in a 40-30-30 ratio. In a nutshell, people gain weight or experience problems if the carbohydrates, proteins, and fats are out of balance. Ironically, if you want to lose weight, you still need some fat in your diet. Fat paces the release of carbohydrates into your bloodstream. Without the pacing insulin levels would spike, cause many of the carbohydrates to be stored as fat, and an hour later leave you with a low blood sugar level and food cravings. Fat sends a message back to your brain that helps curb your appetite. While it contains calories that can be used for fuel, it does not stimulate insulin production, which is necessary to covert food to fat that is stored in your body. (And fat is also essential to using fat soluble vitamins, building cells, and many life functions.) You also need an ongoing, paced consumption of protein to repair and maintain your body, build muscles, and keep your immune system functioning well. Carbohydrates, particularly fruits and vegetables, are essential sources of nutrients and fiber. However, high levels of carbohydrates cause an overproduction of insulin and storage of foods as body fat. With zone eating habits, the key is healthy eating and keeping insulin levels stable 24 hours a day. Details are available in Sears' books, *The Zone, Mastering the Zone,* and *The Anti-aging Zone,* and on his web site: www.Eicotech.com.

Cardinal rules for your diet

Since the word diet has a lot of negative connotations, you want to make the word diet have positive connotations for you. Whenever you hear, see, or say the word diet, give yourself a comforting feeling that you have wisely evolved beyond self-destructive torture games. For you, diet just means what you eat and drink. Your diet needs to:

- be easy and enjoyable to follow for a lifetime
- give you good energy levels all day long (vs. spurts of energy and sputtering periods of low energy)
- make it easy to achieve and maintain your desired weight
- enhance your health
- include a wide variety of foods
- foster a spiritual awareness (this might come from saying a blessing before you eat, deriving a feeling of connection with nature by being a vegetarian and/or choosing organic foods, or just a sense of awe and appreciation)
- give you a good, confident feeling that your diet is helping you be healthy (placebo vs. nocebo effect)
- be judged by its results

The one true diet–Alice in Wonderland

There is no shortage of gurus telling you about a special diet you should follow for health, youth, vitality, and possibly spiritual benefits. It becomes as confusing as Alice felt in Wonderland. Here are some examples of health-oriented diets (as opposed to weight loss diets):

Vegetarian Many vegetarian diets are strongly tied to spiritual disciplines. There are several varieties of vegetarian diets. Vegans eat no animal products. Lacto-ovo-vegetarians eat milk and eggs but no meat or fish. Some vegetarians eat fish and dairy. Vegetarians need to be knowledgeable about their nutrition so they are sure to get the vitamins and amino acids that are primarily available from animals. In 1988 the U.S. Surgeon General's report on nutrition urged Americans to reduce their intakes of animal fats because they increase the risk of obesity, coronary artery disease, high blood pressure, diabetes, and colorectal cancer. Most current centenarians, however, eat a wide variety of foods including meat.

Ayurvedic Ayurvedic practices are based on a 5,000-year-old refining of Indian beliefs about health and mind-body balance. Ayurvedic practices were popularized in the West by the Maharishi Mahesh in the 1980s and Deepak Chopra in the 1990s. Ayurvedic medicine matches three body types (vata, pitta, and kapha) and seven mixed types with recommended vegetarian diets and yoga exercises. It is a very holistic approach and includes breathing exercises and even instruction in how we should eat.

Hypoglycemic People who are hypoglycemic experience wide swings in their blood sugar levels. When they eat a candy bar, their blood sugar levels shoot up (higher than other people's would) and they have a burst of energy. An hour later their blood sugar level plummets (lower than other people's would) and they are lethargic, depressed, irritable, and crave carbohydrates. And thus the cycle continues. Alcoholics are especially prone to hypoglycemia as the body readily converts alcohol to sugar. A *hypoglycemic* diet levels out fluctuations in blood sugar levels with a diet that emphasizes complex carbohydrates, protein, and eating several small meals throughout the day. It advocates minimal caffeine, nicotine, and alcohol as these spike blood sugar levels and contribute to the large fluctuations in blood sugar levels. While a hypoglycemic diet is a necessity for hypoglycemics, it is also a healthy diet for most people.

Food combining In 1902 Dr. Herbert Shelton wrote about food combining, favoring water rich foods and detoxification. Food combining refers to not eating fruits or vegetables or proteins at the same meal. The theory is that when these food groups are combined, they require more energy to digest and digest incompletely, leading to "putrification" of food in your digestive system. This is a vegetarian diet. It was popularized by Harvey and Sheila Diamond's book, *Fit for Life*.[23] Motivational speaker Tony Robbins advocates the diet in his books, seminars, and tapes as offering health and boundless energy. This is a demanding diet. It may cause unstable blood sugar levels for people whose blood sugar levels spike easily.

Blood type The *Eat Right for Your Type*[24] diet is based on the belief that the four different blood groups (O, A, B, and AB) evolved with different dietary habits and needs. For each group the program lists foods that are highly beneficial, neutral, and to be avoided and physical exercises for the blood type. To give an example, D'Adamo says the O blood types historically were hunters. O types thrive on meat, have difficulty with carbohydrates, do best with vigorous aerobic exercise, and are at risk for inflammatory diseases such as arthritis.

Balancing hormones Sports medicine physician Karlis Ullis[25] prescribes different diets according to which neurotransmitter (acctylcholine, dopamine, or serotonin) is out of balance. When it is acetylcholine, mental faculties slip. Ullis' dietary recommendations include fatty acids, antioxidants, and avoiding saturated fats. His physical exercises emphasize mind-body coordination. When it is dopamine, passions are muted. Ullis' recommends a high protein/low carbohydrate diet and exercises that emphasize posture, balance, coordination, and weight resistance. When it is serotonin emotions are volatile. Ullis recommendations include proteins in the morning, carbohydrates later in the day, and low intensive, meditative exercises. Ullis includes an extensive use of vitamins and nutritional supplements tailored to the types. In *Age Right* he reports on athletes' use of human growth hormones and how their use will become commonplace in the first few years of the 21st century. In *Super "T"* he gives a detailed program for men and women on how to use over-the-counter prohormones like adrostenedione to increase testosterone levels and thereby develop muscle, lose weight, and increase sexual drive.

Macrobiotics A macrobiotics diet is a vegetarian diet based on holistic Oriental beliefs and practices. The diet emphasizes organic foods to achieve balance and harmony among mind, body, and spirit. It also emphasizes energy fields, deep breathing, yoga or tai chi, cleansing, and locally grown foods. The diet is 50-60% whole grains. Proteins only constitute 6% of the diet. The macrobiotic diet gained a lot of recognition in the U.S. as a therapy for cancer patients.

Zone *The Zone,*[26] mentioned in a previous section, treats food as "a drug" and focuses on keeping the hormone insulin in a tight "zone." It attributes much of aging and excess weight to elevated insulin levels. Barry Sears, Ph.D., a medical researcher, developed the diet when he was trying to develop a drug for cardiovascular and diabetic patients. Compared to other diets, the Zone emphasizes a high ratio of proteins and low levels of carbohydrates. Sears says the carbohydrate-rich "food pyramid" is good for fattening cattle but not good for people. Rather than the U.S. Department of Agriculture's Food Pyramid, Sears advocates that 40% of our calories should be from carbohydrates, 30% from proteins, and 30% from fat (keep in mind that one gram of fat has nine calories while one carbohydrate or protein gram has four calories). The Zone diet is a close relative of hypoglycemic diets. One important difference is that the Zone calls for low levels of carbohydrates while hypoglycemic diets approve of carbohydrates as long as they are complex carbohydrates (e.g., whole grain bread vs. highly processed, bleached white bread). Vegetarians can follow the Zone diet.

Atkins Robert Atkins advocates avoiding carbohydrates to avoid weight gain. Thus, the diet is high in proteins and fats. It received a major revival in the late 1990s with the updated version of his diet in *Dr. Atkins' New Diet Revolution.* The diet appears to help a lot of people lose weight. Since it goes against conventional wisdom, critics have been ballistic. Their criticisms have focused on it not being a sustainable diet. This is a problem for any diet and Atkins' diet is a lot easier for most Americans to follow than traditional diets. Critics point out that it is hard on kidneys, might cause cardiovascular problems, and requires a healthy gall bladder. Sears[27] argues that low carbohydrate diets initially dehydrate the body to excrete ketones effected by metabolizing excess proteins, and eventually break down muscle tissue to carbohydrates and store protein as fat. If the priority is losing weight, the Atkins' diet might be tried in moderation. It was not designed, however, to be the ideal diet for health.

Milk and Cookie Diet With this diet you can eat all the milk and cookies you want but just one day a year. Despite causing obesity, it promotes longevity. The chief proponent is an S. Claus but little else is known about the diet.

Chewing Gum Diet Researchers have calculated that chewing gum consumes about 11 calories an hour. If you chewed gum virtually all of your waking hours for a year, you would lose 11 pounds.[28]

Why so many contradictory diets?

Each diet has ardent advocates and supporters. There are several reasons for the diversity:

- **Validating values** Choosing a macrobiotic diet is choosing to pursue and endorse a holistic Eastern philosophy and lifestyle. Choosing the Zone diet endorses a scientific approach to life's issues. Choosing Ullis' hormonal balance diet emphasizes peak performance and a sports medicine approach to life. Some diets, e.g., Ullis' hormonal balance, advocate an aggressive program of vitamin and nutritional supplements while others, e.g., macrobiotic and some vegetarian diets consider supplements blasphemy. Choosing to follow some diets might put you out of step with joining friends for coffee, alcohol, or pizza. A diet that is out of step with your values is a hard one to follow (unless you change your values).

- **Marketing** Every diet has its products–books, foods, pills, seminars, retreats, etc. So we get the weight loss diet of the month with the author making the rounds of radio and television talk shows promoting his or her new book. Converts might go to the diet with the most effective marketing as opposed to the diet that is the healthiest. While we would like to think of research and justice as blind and objective, advertising selectively reports research to sell products. Pharmaceutical companies in particular spend millions funding research that supports their products. Testimonials and celebrity endorsements appeal to our emotions rather than to an objective analysis.

- **The placebo effect**   The standard for testing a new drug is a double blind test with a placebo. That means that some of the participants receive the real drug and some receive a placebo (fake) pill. Usually about a third of people receiving the placebo report benefits and/or side effects. The effectiveness of the drug is judged by how the benefits and side effects of the experimental drug compare with the benefits and side effects of a placebo. Even the size and color of a pill influence research subjects' reports about how effective a pill is. Pharmaceutical companies spend millions of dollars researching what size, color, and packaging subliminally suggests effectiveness for a particular product. Since one-third of people benefit from placebos, you could say that placebos are the most effective, least expensive, safest treatment in the world. Richard Bandler jokes that he tried to patent a "medication" called placebo plus–with 50% more inert ingredients a than regular placebo. Any diet will obtain converts from the placebo effect.

- **Prompting healthy lifestyle changes**   In his book, *Anatomy of an Illness*, physician Norman Cousins described how he cured his cancer with humor, watching movies with Laurel and Hardy and other comical actors. Robert Dilts[29] describes how he helped his mother, who had terminal cancer, change her beliefs and lifestyle and rid herself of the cancer. He says her cancer went into remission when she *re-missioned* her life and made a lot of career and personal lifestyle changes. The list could go on and on with extremely diverse approaches reporting cures and successes.

  There are probably two factors causing these results. First is the placebo effect which fosters belief in the treatment and hope. Belief and hope can change the body's chemistry. The second effect is that the belief, hope, and the program prompts people to make lifestyle changes, e.g., laughing more, changing careers. A macrobiotic diet, for example, prompts people to exercise, meditate, become more spiritual, and use less caffeine, alcohol, and tobacco. With prompting so many healthy lifestyle changes, is it surprising that following a macrobiotic diet and lifestyle helps cure cancer?

- **Only reporting interesting and significant results**
Professional journals and the news media are more likely to publish or report something happening than something not happening. Thus, a finding that electric power lines did not cause health problems for residents is less likely to be published than a finding that electric power lines caused health problems.

  In research the usual standard is that the statistical probability of the results being due to chance must be less than 5%. If the study measures several variables, the odds of a chance finding of statistical significance increases. Consequently, as many as one in twenty variables or studies might be statistically significant by chance.

  The popular media seem oblivious to considering the base rates of events. For example, when hundreds of women with silicone breast implants developed health problems such as chronic fatigue syndrome, the media were quick to blame the manufacturer, Dow Corning. When these women were compared with other women with similar ages and backgrounds, comparison groups that did not have breast implants had the same rates of health problems. Thus, it appears that the implants did not cause health problems.

  Finally, there is a surprising amount of research in prominent medical journals that is based on very small numbers of patients and/or has poor statistical design. In sum, while most research is well done, there is still quite a bit of bad research that gets published and publicized. One study does not make a fact. A fact in fact (e.g., the earth is flat or the earth is round) is only a belief. The best course is to only consider research results as possibilities unless and until several studies find similar results and the results are of a large magnitude, e.g., you are 29 times more likely to get lung cancer if you smoke cigarettes vs. a statistic that finds a few percentage points of difference.

- **Individual differences** The biggest reason no one diet works for everyone is the enormous individual differences among human beings. A diet that works well for one person might make another ill. If one diet really were superior for everyone, researchers would have convincing data by now. Some of the diets (e.g., blood type, hormone balance, Ayurvedic) do try to recognize individual differences with different groupings of people. Research on patients who have cancer, diabetes, and other diseases might lead the way to effective individualized dietary recommendations. One recent and interesting approach focuses on keeping the blood pH at an optimal level and using blood tests to determine what foods will keep your pH in balance.[30] These approaches to individualizing diets seem to be on the right track but have a long way to go. There are also numerous books on special diets for people with particular health problems or food intolerances.

Natural foods

While there is enormous controversy among the health-oriented diets, most health advocates concur that it is healthier to eat natural foods whenever possible. By natural I mean the less processed the better. The ideal is organic food. Most health advocates advise avoiding or restricting food additives such as olestra and aspartame (Nutra Sweet). They encourage consumption of tea because of its antioxidant benefits (though some eschew caffeinated tea). They advise avoiding or moderating caffeine consumption. I mention caffeine in particular because so many people are getting high levels of caffeine from coffee, soft drinks, chocolate, tea, caffeine pills, and medication additives (e.g., Excedrin). It is even being added to some chewing gum and bottled water. Caffeine certainly gives an energy boost and helps people concentrate. It increases the levels of circulating fatty acids, making quick energy more available. Studies have even found lower suicide rates for coffee drinkers. Problems with caffeine can include insomnia, increased stomach acid, decreasing bone mineral density (osteoporosis) at all ages, insulin and blood sugar imbalances, nervousness, decreased sperm motility, and birth defects. It is also a diuretic (causes you to urinate) and makes it difficult to be adequately hydrated. In excess it is taxing on your kidneys.

Caloric restriction with adequate nutrition (CRAN)

Research with mice, rats, water fleas, spiders, guppies, and Rhesus monkeys all found that reducing their caloric intake 30-40% below unrestricted consumption resulted in the animals being healthier, more agile, and living about 30% longer.[31] [32] With caloric restriction great care is taken to make sure you (or the research animals) receive adequate carbohydrates, proteins, fats, vitamins, and minerals. The diet effects a lower, more efficient metabolism and lowers the body temperature about a degree (most of our calories go to keep our bodies at 98.6 degrees).

Theories about these results include: less wear and tear on the body in digesting food, less free radical damage as fewer calories generates fewer free radicals, lower insulin production, and lower blood glucose levels. A number of researchers believe the benefits apply to humans as well. Ray Walford[33] [34] [35] and his daughter Lisa are major caloric restriction researchers and advocates and follow caloric restriction themselves. Walford was the physician for the Biosphere II experiment. Once in the Biosphere, participants found the Biosphere was not able to produce enough food to feed them. Rather than sending out for pizzas they agreed to try a caloric restricted diet and found it improved their health.

Possible benefits include good health and longevity, needing less sleep, a trim physique, increased alertness, lower blood pressure, lower insulin levels, lower blood glucose levels, lower cholesterol levels, and lower risk of cancer, heart disease, and diabetes. Possible disadvantages of caloric restriction include often feeling hungry, increased sensitivity to heat and cold extremes, cold hands and feet, decreased levels of testosterone and other sex hormones, decreased sex drive, weakness, lack of energy, hemorrhoids, depression, and possibly decreased fertility.[36]

So much of our socializing is centered around food that caloric restriction can make social events awkward. The results with more than 200 species of mammals are very convincing. Whether the results generalize to longevity for humans is yet to be demonstrated. Apparently most people who pursue caloric restriction are vegetarians. People who choose caloric restriction for health reasons are probably a select population that is extremely motivated and conscientious and might show impressive health benefits with other strategies as well. Fewer than 200 people worldwide are known to be following Walford's plan.[37] Note that caloric restriction with adequate nutrition (CRAN) does not advocate fasting.

If caloric restriction would be torture for you, the stress and unhappiness would do more harm than good. If you find it relatively easy to be disciplined about food consumption and the idea appeals to you, it is worth considering. Barry Sears endorses the concept and believes zone eating behaviors will prevent feeling hungry. Even if you are not interested in trying it, it demonstrates that we can live healthily on fewer calories. With the human "experiments" still at an early stage, pursuing CRAN should probably be done with moderation (e.g., 10% or 15% as opposed to the extremes of 30%) if pursued at all.

CRAN charts a narrow course between health and malnutrition. Even occasionally missing the mark can be very unhealthy and counterproductive. It is not to be tried whimsically. Unless you are very careful with the nutritional and health practices, it would be easy to become deficient in nutrients, hormones, white blood cells, etc. One way to view CRAN is that it is slowing maturation. Puberty comes at an earlier age to children who have a good diet and a later age to children who have a restricted diet. Leonard Hayflick[38] demonstrated that our cells can only reproduce approximately fifty times. CRAN would delay how frequently cells reproduce and consequently extend the life span. If, however, there is a way around the Hayflick phenomenon, there is no need to go to Spartan lengths to slow maturation. Telemere research (discussed in Chapter 17) is one example of how the Hayflick phenomenon might be overcome.

What's overweight anyway

The Metropolitan Insurance Company's height and weight tables have been the standard that everyone has used for decades. The tables are designed to predict the risk of death. The tables use height, weight, and sex to calculate ideal body weight. Reuben Andres[39] found that people normally increased their weight with age up to 65 and the increased weight did not increase their risk of mortality. After 65 people tend to lose weight. He concluded that the Metropolitan tables were accurate for ages 40-45 but too liberal for younger people and too restrictive for people in their 50s and 60s. He also found that sex was not a pertinent factor and there was no need to have separate tables for men and women.

To illustrate, for ages 25-59, the Metropolitan tables indicate that at 5 feet and 8 inches, a man should weigh between 137 and 171 and a woman between 126 and 167. Andreas' study recommended that a 25-year-old should weigh between 116 and 153 while a 65-year-old should weigh between 158 and 196. His study was based on data from 25 life insurance companies in the U.S. and Canada, 4.2 million policies and 106,000 deaths. He also reviewed studies from 20 countries, including the U.S., and found that many studies favored an adjustment according to age and not a single study favored non age adjusted tables. Heymsfield and Allison[40][41] studied 70-year-olds and found that being 20 pounds overweight did not lower life expectancy while being underweight did. Their research excluded people who were known to have diseases that would cause them to lose weight.

The normal pattern is for people to gain some weight between 30 and 60 and start losing some weight after 65. So if you are in your 50s or 60s, carrying an extra twenty pounds might not shorten your life span. Quality of life is another consideration. A study[42] of over 40,000 nurses found that weight gain over time was accompanied by significant declines in physical functioning, vitality, mental health, and freedom from pain (except for some women who were already very thin). The difference was three times as strong as the decline in physical functioning from smoking cigarettes. If an extra 10 or 15 pounds makes you sluggish, impedes you from being active and doing what you want to do, or makes you look or feel unattractive, it is worth the effort to lose the extra pounds.

What to do

Someday the answers might be clear. Until our understanding of nutrition is more sophisticated, the best course is to judge diets by their results. If a specialty diet makes sense to you and appeals to you, put it to the test. Since it is easy to lose perspective or make decisions on the basis of emotions or what we think makes the most sense, it is important to keep data. At a minimum, chart energy levels, how you feel physically, and how you feel emotionally in the morning, afternoon, and evening on scales of one to ten. Start the chart two weeks before changing your diet and keep the charts for two to four weeks after going off the diet (assuming you go off it). Note any unusual events that would affect results, e.g., highly stressful events, major good or bad news, major holidays. Do not make other major changes in your diet or habits during the experiment (e.g., changing vitamins/minerals/nutritional supplements). Then put on your scientist hat and study the data to see what patterns you can detect.

If you do not have a diet that works well for you, I would suggest trying the Zone diet as it is compatible with most Americans' eating habits, is reasonably easy to follow, keeps blood sugar levels stable, and helps prevent diabetes. I am also impressed with the Zone because it is based on scientific research with a wide variety of populations including healthy people, diabetics, overweight patients, HIV patients, and athletes. Whatever your diet, try to avoid highly processed foods, hydrogenated or partially hydrogenated oils, and consuming a lot of saturated fats. Fortunately, the U.S. Food and Drug Administration required food producers to list the amount of trans fatty acids in food beginning in 2000. Trans fatty acids (often in the form of partially hydrogenated vegetable oil) increase Low Density Lipids (LDL) cholesterol ("bad cholesterol"). The labeling will prompt consumers to avoid these foods which in turn will prompt food processors to find formulas without trans fatty acids.

Water: Evian backwards spells naive

Our bodies are 80% water and water is the primary vehicle for our bodies to circulate blood, lymph, hormones, cerebral spinal fluid, etc. and eliminate wastes. Not drinking enough water starves our cells, taxes our kidneys, and keeps toxins in our bodies. Thus, the most important thing about water is to drink enough of it–at least eight glasses (64 ounces) a day. If you find that you just cannot seem to get yourself to drink that much water, try some close alternatives. One alternative is to put some lemon juice in the water to give it a little more flavor. Diluted orange juice is an alternative. Another is to drink a lot of tea or iced tea. The tea also gives you antioxidant benefits. If you choose tea with caffeine, consider how much caffeine you are consuming and how it is affecting you. (Herbal, black, and green tea all also have unique health benefits.) Often when people feel hungry, they are really thirsty. About 37% of our daily water intake comes from food. Fruits and vegetables are 70% to 95% water, cooked meat is 50% to 60% water, and even bread is 35% water.

The Natural Resources Defense Council tested 103 brands of bottled water and found that one-third of them did not meet California standards and guidelines for bottled water.[43] Bottled water in most states only needs to meet the same standards as municipal drinking water. The NRDC study found some of the bottled water contained: bacteria, arsenic nitrates (from fertilizer run off), chloroform, plastic chemicals, chlorine, and substances associated with cancer or spontaneous abortions. Overall they concluded that the safety of bottled water is on a par with tap water. Bottled water, whether in individual bottles or water cooler bottles, can meet federal standards when it leaves the bottling plant, but sit in warehouses for weeks or months at room temperature or hotter temperatures, providing a breeding ground for bacteria. The NRDC report notes that several studies have found there can be substantial growth of bacteria in bottled water in as little as one week of storage. Federal standards do not require any expiration date on bottled water. Several major bottled water companies have had to issue recalls because of bacteria in their water. Another problem is that the water might leach plastic from the bottle. Finally, while bottled water names and labels suggest pristine natural sources, 25% of bottled water is from municipal drinking water (with additional filtering, treatment, or distillation).

Perhaps the best analysis comes from a 13-year-old eighth grade girl in Anderson, Illinois. Her winning science fair project–"Health or hype? Is bottled water really safe?" examined six brands of bottled water. She found that hard water (mostly from calcium and magnesium) made water taste better. Mineral water (Zittell in her study) was the hardest and tasted the best followed by spring water (Evian in her study). She found Evian also contained "traces of chlorine." Only one brand, Cool Blue, contained fluoride. Her conclusion to the study was that "people shouldn't have to pay money for their water but it is not bad to drink bottled water." The amount of minerals in municipal water will vary but will be higher than many of the bottled waters and certainly the distilled bottled waters.[44]

A British study gathered a group of food, wine, and water quality experts and had them blindly rate and describe tap water from London and five other cities and five bottled waters. The city of Kent's tap water tied with Evian. Four of the five panelists believed Kent's water was bottled. Kent's water and Evian were closely followed by Glouster's tap water. Overall, panelists could not distinguish between bottled water and tap water.[45]

Most city tap water is satisfactory. We can make it healthier by removing the chlorine before drinking or bathing. Removing the chlorine also makes the water taste better. Municipal water companies have added chlorine since the 1890s. It is an inexpensive way to kill cholera, typhoid, and many other water borne diseases. Chlorine, however, reacts with many decaying organic substances and can produce toxic chemicals such as formaldehyde. Your colon's primary job is to extract water from the decaying digestive byproducts from your intestine. Otherwise, you would have to drink a lot more water. Thus it is no surprise that chlorine is associated with higher colon cancer rates. Chlorine is also irritating to your eyes and skin, as you have noticed after swimming in a chlorinated swimming pool. You could remove chlorine by simply putting an open pitcher on the table or counter for about 24 hours and the chlorine will evaporate. The water will collect some bacteria but it would be healthier than chlorinated water. You could put a pitcher of water in the refrigerator for three or four days. With the cooler temperature it would take three or four days for the chlorine to evaporate but it would contain fewer bacteria than the pitcher at room temperature for 24 hours. It is preferable to use unchlorinated water in your sinks, bathtubs, and showers. This is both to avoid the chlorine irritating your skin and to avoid breathing chlorine gas as it evaporates (especially in a hot shower).

Most municipal water has had fluoride added to prevent tooth decay. Voluminous research indicates that it reduces cavities by 50-60%. The American Dental Association's web page (www.ada.org) indicates that even adults benefit from fluoridation, particularly when their gums recede exposing lower parts of their teeth. Most bottled waters contained only a small fraction of recommended levels of fluoride and some do not contain any fluoride. Distilled water has no fluoride. Filtered water may or may not have fluoride depending on the type of filtering system. If most of the water you or your family members drink is not fluoridated, consult with your dentist about fluoride supplements. Ways of supplementing fluoride include mouthwashes, rinses, tablets, drops, lozenges, and toothpaste. Ingesting fluoride is more effective than topical fluoride treatments as the fluoride strengthens your whole tooth as opposed to just the enamel.

Distilling water removes virtually everything from water but the water and leaves the water tasting flat. Since your body has more minerals than distilled water, distilled water leaches minerals from your body. Thus, I do not recommend distilled water for your usual drinking.

Filtering water is easy and inexpensive. Most water filters run the water through paper filters and a variation of activated charcoal. Most filtering removes chlorine and other chemicals but leaves in most minerals. Filtered water also tastes better than chlorinated water. Many faucet water filters only work on cold water. Some include activated charcoal to filter out heavy metals and contaminants. Filter options include:

- **Units attached to the faucet** Many swivel on for drinking water and off for water for other purposes. Many have instructions not to use them with hot water. Their extra weight, maneuvering them, and slowing the water flow might place extra wear and tear on your faucet. (less than $50 + periodically replacing filters)
- **Units attached under the sink** These usually only service the cold water. Most have filters and activated charcoal ($100-$200 + periodically replacing filters and activated charcoal)
- **Whole house units** Whole house filters are an ideal solution and their economy of scale makes their maintenance costs about the same as two faucet units. The units may lower your water pressure a little which can be a problem if you already have low water pressure. (There are units that cost thousands of dollars for softened and/or distilled water. Units that just filter the water start at $400 plus $200 or more in plumbing costs + periodically replacing filters and activated charcoal)
- **Portable units suitable for traveling** (less than $50)

- **Refrigerator ice maker units** These units are available as an add on and are likely to become a common feature on higher priced refrigerators.
- **Shower head attachments** These solve the showering/bathing issue. They usually need to be replaced in two or three years. ($30-$40 each)
- **Bottled water coolers** The supplier delivers five gallon bottles to your home. For renters or people who move a lot, this can be a good alternative to having your own filtering system. ($10-$30 a month)

Note that there is a maintenance cost for periodically replacing filters and possibly activated charcoal. The ideal solution is a whole house water filtering system if it is feasible where you live. I am impressed and pleased with the one I obtained from Pure Earth Technologies.[46] Its cost was $400 plus $200 for a plumber. Their filter materials cost about $100 a year. (I obtain no consideration for recommending them.) You might also check to see if *Consumer Reports* has a recent review of water filters.

Issues in choosing water

- Generally, minerals in your water are a good thing and improve the taste. Distilled water has no minerals and leaches minerals from your body. Thus, filtered water, dechlorinated tap water, or bottled water is healthier than distilled water. Women in particular benefit from extra calcium in the water. Some rural areas have water with very high mineral content and the water tastes bitter.
- In most cases you want your water to contain calcium, magnesium, and potassium, but not contain the heavy metals, e.g., lead, iron, cadmium, aluminum.
- Fluoride is very helpful in preventing tooth decay and should be in your water or some form of supplement. Your dentist can advise you about supplements.
- Water with a lot of minerals or "hard water" impairs the effectiveness of soaps and detergents. If you have hard water, you might need a water softener to help with laundry, dishes, and even

bathing. Water softeners can be used in the washing machine or dishwasher or in a whole house system. Hard water does not necessarily mean the water is not good for drinking.

- If you cannot filter water, let it sit out for up to 24 hours so the chlorine can evaporate.
- Some people reuse the plastic bottles from bottled water. The bottles were only designed to be used once. The bottles' narrow mouth openings make them difficult to clean, providing an easy breeding environment for bacteria. The plastics can deteriorate with repeated use and be absorbed into the water or contents of the bottle. Refilling bottles needs to be limited to wide mouth heavy duty plastic bottles made for reuse (e.g., sports bottles, bicycle water bottles).[47]
- NSF (National Sanitation Foundation) certification is the most credible standard for certifying bottled water, filtration systems, and even plumbing. Products they inspect and approve have an NSF label. Their web site is: http://www.nsf.org.
- Water filters that distill water are expensive, slow, costly, and prone to maintenance problems. They also greatly restrict water pressure.
- You might want to gather information on your water before deciding what kind of filtering system you need. The water department or governmental agencies might be willing to provide data on request. While their data might not tell you exactly what is in the water in your home, it can give you an idea of what problems are likely. Having your water tested is expensive. Do it yourself kits can lower the cost. With thousands of possible contaminants it is only feasible to test for the most likely problems. Even a fairly comprehensive test is only a snapshot and might not indicate what is in your water at different times of the year when the temperature, pH, and water tables might vary.[48]
- While individual bottles of bottled water might be chic, they do little to improve our health. The four billion dollars spent on bottled water in 1998 could have done a lot of good if spent on more useful purchases. The bottled water industry's consumption of plastics and transportation resources is an ecological setback.

Alcohol

There is a dietary supplement that can, if taken in the proper dosage, reduce your risk of heart disease, colon and rectal cancer, hepatitis, macular degeneration, and depression. It helps people relax and handle stress. It increases estrogen production 327% in women who are taking estrogen (lessening the amount of estrogen they need to take), might improve cognitive functioning, and in some forms aids digestion. Normally advertisers would deluge us with promotions for this miracle substance. Physicians and the government, however, are reluctant to allow promotion of the health benefits of alcohol for fear it will encourage people to drink and many would drink too much. Can't you hear the alcoholics quoting their doctors saying drinking is good for you? I do not want to encourage drinking either. There is a considerable body of research, however, that indicates moderate drinkers live longer than either teetotalers or heavy drinkers. It holds true for wine, beer, and liquor.

Life is full of paradoxes. The French diet is rich in fat and wine but the French have longer than average life spans. Indeed the oldest person on record, Jeanne Calment, was French. Many have debated the "French paradox." Why do the French get long life, great food, and France too? They have fewer deaths from cardiovascular problems or cancer (though more deaths from cirrhosis of the liver). Part of the French paradox could be that the French do much of their drinking with meals. Perhaps it is that they follow a Zone diet with meat being part of the meal but not the main course. Wine in particular appears to have additional benefits beyond other forms of alcohol. It could be genetic. As the French have been adopting a more American style of eating, however, their longevity is now approaching American longevity, casting doubt on a strong genetic role.

Researchers really don't understand the mechanisms that make alcohol salubrious. Perhaps it is chemistry. It is believed to cause hormones to keep blood platelets from sticking together. Perhaps it is that alcohol gives us an excuse to slow down, relax, and take our minds off the stresses of the day. Finally, there is the possibility that some of the apparent benefit is a selection factor–i.e., perhaps people who choose moderate drinking are more flexible and better at handling stress than teetotalers. Barry Sears[49] concludes that modest to moderate alcohol consumption produces "good" eicosanoids (a class of "master hormones") and excessive alcohol produces "bad" eicosanoids. Thus, alcohol helps keep these master hormones in "the zone." In any case, modest alcohol consumption appears to be good for your health. Red wine (perhaps because of resveratrol in the grape skins or flavinoids in the juice) might be a little more beneficial than other forms of alcohol. This is not to say you must drink for longevity. Mormons and Seventh-Day Adventists advocate abstention from alcohol, as well as many healthy lifestyle practices, and have longer than average life spans.

Conclusions

The key to nutrition is balance and common sense. Today's centenarians have not been following extreme diets. They aren't worry warts who fret about whether their meals have too much of the wrong kind of cholesterol. Rather they have a sense of good nutrition and enjoy eating and enjoy life. For many current centenarians, their enjoyment of life often includes modest liquor consumption.

To summarize key points:

- Find a diet that works for you and fits with the previously mentioned Cardinal Rules for Your Diet. If your current diet isn't working for you consider the Zone diet.
- Choose healthy foods most of the time.
- Drink eight glasses of water a day and try to make most of the water you consume filtered water. If drinking eight glasses of water is difficult, substitute decaffeinated iced tea or diluted fruit juice, or water with lemon.
- Keep alcohol use modest–no more than two drinks a day.
- Consider the vitamin, mineral, and other supplements discussed in the next chapter.
- Periodically review your eating habits but don't second guess them on a daily basis.
- Once you have a healthy diet in place, relax and enjoy life. More harm is done by worrying about how much cholesterol is in your food or whether that glass of iced tea has filtered water than the possible harm from the cholesterol or chlorine.

Chapter 13

Supplemental Vitamins, Minerals, and Hormones

Do we need more vitamins and minerals?

The case for taking vitamins grows so persuasive that not taking
them is an invitation to reckless aging and premature death.
–Jean Carper[1]

Some health food advocates say that people who eat healthy, balanced meals with lots of fresh fruits and vegetables get all the vitamins and minerals they need to be healthy. They note, however, that the soil in many countries has become so depleted that this is no longer the case unless the food is organic. Before electric refrigeration, which became common in the 1920s, it was difficult to have fresh fruits and vegetables in temperate climates. Today a large proportion of American fruits, vegetables, and other foods come from other countries. Many of the most health conscious individuals are vegetarians and they have an even more difficult task of getting all the vitamins, minerals, and amino acids they need without supplements. Even if it is possible to derive all the vitamins and minerals you need from your food, how many people really consume an ideal diet with a wide variety of foods?

There is another problem. The "you just need a healthy diet" argument is usually based on the Food and Nutrition Board of the National Research Council's list of minimum daily requirements (MDR) for vitamins and minerals. These are minimum requirements for preventing disease. Our goal, however, is optimal health and Optimal Daily Allowance (ODA) dosages. Optimal health calls for vitamin levels that give you improved health and longevity without excesses that cause side effects, overwork our livers or kidneys, or waste money. The answers change as research accumulates. Consider a few examples. We are admonished to lower our cholesterol levels to reduce our risk of heart and circulatory disease. Lowering cholesterol, however, reduces our body's production of Coenzyme Q-10, one of the top antioxidants. Beta carotene is another of the highly touted antioxidants that reduces the risk of cancer and other diseases.

For smokers and heavy drinkers, however, beta carotene appears to increase the risk of lung cancer.

The wisest course is to seek a fairly conservative approach that does not overreact to headlines about a single study but changes as a preponderance of evidence accumulates. In Jean Carper's *Stop Aging Now!* prominent researchers and authors in health, alternative health, and aging briefly list what vitamins and supplements they use on a daily basis. Seven of the eleven reported only taking what would be included in a multivitamin that includes minerals and beta carotene. Three took a multivitamin and Coenzyme Q-10. One took a multivitamin, Coenzyme Q-10, *Ginkgo*, and garlic. Carper's own recommendation was for the equivalent of a good multivitamin (with minerals and beta carotene) and Coenzyme Q-10. She then listed several optional supplements (fish oil, garlic *Ginkgo*, glutamine, and glutathione). Michael Roizen in *Real Age,* a book which is carefully based on research data, advised taking a daily vitamin with minerals but concluded the jury was still out on other supplements. Andrew Weil,[2] whose books include *Natural Health, Natural Medicine,* and *Spontaneous Healing*, advocates supplements (specifically vitamins, carotenes, selenium, zinc, and Coenzyme Q-10).

What to do about vitamins and minerals

- The best solution is to choose a well-researched multiple vitamin. Some low-priced multiple vitamins might be formulated on the basis of economics. Most pharmaceutical companies, however, have given careful consideration to optimal health, balancing the proportions of vitamins and minerals, and including antioxidants such as beta carotene. My personal preference is the Life Extension Foundation's "Life Extension Mix." (I do not receive any consideration for recommending them.) I am impressed with their careful, researched-based consideration of what goes into the product and their updating of the product annually. The current formula contains the usual vitamins and minerals, and a variety of antioxidants, vegetable extracts, and amino acids too long to list.[3] There is so much loaded into the vitamins that the recommended dosage is three pills, three times a day. A comprehensive vitamin is less expensive than purchasing vitamins and minerals piecemeal. It also avoids the risk of getting vitamins out of balance so they do not work well together; for example, too much vitamin C impairing the use of vitamin B-12.

- Most people, especially if they eat meat, obtain enough iron from their diets and do not need it in their vitamins. (Exceptions often include women who are menstruating and blood donors.) You don't want too much iron as it combines with free radicals and does some of the worst free radical damage. If you do need to take iron, it should be ferrous fumarate, ferrous citrate, or ferrous gluconate, not ferrous sulfate (which destroys vitamin E).
- Women need more calcium and vitamin D than men to prevent osteoporosis.
- With a multiple vitamin, the question becomes whether there is anything unique about your health that indicates modifications to the multiple vitamin.

When to take vitamins, minerals and supplements

Generally, your body will absorb vitamins, minerals, and supplements whenever you take them. Timing is merely a question of getting the full effectiveness of dosages.

- Oil soluble vitamins (A, D, E, and K) need to be taken with food that contains some fat or oil to help with their absorption.
- Water soluble vitamins (C and the B vitamins) should be taken two or three times a day as their half life is short.
- If you take amino acid supplements with food, your stomach will secrete stomach acids and digest a lot of the amino acids as food. If you take amino acids on an empty stomach, they are more likely to be absorbed into the blood stream and converted into neurotransmitters (the usual reason for taking amino acid supplements).
- A high dose of vitamin C can impair the absorption of vitamin B-12.
- A high dose of vitamin C is wasted as the body excretes whatever it cannot use. If you want a lot of vitamin C, take it several times a day.
- Supplements that tend to increase energy, such as *Ginkgo*, ginseng, and teas with caffeine should be taken early in the day.

- Fiber can inhibit the absorption of minerals as the minerals can bind to the fiber and pass through the gastrointestinal system without being absorbed.
- Calcium levels drop during sleep. Some experts believe the ideal time to take calcium supplements (with its partner vitamin D) is on an empty stomach before going to bed.
- Supplements that are sleep inducing, such as melatonin, should be taken close to bedtime.
- Coffee or tea can impair the absorption of some minerals.

Herbal supplements: Nature's wisdom?

Until recently, physicians have largely snubbed herbal approaches, leaving consumers to fend for themselves in a largely unregulated market. Nevertheless, Americans have flocked to herbs for several reasons:
- the appeal of a natural lifestyle
- disenchantment with conventional medicine
- concern about side effects from conventional medications
- a desire to promote health and prevent disease
- not wanting the expense and hassle of getting a prescription
- wanting to be in charge of their own health

We can roughly divide the top ten herbs into those that are believed to:
- promote health; for example, *Ginkgo* and garlic to promote circulation, and ginseng, a stimulant which increases adrenocorticotrophic (ACTH) release
- prevent/treat disease, e.g., saw palmetto to prevent/treat prostate cancer, cranberry extract to prevent/treat urinary tract infections, echinacea to prevent/treat colds and flus
- treat specific problems, e.g., St. John's wort for depression, valerian and kava for anxiety and insomnia, black cohosh for menopausal problems

The ten most frequently used herbs[4] (each mentioned in the bullets above) have received considerable research attention, especially in Europe. Overall, research found some support for their effectiveness and generally only modest side effects. However, it is a buyer beware market. Many herbs have not been standardized and have not been tried on various age groups. Many have several varieties that presumably vary in effectiveness. There is some outright fraud in supplements that do not have the advertised ingredients. Of the top ten herbs, ginseng and echinacea currently have the least research support.

What to do

- Since research on herbs is limited and taking a lot of herbs might have unknown interactions with other herbs, supplements, medications, etc., it is best to be cautious and conservative in their use.
- Piecemeal articles abound on the herbal wonder of the month, and should be taken lightly as they do not look at the big picture. There are at least four alternatives to the piecemeal problem:
    - Periodically (perhaps whenever a new edition appears) take a look at an objective review of herbs, e.g., the latest editions of *Tyler's Herbs of Choice*[5] and/or *Tyler's Honest Herbal.*[6] Tyler's books are written by pharmacists and are the authoritative standard. They meticulously consider research on each medicinal herb.
    - Look for reviews that rank which herbs and supplements are the most important. The Life Extension Foundation, for example, lists their top ten supplement recommendations[7] each year and the list includes several herbs. Their most recent top ten recommendations had *Ginkgo*, saw palmetto, garlic, and their "herbal mix."
    - Use a well-thought-out mix of herbs, which makes sense to you after considering the ingredients. For example, some herbal mixes include echinacea despite research indicating that it should be taken as needed, and not on an ongoing basis. Mixes might contain substances that can cause allergic reactions in some people (licorice, for example, causes some people's blood pressure to shoot up).
    - Choose a comprehensive program that is integrated with vitamins and other supplements as opposed to a piecemeal

approach. One of the best integrated, very aggressive programs is outlined in Dharma Singh Khalsa's *Brain Longevity.*

- Consider any documented side effects. Of the top ten herbs mentioned, only saw palmetto, cranberry, and black cohosh had no significant adverse effects reported with normal doses. Garlic and *Ginkgo* were safe as long as blood thinning is not a concern (e.g., if you are undergoing anticoagulant therapy or have a problem with bleeding).
- Observe whether you experience any side effects.
- Only purchase products from well known, reputable manufacturers.
- Only purchase products that list all the ingredients and their dosages.
- If you choose to only use a few herbs, current research suggests garlic and *Ginkgo* as the safest and most efficacious. Men might also consider saw palmetto to reduce the risk of prostate growth and prostate cancer. Specific herbs might also be used for specific problems, e.g., cranberry extract to prevent/treat urinary tract infections.

Miscellaneous supplements

Aspirin is a curious medication. It was used by ancient Greeks and American Indians. If it were discovered today, the U.S. Food and Drug Administration would be reluctant to approve it because of its possible side effects such stomach irritation, stomach bleeding, iron deficiency, and Reye's syndrome in children. It is a wonder drug for everything from headaches to arthritic pain. Even in low doses (e.g., 1/4 of a 325 mg tablet), it thins the blood, which helps prevent blood clots. If you have a heart attack, you are given aspirin as soon as possible. Subsequently, you would be advised to take low doses of aspirin daily. A number of health and longevity experts recommend routinely taking a low dose aspirin once a day with a meal as a preventive measure against heart attacks and strokes. The research is not in yet on the effectiveness of routinely taking aspirin to prevent strokes and heart attacks in people who have never had one. Taking aspirin as a preventive measure seems reasonable, especially if you have a family history of cardiovascular problems and you do not have contraindications, e.g., problems with blood clotting, stomach irritation from aspirin, ulcers, aspirin allergy. If you take aspirin, take it with food to prevent stomach irritation.

Coenzyme Q-10 became one of the top supplements in the latter part of the 1990s. Primarily touted as an antioxidant, research has also found it helps prevent atherosclerosis, might help prevent breast or prostate tumors, and helps prevent dopamine (a neurotransmitter) depletion. It also prevents oxidation of LDL cholesterol and reduces periodontal disease. It also is appearing in skin care creams. Given its strong research support, taking a Coenzyme Q-10 supplement is advisable, especially if you have reason to be concerned about cardiovascular problems.

Soy, a legume, is a principal source of protein for vegetarians. Soy meat substitutes are becoming more and more palatable and available. Soy milk is also becoming a popular alternative to milk. Whole soy beans can be roasted, boiled, or frozen and eaten by themselves or with other foods. Soy is also available as a flour, tofu, and textured meat substitute, and miso. Soy pills and powders are also available. Soy is an antioxidant, inhibits LDL cholesterol oxidation, lowers cholesterol, is a good source of choline for neurotransmitters, and helps prevent atherosclerosis and cancer including breast, ovarian, and prostate cancer. It has been used, in large doses, as an adjunct cancer treatment. It is especially important for women as it helps replace estrogen in some menopausal women, moderates estrogen levels, stimulates bone formation, and helps to prevent gallstones. Soy's benefits are believed to be due to the chemicals genistein and daidzein. Switching from animal proteins to soy proteins will result in somewhat lower testosterone levels. Weight lifters often use soy whey powder drinks after their workouts to build muscles. It makes more sense to eat soy than to take it in pill form. If your diet has little or no soy, however, soy supplements might be helpful.

Hormonal supplements–almost ready for prime time

What if you could take a single hormone that would cause you to:
• lose fat

- increase muscle mass 8.8% without extra exercise
- lower blood pressure
- strengthen your immune system
- strengthen your bones
- reduce wrinkles
- give you thicker hair
- sharpen your vision
- enhance your mood
- improve your memory
- improve your sleep
- heal wounds faster
- increase the functioning of your heart, liver, spleen, kidneys, and other organs
- increase your energy level
- improve your sexual functioning, and
- slow aging?

There is such a hormone. But before you sign up, there are, of course, some catches. Currently, you would have to inject the hormone several times a week at a cost of $10,000 a year. There are some risks of joint aches and pains, insulin resistance, diabetes, fluid retention, and carpal tunnel syndrome (pain, tingling, and/or numbness caused by swelling of the wrist which presses on a nerve). There also is a risk that your body might cease producing its own and you would become dependent on the hormone supplement.

The hormone is Human Growth Hormone (HGH), which your pituitary gland secretes in minute quantities primarily while you sleep. Since the 1980s, thousands of very short children received HGH to help them grow to a more normal height. HGH had to be derived from the pituitary glands of cow cadavers and was extremely expensive. When three children (later fifty children) taking HGH developed "mad cow disease," the cadaver source could no longer be used. In 1985 and 1986 Genentech and Eli Lilly developed synthetic HGHs, reducing the cost to of HGHs to $14,000-$30,000 a year and ending the need to harvest HGH from cadavers. Today the price is around $10,000 a year and going down. In June 1999 Genentech announced that it completed clinical trials on a slow release HGH injection and is applying for FDA approval. The slow release would only require one or two injections a month.

Most of our hormones, including HGH, peak in our twenties, begin declining by age thirty, and by age seventy are at less than half of their previous levels. Daniel Rudman[8] believed that replacing the lost HGH would reverse aging. He gave 12 healthy men, ages 61-80, three injections a week for six months and obtained the results cited in the list at the beginning of this section. He described it as the equivalent of reversing 10 to 20 years of aging. HGH also increases your body's production of B-endorphins, which helps you feel better and counters depression. Of course looking and being healthier helps you feel better as well. Unfortunately, Dr. Rudman died in 1994 of a pulmonary embolism at age 67 and was not able to continue his research.

European researchers used HGH with patients who lost their pituitary glands from disease and/or surgery and obtained results similar to Rudman's results. Edmund Chein[9] used HGH with more than eight hundred mostly healthy adults and reported excellent results with only mild side effects–mild joint pain and fluid retention which cleared up after a few months of treatment. Chein's treatment differed from Rudman's in that he had patients self-inject two small doses twice a day, six days a week.

HGH remains in your blood stream for only a few minutes. Your liver converts it into growth factors including IGF-1 (insulin-like growth factor). In your prime, IGF-1 levels are about 350 nanograms per milliliter. While early researchers attempted to restore IGF-1s to this level, Ullis[10] reports that current research is showing that the risk of prostate cancer rises dramatically above 185 nanongrams. Consequently, he recommends not exceeding that level until more is known. This requires periodic blood testing. Research also is finding that several compounds are involved in what was thought to be just HGH.

In 1996 the U.S. Food and Drug Administration (FDA) approved HGH for adults. Dr. Ronald Klatz, president and founder of the 8,500 member American Academy of Anti-aging Medicine, has been promoting the efficacy of HGH and has written two books on HGH, *Grow Young with HGH* and *Ten Weeks to a Younger You.*[11] [12] As we learn more about HGH, the risks of using it, and as the costs come down, HGH will eventually become an option for healthy adults who want to reverse the effects of aging. Currently, HGH is only available by prescription and injection and requires several months of treatment to be effective. Treatment is contraindicated for people who have cancer, chronic edema, carpal tunnel syndrome, uncontrolled hypertension, blood sugar regulation problems, or are pregnant. As previously mentioned risks include joint aches and pains, insulin resistance, diabetes, fluid retention, and carpal tunnel syndrome. Another risk is that your body might lose its ability to produce its own HGH and you would become dependent on supplements for your current level of HGH production. To try to avoid this, physicians often cycle administration; for example, Chein has patients use injections only six days a week and some physicians discontinue treatment every six months.

Here are some less drastic and less expensive measures to increase your body's level of HGH:

- Exercising induces a release of HGH. High intensity exercise like weight lifting boosts IGF-1 levels 200-400%.[13]
- Since insulin inhibits the release of HGH, a diet that keeps insulin levels stable supports HGH secretion. The Zone eating program is specifically targeted at keeping insulin levels stable.
- Especially when exercising, avoid consuming anything that would spike your insulin levels as insulin inhibits the release of HGH. A small amount of food during exercise, however, is OK to allow insulin to move amino acids into muscle cells.
- Avoid eating foods that will spike your insulin levels before bedtime as most HGH is released while you sleep and the increased insulin would inhibit its release.
- There are a number of supplements that purport to increase HGH release. Sports physician Karlis Ullis[14] says that in his experience arginine and lysine are ineffective but the amino acid L-glutamine works for some people.
- There is disagreement about when to eat. Insulin suppresses HGH release. Klatz[15] concluded the longer it has been since we have eaten, the more HGH will be released into your system. He even advocates fasting to increase HGH. Sears, who emphasizes keeping insulin and blood sugar levels in a stable zone 24 hours a day, believes that stable insulin levels will ultimately effect

more HGH in your blood plasma. In either case, avoiding excess insulin helps.

Most people are more likely to consider secretagogues than HGH injections. A secretagogue is a substance that induces other cells to secrete something. In common usage it often refers to substances that cause the body to secrete HGH. In 2000 over a hundred products purporting to raise HGH were on the market (many on the Internet). These include homeopathic products that use minute amounts of chemicals to prompt a counter response from the body. It is a buyer beware market. The American Academy of Anti-Aging Medicine compares many of them on its web site www.worldhealth.net. In 1999 Ullis[16] [17] concluded that the only credible alternative to injections of HGH is the orally administered secretagogue MK0677, but that several secretagogues should be available in 2000 using pills or patches. Merck has MK0677 in phase three clinical trials. Six major pharmaceutical companies are developing secretagogues.

Ronald Klatz also reports that a Japanese study with weight lifters found that injecting GHB (gamma hydroxybutytrate) quickly made HGH levels rise to nine times higher and stimulated the slow wave sleep associated with release of HGH. GHB is usually consumed with a beverage at bedtime. Due to its abuse by teenagers seeking a high and supposed possible use as a date rape drug, it requires a prescription. A related chemical, 2 (3H) Furanone di-dydro apparently has similar but weaker effects and its use might also become limited by federal or state governments.

Yet another future possibility is IGF-1 itself.[18] It appears to be even more potent than HGH and is better at regulating blood sugar levels (note the name insulin-like growth factor). It is still in early stages of clinical study.

Testosterone

Research reported in the prestigious *New England Journal of Medicine*[19] studied men ages 19 to 40 who had previous weight lifting experience. They were divided into four groups. Their gains in fat free mass were as follows: placebo group 0.8 kg, placebo and exercise group 2.1, testosterone injections only group 3.2, and exercise and testosterone injections group 6.1. On measures of triceps, quadriceps, bench press, and squats, the placebo/exercise group's weight lifting and muscle size gains were about the same as the testosterone only group's gains. The exercise/testosterone group's gains were much higher than the other groups. Thus, even without exercise, testosterone builds muscle. With exercise testosterone builds even more muscle (and reduces fat).

Testosterone is the principal male hormone, and is an important hormone for women as well. It enhances the sexual drive of men and women, builds muscle, elevates mood, prevents osteoporosis, improves memory, lowers cholesterol, and protects against heart disease. By age 70, men's testosterone levels are at less than half of their teen/young adult levels. Resistance exercises like weight lifting increase testosterone levels. Testosterone supplements increase the level of IGF-1 in both men who had low levels of testosterone and men who had normal levels.

In the early 1990s, the only testosterone treatments were injections. Then the U.S. Food and Drug Administration approved a patch applied to the scrotum and approved skin implants. The FDA has now approved a patch that can be worn on the buttocks or back, gels, lozenges, suppositories, and pills. Ronald Klatz[20] advises that the pills are ineffective and synthetic testosterone can cause liver toxicity. (Testosterone is not patentable so the pharmaceutical companies have focused on synthetic versions that are patentable.)

The number of men taking testosterone supplements is increasing rapidly. *Newsweek* magazine had testosterone as its cover story on September 16, 1996. The benefits of testosterone therapy typically become apparent within a few weeks. Testosterone supplements decrease the risk for heart disease, atherosclerosis, hypertension and obesity and decrease LDL "bad" cholesterol levels. Supplements improve autoimmune system functioning (e.g., rheumatoid arthritis, lupus) but decrease other immune functioning. Physicians watch for increased Prostate Specific Antigens (the PSA test) and increased hematocrit (indicating the blood is getting too thick and might have difficulty circulating). Contraindications to testosterone replacement for men include prostate concerns, low HDL cholesterol, and blood circulation problems. There are possible long-term risks with supplements including atrophying of testicles, high red blood cell and hematocrit counts, depression, fluid retention and a reduction in sperm count, semen volume, and HDL "good" cholesterol. There is also the risk that the body might reduce its own production of testosterone, creating a dependency on the supplements. Some physicians recommend cycling on and off the supplements to reduce the risk of dependency. Note that stress impedes your body's ability to produce testosterone.

Men's estrogen levels do not decline with age. There is some evidence that the increased ratio of estrogen to testosterone in men effects an increased risk of cancer (thus making testosterone replacement likely to lessen the risk of prostate cancer). Ullis[21] disagrees with the popular belief that testosterone contributes to prostate cancer. He points out that if this were the case we should see high rates of prostate cancer in teenagers and young adults as they have the highest testosterone rates. Rather prostate problems typically begin when testosterone rates are dropping and men have a lower ratio of testosterone to estrogen (which does not drop for men). Thus, testosterone supplements for men might help prevent prostate cancer.

Just using testosterone supplements doesn't necessarily work. Older men's bodies often convert testosterone into estrogen. The estrogen then uses testosterone receptors in the body, making them unavailable for testosterone. Excess estrogen also increases the production of SHBG (sex hormone-binding globulin), which binds to testosterone and makes it unavailable. For testosterone to do its job it needs to be free so it can attach to testosterone receptors. The Life Extension Foundation reports[22] that several herbs, chrysin, muira puama, and neetle root extract increase free testosterone by blocking the conversion of testosterone to estrogen and/or binding to SHBG so less SHBG will be available to bind with testosterone. The Life Extension Foundation has conducted three small studies and is conducting clinical trials on how well these herbs increase free testosterone levels.

Women produce testosterone in their ovaries and their adrenal glands. Most women's ovaries cease testosterone production by age 40 (before they cease producing estrogen).[23] Women need some testosterone to have a healthy sex drive, good energy level, strong bones, and to develop muscles as opposed to fat. Women who take estrogen supplements can end up with their ratios of testosterone to estrogen badly out of balance. The consequence is an increase in fat tissue. Consequently, some women take small doses of testosterone (or testosterone precursors) to avoid these problems and to lessen menopause problems. At higher doses testosterone would tend to masculinize them.

Testosterone precursors ("T-boosters")

When a reporter happened to notice a bottle of androstenedione in baseball home run king Mark McGuire's locker, the supplement became the subject of thousands of news stories. What McGuire took was an over-the-counter supplement that is a chemical precursor of testosterone. Currently the definitive source of information on testosterone precursors is sports physician Karlis Ullis' book, *Super "T": The Complete Guide to Creating an Effective, Safe, and Natural Testosterone Supplement Program for Men and Women.*[24] He outlines the different types of testosterone precursors and the advantages and disadvantages of each. His program includes cycling on and off the supplements to lessen the risk of your body becoming dependent on them. The program is aimed at increasing lean body tissue, decreasing fat, and obtaining the other benefits that go with increased testosterone levels. His book also has fascinating discussions on enhancing sexual performance.

Using testosterone precursors can be helpful to women and men. A touted safety factor is that because your own body produces the testosterone, your body will not produce more than it needs. The testosterone precursors boost testosterone for about two to three hours.

His program for women uses far less testosterone and has more complicated options. For simplicity I will describe his basic program for males. Men would take 100 or 200 mg of 4-Androstenedoil thirty to sixty minutes before their weight training workout so they could challenge their muscles more by lifting more than usual. His program for serious athletes has the athletes taking the supplements three times a day and cycling off every six to eight weeks. During the off cycle he recommends using creatine monohydrate, a fairly safe over-the-counter supplement that facilitates quicker replenishment of ATP. ATP (adenosine triphosphate) is a key chemical in energy transfer in muscles (and all cells of the body). All things considered, the testosterone precursors appear to be a much safer and less expensive than HGH or testosterone supplements. The price of supplements has come down to about fifty cents a workout and there are a number of suppliers on the Internet.

When athletes started using anabolic steroids, the American Medical Association said they were dangerous and they did not work anyway. The did not work anyway part was ludicrous to many athletes who had huge strength and performance gains from using them. The "did not work claim" undermined the credibility of the AMA's appropriate warning that anabolic steroids are very dangerous. The AMA is now saying the same about androstenedione- -it doesn't work and it is dangerous. Taken in moderation and with cycling it appears to be reasonably safe. The standard should not be whether someone can find one individual who had a problem with it but a consideration of the risks and benefits of using it vs. not using it (e.g., having more fat tissue and less muscle). An article in the *Journal of the American Medical Association* concluded that androstenedione does not increase testosterone levels or muscles at a statistically significant level.[25] The article is being widely cited. Certainly there is the possibility of a placebo effect and good studies are needed. The *JAMA* study, however, had a small number of subjects and such abysmally poor experimental design that the research is worthless and never should have been published. An excellent critique is available on the Internet.[26]

Estrogen

Estrogen is the principal sex hormone for women but also is an important hormone for men. With menopause, women's decline in estrogen is more abrupt than men's decline in testosterone. Estrogen enhances sexual functioning, sharpens thinking, enhances mood, and resists osteoporosis, colon cancer, heart disease, and Alzheimer's disease, and improves skin quality. With declining estrogen levels, women's heart disease risk approaches that of men. Estrogen is an antioxidant and it strengthens blood vessels. In the menstrual cycle estrogen rises to prepare the uterus for an egg. Then estrogen drops and progesterone increases until the end of the cycle when progesterone declines too.

Estrogen replacement is more than 40 years old. Premarin is one of the most widely prescribed drugs in the U.S. While estrogen replacement helps protect against heart disease and osteoporosis, there is some trade off in an increased risk of breast and uterine cancer. In 1997 Evista became the first "targeted estrogen" or selective estrogen receptor modulator (SERM). It appears to have the benefits of estrogen without the increased risk of cancers. Another option is Estradiol[27] and related hormones that more closely match the human estrogen our bodies naturally produce. Estradoil is used extensively in Europe but not much in the U.S. Because Estradoil cannot be patented, pharmaceutical companies have little incentive to promote it as competition keeps their price markup slim and there is more profit in patentable variations. Soy foods tend to foster the natural production of estrogen. There also are more natural alternatives to Provera progesterone supplementation. Ullis[28] reports that with dietary and herbal alternatives most women can delay estrogen and progesterone replacement therapy up to age 60 if there are no cardiovascular problems or family history of Alzheimer's disease. The natural alternatives do not promote fat storage or increase the risk of breast cancer.

Men also need estrogen. Boys need it to grow bones and older men need it to prevent bone loss. Too much estrogen (in proportion to testosterone), however, causes a man to lose muscle tone, become obese, develop an enlarged chest, experience a decreased sexual drive, and develop connective tissue disorders. Because women cease producing estrogen and men do not, most 55-year-old men have more estrogen than most 55-year-old women who are not taking estrogen supplements. The National Osteoporosis Association reports that about 20% of the 28 million Americans with osteoporosis are men.[29] They report that a man over 50 is more likely to develop an osteoporosis-related fracture than to develop prostate cancer.

DHEA

Dehydroepiandrosterone (DHEA) is a steroidal hormone that your body naturally produces in abundance. Like most of our hormones, the quantity in our bodies decreases when we pass age 30. DHEA is a precursor of testosterone and estrogen. The idea is that if you take DHEA you will produce more testosterone and estrogen. The possible benefits include increased energy, sexual drive, and memory, improved immune system functioning, and decreased skin wrinkling, risk of cancer or heart disease, and less body fat. DEHA has been available as an inexpensive over-the-counter pill or skin cream since the mid 1990s. There has been an enormous amount of research on DHEA. So why isn't everyone taking DHEA? There are several reasons:

- Many individuals don't show much response to it.
- If it does stimulate estrogen and testosterone production, it would have some of the same possible side effects as increased HGH. (The only risk that is well documented is an increased risk of prostate cancer.)
- It is difficult to determine what the appropriate dosage should be without taking blood tests and most people are not willing to endure the time, out-of-pocket expense, and discomfort of blood tests.
- Karlis Ullis[30] warns that DHEA promotes the production of both estrogen and testosterone and in some men DHEA might be counterproductive by producing more estrogen than testosterone.

Pregnenolone

Pregnenolone is known to enhance memory and concentration, reduce fatigue, and relieve arthritis. It is a precursor to DHEA and progesterone. It would seem that if you took pregnenolone it would naturally produce DHEA. Along with our body's decline in DHEA, however, is a decline in the enzyme necessary to change pregnenolone to DHEA. Pregnenolone is available over the counter but has not received the recognition that DHEA has received.

Melatonin

Melatonin is produced by the pineal gland, "the body's clock." Melatonin regulates sleep cycles, is an antioxidant, reduces the risk of heart disease and cancer, strengthens the immune system, enhances sexual vitality, counters the effects of stress hormones (corticosteroids) and might play a role in regulating aging. Melatonin is sold over the counter and is popularly used as a sleep aid, a treatment for jet lag, and an anti-aging supplement. Since it causes drowsiness, it should only be taken before sleep. If the dose is too high, it will cause drowsiness on awakening. If you experience depression when there is less sunlight in the winter (seasonal affective disorder or SAD) be cautious about using melatonin during the winter.

If you are considering hormonal supplements

- Do you have reason to believe you have abnormally low levels of the hormone relative to your age? Being deficient increases the advisability of supplementing the hormone.
- How much research is available on supplementing this hormone? Estrogen supplements have a vast amount of research and the issues in deciding whether to use them are fairly well understood. Testosterone supplements are not as well understood but a lot of data will be generated in the next ten years (by 2010). Human growth hormone is riskier as there is far less research and far fewer people taking it.
- What are the side effects? Every medication and every supplement has side effects.
- How much does it tax your liver? Almost any supplement taken orally gives the liver one more thing to detoxify. Creams avoid taxing the liver but are harder to dose. Patches (e.g., estrogen, testosterone) provide a steady, measured dose without taxing the liver.
- Are you willing to monitor blood levels? The safest way to take supplements is to have your physician periodically test blood levels of the hormones and other indicators, consider whether the dosage is optimal, and prescribe the amount of hormone to take. Many people, however choose not to incur the time and expense of doing this. The Life Extension Foundation[31] publishes a directory, for its members, of physicians who are especially interested in and knowledgeable about longevity (and hormone supplements). It also has a mail order blood testing program for

members. Their web site is www.lef.org. The American Academy of Anti-Aging Medicine[32] has a free list of physicians interested in anti-aging therapies. Their web site is www.worldhealth.net.

- What is the source of the information? The pharmaceutical industry makes money by selling its products. Their sales representatives make the rounds of doctors' offices, giving free samples, a sales pitch for their products, and favors such as lunches and presents. While few physicians are likely to be bribed by the process, having samples and current information makes it easier for them to prescribe those products. The pharmaceutical companies produce the research to meet FDA approval and to promote their drugs. Reports periodically surface of pharmaceutical companies suppressing reports of research results which are unfavorable to their products. Medications which are not patentable receive little research attention or marketing as a competitor could capitalize on a pharmaceutical company's research and produce a generic version. When supplements are sold by nonpharmaceutical organizations it is even more difficult to verify the quality and claims for the supplement.
- What formulation is the best choice? For example, Premarin and Provera vs. supplements that more closely match human estrogen and progesterone.
- What does it cost? If you have deep pockets–no problem. For many people, however, cost is a consideration.

What to do about hormone supplements

In life we have to make decisions on incomplete information. My best judgment at this time is:
- Estrogen/progesterone supplements are advisable for most women when they reach menopause. Consideration should be given to estrogens and progesterone that closely match human estrogens and progesterone and to foods, like soy, that tend to induce estrogen production. For estrogen replacement the reduced risk of heart disease, osteoporosis, and Alzheimer's disease outweighs the increased risk of breast cancer for most women. Physicians can help assess whether this is advisable for you.

- If you are in good health, it probably is wisest not to take hormonal supplements or secretagogues until more is known about them. By the middle or end of the decade (2005-2010) we should know enough to make good decisions about whether to take hormone supplements other than estrogen and progesterone. Currently, it appears risky to be guinea pigs.
- If your hormone levels are low for your age, consider a supplement.
- If you decide to take any of these hormone supplements, chart your target behaviors for a month before starting the supplement, introduce just one new supplement, and chart the target behaviors for as long as it is supposed to take for the supplement to show results. Note any other changes in your health, even if they seem unrelated. If you think you want to continue the supplement, consider going off it and repeating the experiment to make sure the change you saw was not a coincidence.
- If you use a hormone supplement, consider cycling on and off it.
- The risk/benefit ratio for testosterone precursors appears to justify considering them on a limited basis (e.g., three times a week with cycling on and off).
- The most intelligent way to take supplements is by having your physician periodically test blood levels, consider whether the dosage is optimal, and prescribe the amount to take.
- If you are particularly concerned about breast cancer or prostrate cancer, *Life Extension* magazine has excellent protocols for prevention and treatment in their May, 1999 and November, 1999 issues.

Conclusion

When it comes to vitamins, hormones, and supplements, there are many advocates who seize on a particular issue or supplement and treat it as if it were the only issue. Our bodies, however, are very complex, interrelated systems. Adding a vitamin or supplement can cause repercussions throughout the system. Permit me to use a football analogy. If the other team completes a pass, it is tempting to pull more players back to defend against the pass. Unless it is late in the game and your opponent is far behind, your opponent will probably take advantage of your changed defense and run the ball. There are times when changing the defense makes sense and there are times when it just creates new problems. Great coaches stick with the fundamentals and know when to deviate from the play book and when not to deviate. You are the coach and your body comes with an incredibly brilliant, complex book of fundamentals. Be sure you know what your are doing before you call any Statue of Liberty plays or throw any Hail Mary passes.

It is difficult to obtain all the vitamins and minerals we need from our food. Consequently a multivitamin with minerals is certainly indicated. There are a few herbs and supplements that are worth considering but there is a point of diminishing returns. Indeed, every additional supplement intended to help one system or function runs the risk of unbalancing another system or function. Currently the supplements most worth considering are garlic, *Ginkgo*, and soy. Garlic and soy can be obtained from your food without a supplement. Also worth considering are Coenzyme Q-10 and low dose aspirin. Men might also consider saw palmetto.

For hormonal supplements, natural estrogen/progesterone replacement is advisable for most women at or after menopause. It is reasonable for men and women to consider using testosterone precursors on a very limited basis (e.g., up to three times a week with cycling on and off every six to eight weeks). For other hormones we are in the early stages of a revolution. The calvary should arrive before the end of the decade (2010). Rather than being a guinea pig and experiencing the mistakes that go with new medications or supplements, it is prudent to wait a little longer.

Resources

Books recommending vitamins and minerals are ubiquitous. The most helpful ones consider the whole picture rather than just listing vitamins and their benefits with no discussion of interrelationships. *Tyler's Herbs of Choice* and *Tyler's Honest Herbal* are well researched and balanced resources for evaluating herbs. Independent analyses of the quality of brands of herbs and supplements are appearing on www.consumerlab.com. Dharma Singh Khalsa's *Brain Longevity* presents an aggressive approach to supplements with an emphasis on cognitive functioning. The Life Extension Foundation's *Life Extension* magazine is a good way to stay current on supplement and anti-aging treatments. The magazine and a 25% discount on LEF products come with the annual $75 membership. Ronald Klatz's *Ten Weeks to a Younger You* gives an excellent overview of anti-aging with an emphasis on HGH and other hormones. Karlis Ullis' *Age Right* gives an excellent overview of hormone supplements and how to individualize treatment according to your needs. His *Super "T"* gives a detailed program for using supplements that boost testosterone. Hormonal therapy is developing rapidly and books on the subject will become dated within a few years so look for books with the authors' most recent copyrights.

Chapter 14

Fitness: Emotional vs. Outcome-based Choices

When you had to pump water, it was necessary to
prime the pump by putting a little water in the pump.
Physical activity is the primer that gives you energy and health.

After engaging in a regular exercise program for one year,
your body reacts as if you've been exercising your entire life.
–Edward Jackowski[1]

If you don't have time for fitness, you will have time for illness.

If you rest, you rust. –Helen Hayes[2]

I use the word fitness as opposed to exercise because fitness is a broader, more positive term. For living a vital healthy life for 150 years, you need to engage in optimal amounts and types of fitness activities. Optimal fitness outcomes involve:

- engaging in sufficient aerobic, strength, stretching, relaxing, and other fitness activities to achieve strength, flexibility, cardiovascular fitness, strong bones, good energy, good posture, good breathing, and relaxation responses
- not overdoing exercising, which can cause poor health, injuries, and produce an excess of free radicals
- avoiding injury and undue wear and tear on your body
- making sure that your body will be strong and flexible when you are in your hundreds
- achieving your goals (e.g., weight loss, building strength, effecting growth hormone or testosterone release)
- targeting your most likely health problems (the weakest link in the chain)

The weakest link in the chain

A chain is only as strong as its weakest link. You need to identify and target the weakest link or links in your physical fitness.

Ask yourself:
- When I get sick, what kinds of illnesses do I usually get?
- When my body hurts, where does it usually hurt?
- If I get and injury, where do I get injured?
- What does my annual physical say is the weakest part of my physical health?
- How good is my posture when standing and when sitting?

Check which of the following health problems are an issue for you. Then rank in order the ones you checked.

___back pain   ___depression
___insomnia   ___frequent colds
___constipation   ___unhappy with appearance
___overweight   ___low energy
___difficulty relaxing   ___pain
___vision getting worse   ___other:
___cardiovascular problems   ___other:

Considering your answers to the questions and the items you checked and ranked, what are your weakest links? You need to do whatever it takes to strengthen the weak links because the weak link or links jeopardize your longevity. The weakest links need to be your priorities. If you have to skip some fitness activities, make sure the weakest links are last on the skip list.

If you have sinus problems, you need to emphasize fitness activities that clear the sinuses, e.g., aerobic activities to move mucus and lymph, irrigating your sinuses with salt water, yoga postures such as inverted postures and the lion pose. If you have low back pain you need to determine what is causing the pain, e.g., poor posture, walking on the wrong part of your feet, lack of flexibility in the hip and spine. Then take appropriate action, e.g., flexibility activities, posture exercises, therapeutic massage or manipulations to improve alignment and functioning. If you tend to dislocate your shoulder playing baseball, get a good diagnosis for what is causing the injury and take appropriate actions; for example, warming up and cooling down first, strengthening certain muscles, or discontinuing the activity because it is not good for your body. If your annual physical says your blood pressure is high, look into what fitness activities (and eating habits and supplements) will help you lower your blood pressure (hopefully without medications).

Intelligent fitness

Your body's metabolism, muscles, and other systems follow rules. If you know the rules and follow them, you will be much more effective at meeting your fitness and longevity goals. You could complain and rebel, objecting that you already have too many rules in your life. Or you could be happy to be part of the elite minority who understand and use the rules to achieve great results. Knowing and following the rules means being in harmony with nature and life. Make sure your metaphors support your appreciating, revering, and following the rules.

One of the most important rules came from Aristotle 2500 years ago in his philosophy of the Golden Mean. Simply stated, he advocated for all things in moderation. It is certainly true for fitness. At one extreme we see people who don't want to turn off the television and do something. They rationalize. They grumble that if you subtract the time you spend exercising, it would cancel out the few extra years you would add to your life by exercising. At the other extreme are joggers who run a hundred miles a week despite health problems, weight lifters who take steroids to have huge muscles, and people who are addicted to dangerous or "extreme" sports (e.g., hockey, football, sky diving, white water rafting, skate boarding). People who are likely to live the longest are those who engage in a reasonable amount of fitness activities and meet all of their fitness needs.

Clearly, moderate fitness activities effect greater health, energy, immune functioning, appearance, and self-esteem. But, many Americans aren't moderate. Each year 17 million Americans have at least one notable injury as a result of exercise. Research indicates that there is an optimal golden mean for physical activity. In a study of 17,000 male Harvard graduates, death rates were 1/4 to 1/3 lower for those who expended 2,000 calories a week in exercising. After 3,500 calories per week, however, the death rates started increasing.[3] Athletes learn, often the hard way, that overtraining results in deteriorating performance and increased health problems and injuries.

More isn't better if it consumes the host. As in Aesop's fable of the tortoise and the hare, the tortoise wins.

One of the "rules" is that your body seems to have a set point for fitness.[4] An inactive person's body will quickly show improved fitness with increased activity. There comes a point, however, where you are fit and there are diminishing returns or even a loss of fitness with increased activity. At that point it takes a lot of extra effort to achieve modest gains and the gains are easily lost if you do not keep up the high level of activity. If you are overtraining, your fitness actually deteriorates because your body does not have the time, nutrition, and rest to recover and rebuild tissue. When athletes hit a plateau, they go to great lengths to trick their bodies beyond the plateau by changing their routines, nutrition, supplements, and cycling interventions. If a stuck point prompts you to improve your nutrition, great. However, unless your objective is to be a competitive athlete, it is wiser to respect your set point and not fight it by increasing your activity level. Another option when you hit a plateau is to put any extra effort into other aspects of your fitness; for example, if you are primarily doing strength training, you could emphasize flexibility, aerobics, posture, or breathing.

If we project ahead to fitness needs when we are in our hundreds, we find that key issues are:

- maintaining an active lifestyle
- having strong bones to avoid osteoporosis and avoid breaking bones
- having a flexible body (as opposed to arthritis and joint problems)
- having the strength and balance to avoid falling and breaking a hip (the demise of many out-of-condition elderly people)

Why do people choose one fitness activity over another?

Common sense is rare when it comes to fitness activities–and for good reasons. Sales experts tell us that people buy on emotion and justify their decisions with logic.[5] The emotional reasons people choose particular fitness activities or sports might not be a good fit with their longevity goals.

Emotional reasons include:
- looking attractive
- making a particular part of your body more attractive, e.g., abdominal muscles, biceps
- socializing with friends
- being part of a social group that shares similar values (or business interests)
- emulating movie stars, athletes, or other role models
- avoiding health problems, e.g., fear of a heart attack
- making a team
- enjoying competing
- winning awards, recognition, publicity, money
- defending yourself
- feeling good
- getting an endorphin high
- achieving a meditative state
- relaxing
- fostering good health and longevity

Your longevity outcomes

For longevity purposes, emotional reasons are good as long as they do not conflict with your longevity outcomes. Longevity requires a long-term perspective and outcomes that:

Follow longevity principles:
- Do no harm.
- Engage in all things in moderation.
- Emphasize what your body needs most (target your weakest link).
- Listen to your body.

Address all the fitness needs:
- strength
- flexibility, agility, and balance
- cardiovascular (aerobic)
- strong bones
- energy
- posture
- breathing

- relaxation response/spiritual
- sunlight

Possibly address optional fitness needs:

- massage
- visual improvement
- facial tone
- internal cleansing

Are enjoyable (and possibly create flow states)

The following sections discuss each of these factors.

LONGEVITY PRINCIPLES

Do no harm

I heard on National Public Radio (and I am still trying to track down a written source) that the average life span of an NFL football player is 55. When they were children, NFL football players were some of the healthiest, most physically fit kids in the country. Overdeveloping the body, repeated blows, concussions, steroids, and the emotional pressures take their toll. Their short average life span is sobering. The average career span of NFL football player is only four years. Research on the Green Bay Packers found that two years after retiring from professional football 78% were unemployed, bankrupt, divorced or all three.[6] Like the fable of the Midas touch, it is a lesson to be careful what you wish for.

Jogging has many benefits. It is a great aerobic activity that keeps a person trim, lowers blood pressure and pulse, gets people outdoors and feeling good, and offers competition, athletic and social events, and comradery. Many serious joggers, however, have numerous health problems. Pounding their feet against the pavement is hard on their knees, kidneys, and gastrointestinal tracts. Diarrhea, cramps, rectal bleeding, loss of bowel control, and colds and flus are common problems. Joggers can get an endorphin high from running and often feel depressed when they go a day or two without running. Massage therapists will tell you that joggers are often very unbalanced because they overuse some muscles and underuse others. Joggers sometimes become addicted to the sport and continue running even when their joints are injured or they stop menstruating. If they jog too much, their upper bodies might become emaciated as their bodies do not have enough time to recover between runs and cannibalize protein from upper body muscle tissue.[7] For some, jogging is a sport that becomes self-destructive.

The brain damage boxing can cause is well known and often evident in interviews with veteran fighters. Football, even at the high school level, can result in serious, lasting injuries. Players often try to ignore or deny concussions. Soccer is excellent activity except for head butting the ball. Common sense tells you that the brain is delicate and banging your head against a ball going as fast as twenty miles an hour is not good for your brain. Research data are starting to document subtle brain damage caused by head butting soccer balls.[8] [9] Serious bicycling can irritate a man's genitals and might lower sperm counts. If you engage in sports that pose health problems, it should be in moderation. If you want your children to have long healthy lives, set limits in unhealthy sports (for example my children know they are not to head butt soccer balls). Frequent athletic and fitness activities should be ones that are kind to your body.

Edward Jackowski rates what exercises are kindest to your body and give good fitness benefits. Topping his list is jumping rope. He reports jumping rope has only a seventh to half as much impact on your knees as running because your feet only go about an inch off the ground and your weight is better distributed when you land. Rope jumping burns 600 to 1,000 calories and hour, exercises all the major muscle groups, enhances coordination, is portable, inexpensive, and rarely causes injuries. Six minutes of intense rope jumping can be equivalent to jogging for half an hour. Jackowski recommends quality cross training shoes, a suspended wooden floor (as it has more give), and a plastic or vinyl rope. He advises to be sure to stretch your calves. To determine the length of the rope, step on the rope and have the ends of the rope touch your armpits.

Jackowski also highly recommends cross country skiing, cross country ski machines, and full-court basketball. He recommends stationary bicycles as an excellent way to warm up. His reservations on fitness activities include:

- The nature of swinging a golf club tends to create or aggravate back problems.
- High impact activities, e.g., step aerobics and jogging, are very hard on knees.
- Yoga can be good for flexibility but does not give aerobic or anaerobic benefits.
- Aerobics classes rarely help women look slimmer and often cause injuries because they frequently combine warm up and stretching.
- Walking doesn't reach an aerobic level unless it is very rapid, uphill, or with a backpack and it takes ten times longer to lose weight walking than jumping rope.
- Weight lifting has a high injury rate and, unless you are training for a particular sport, most people need endurance more than they need bigger muscles.
- Walking can place a lot of stress on your knees and back and can cause foot and ankle problems. Warming up and stretching (especially the hamstring muscles) is helpful.
- Over time most runners develop "terrible feet, a bad back, and a very inflexible body."[10]

Hippocrates admonishes physicians to "First do no harm."[11] This should apply to exercise as well. If common sense, objective feedback, or your body tells you that a fitness activity is not healthy for you, heed the feedback. Either reduce the activity to a healthy level or replace it with healthier fitness activities.

All things in moderation

Hand in hand with do no harm is Aristotle's philosophy of the golden mean. Simply stated, he observed that almost anything taken to an extreme becomes problematic. Thus, people need moderation in eating, drinking, fitness, work, etc. His philosophy can be a little difficult to reconcile with the way our society gives huge rewards to the best in almost any endeavor. Thus, our top athletes, entertainers, business people, etc. become millionaires. To determine whether a passion needs moderation, ask what the pursuit is costing, whether it is something that you truly love and enjoy doing, and whether it is doing any harm. In the case of fitness or athletic pursuits, lack of moderation can involve injuries or sapping too much time from family or other priorities.

Emphasize what your body needs most (target the weakest link)

As previously discussed, you need to identify and target your weakest link health problems with a whatever-it-takes attention and determination.

Listen to your body

It would be easier if we could just have a checklist of the ideal fitness activities. Everyone's body is different, however, and has different needs. A sport, fitness activity, or activity equipment that is ideal for one person might be harmful to another person. Ask your body:

- Is this causing pain?
- Is this causing tight muscles?
- Are my muscles more or less balanced after the activity or sport?
- Is this helping or hurting my posture?
- Is the activity or the timing of the activity affecting my sleep?
- Is this helping my breathing, digestion, vision, or other functions not normally associated with fitness?

How to exercise

Edward Jackowski[12] *Hold it! You're Exercising All Wrong* makes a convincing case for the importance of every workout always having warm up, stretching, exercises, and a cool down–and in that order. One of the implications of his recommendation is that fitness activities should be done once a day rather than scattered through the day. Here is why each stage is important:

1. **Warm up (5-15 minutes)** Warming up gradually raises your heart rate. Shocking your heart with sudden intense exertion greatly increases the risk of a heart attack. Warming up gets blood flowing to your muscles and dilates capillaries so muscles will be

ready for the demands you will place on them. Warming up raises your body's temperature so muscles are warmer and can facilitate oxygen entering the muscles and the breakdown of glucose and fatty acids. Intense exercise without warming up dumps more fatty acids into your blood than the muscles can use. The excess fatty acids might end up lining your blood vessels. Warming up gradually loosens up muscles, tendons, and other tissues so they are more flexible and less likely to be torn or injured. Warmer muscles can also absorb a shock or injury better. Your nervous system also warms up and transmits messages more efficiently. A stationary bike with low resistance or briskly walking in place are good warmups. The ideal warm up uses all the muscles the exercising will use.

2. **Stretching (4-7 minutes)**   Stretching increases the range of motion, which enhances circulation to the muscles and flexibility. Many exercises, especially weight lifting and running, decrease range of motion unless you stretch. Stretching involves going just short of pain, breathing, and statically holding the position. Never bounce. Stretching is specific to each muscle. Most injuries occur from not warming up or not stretching.

3. **Exercising**

4. **Cool down (4-8 minutes)** In cooling you gradually decrease the intensity of exercising. It is important for keeping blood from pooling, removing metabolic waste products from your blood, reducing soreness, and lowering the risk of cardiovascular complications.

If your exercise tends to reduce your muscles' range of motion, e.g., as weight lifting or running does, it might be a good idea to do stretching between exercising and cooling down.

FITNESS NEEDS

Fitness for strength

*Strength training is the closest thing there is
to the Fountain of Youth.*[13]

*In every study we've done so far, without exception,
when people become stronger, they become more active.*[14]

As most people age they lose muscle mass. This is partly due to older people moving less than children and teenagers and partly due to decreasing hormone levels. The phenomenon has a name–sarcopenia (literally vanishing flesh).[15] [16]   While there is enormous individual variability, even healthy people who maintain a stable weight tend to lose 20-25% of muscle mass between their twenties and seventies. Muscle tissue shrinks and fat deposits increase. (Note the muscles do not "turn to fat.") Women who do not take hormone replacements for menopause experience a particularly large drop in muscle mass at menopause.

To illustrate how resilient the body is and how responsive it is to strength training, consider a study by Frontera et al.[17] Men 60 to 72 engaged in a three-day-a-week strength training program. Their knee flexor strength increased 227% and their knee extensor strength increased 107%. Their total muscle mass, as indicated by CT analysis, increased by 11.4%. Biopsies showed an increase of 33.5% in type I muscle fiber area and 27.5% increase in type II fiber area. Their oxygen consumption also increased, indicating increased aerobic capacity.

Groundbreaking research at Tufts Center on Aging addressed whether muscle loss was inevitable. Instead of assuming elderly people had to be pampered in the amount of weight they lifted, researchers had participants exercise at 80% of their capacity. In one Tufts project[18] women 50-70 engaged in strength training and exercised twice a week for a year. Participants showed increased muscle mass and a slight gain in bone density. Their muscles became 10-12% larger and 100-175% stronger.[19] The control group showed losses in all areas studied including a 2% loss of bone tissue. In another study, many frail nursing home residents (average age 90.2 years) learned to walk again because of strength training. These residents gained in muscle strength (174%), muscle size (9%), and functional mobility.[20]

Strength training (contracting your muscles a few times against a heavy load or resistance) benefits include:

- increasing strength
- preserving and enhancing muscle tissue (especially "fast twitch" muscles used for quick movement)
- activating the nerve cells to muscles, making the body able to respond faster and better
- preserving and enhancing bone tissue (which in turn prevents osteoporosis)
- enhancing balance
- improving flexibility
- improving coordination
- increasing metabolism both during the activity and for several hours afterwards
- increasing metabolism as muscle requires a higher metabolism rate than fat
- improving posture
- keeping tendons and joints strong and elastic
- enhancing energy
- enhancing mental abilities
- helping with weight management or weight loss
- enhancing mood
- reducing the risk or severity of diseases such as diabetes
- dramatically increasing range of motion for people who have arthritis[21]
- enhancing physical appearance
- enhancing self-esteem
- giving some of the benefits of aerobic activities

Weaker muscles, poorer flexibility, and poorer coordination result in people walking more slowly, more tentatively and with less stability. Weaker bones make falls more likely to cause serious injuries from falls. One-third of people over 65 sustain serious injuries from falls each year–often broken hip bones.

Most fitness experts conclude that free weights give better results than machines as they involve related muscles in stabilizing and guiding the weights, which builds balance and coordination as well as muscle. The fitness industry pushes machines because there is more money to be made from selling the equipment or people having to go to a spa to use equipment. People need a balance in strength fitness, not an overemphasis on beautiful abs, pecs and biceps. The fitness industry, however, tends to sell people what they want rather than what they need.

The longevity objective for strength training isn't to look like Arnold Schwarzenegger, but to have fit muscles, strong bones, and maintain an appropriate weight and healthy ratio of lean to fat tissue. Much of the literature on strength training comes from weight lifting and body building literature. Some of their rules are:

- Always warm up.
- Eat a balanced snack about an hour before your workout, avoiding foods with a high glycemic index (foods which quickly turn to glucose).
- After about an hour, the workout produces diminishing returns.
- Give the muscles you worked at least a day of rest before focusing on them in a workout again.
- For building strength, the norm is three sets of ten repetitions with good form. More muscle is developed from heavier weights than from more repetitions.
- For building endurance, you need a lot of repetitions.
- Always cool down after a workout.
- If you use supplements, e.g., creatine or androstenedione, cycle off them periodically so your body does not habituate to them.

Most adults would like to lose some weight. While an anaerobic workout burns (oxidates) glucose and protein as opposed to body fat, it still helps with weight loss in several ways:

- Your metabolism remains higher for several hours after the workout.
- By adding muscle you increase your overall metabolism as muscles use more calories than fat.

- Anaerobic activities prompt your body to release Human Growth Hormone and testosterone, which effect a more favorable muscle to fat ratio in your body.
- Even if you do not lose pounds (and muscle weighs more than fat), having a more favorable muscle to fat ratio and more toned muscles is healthier and makes you look and feel trimmer.

Fitness for cardiovascular benefits

Aerobic exercise is the key to cardiovascular fitness and weight loss. Despite Americans' obsession with losing weight, it is amazing how few Americans have any understanding of the rules for losing weight aerobically. The rules include:

- At low levels of activity your body burns glucose.
- At high (anaerobic) levels of activity your body burns glucose and protein.
- At moderate levels of activity your body burns body fat and glucose.
- If you engage in aerobic or anaerobic activities and do not consume enough proteins, your body will cannibalize protein from your muscle tissues.
- The rule of thumb for being at a fat burning aerobic level is that you are breathing heavily but can still talk.
- The more fit you are, the more intense the activity will need to be to reach the aerobic fat burning level.
- The more unfit and overweight a person is, the more difficult it is to achieve the aerobic fat burning window between low activity glucose burning and high activity anaerobic activity. Thus, physiologically an unfit, overweight person has a much more difficult time losing weight than a fit person who only needs to lose a few pounds.
- Your body must have some fat and glucose in the bloodstream in order to burn body fat. If you totally avoid fat in your diet, you will not be able to burn body fat.
- When beginning aerobic activity, your body primarily burns glucose. After about twelve minutes your body increases the

release of body fat to the muscles. After twenty to thirty minutes your body greatly increases the release of body fat to the muscles.

- Just as your body adapts to using muscles more by making muscles bigger, the more aerobic activity you engage in, the quicker your body mobilizes body fat for use by your muscles (as opposed to relying on just glucose) and the quicker it produces and mobilizes the enzymes needed to convert fat into energy.
- Where you accumulate fat and where you lose it is genetically programmed. Exercising your abdominal muscles (or any other particular muscles) might tone the muscles and make them look trimmer, but will not override your genetic program for where you lose fat.
- In addition to the calories you burn during an aerobic activity, your body maintains a higher metabolism and burns extra fat for several hours after the activity as it uses body fat to replace the glycogen that was consumed.
- The heat you feel a couple hours after aerobic (or anaerobic) activities is from your body synthesizing glycogen to replace the glycogen that was depleted.
- The reason you continue to breathe heavily or deeply after aerobic activities is that your body needs the oxygen to recover and rebuild.
- Always warm up and cool down (for the same reasons cited in the section on strength fitness).
- Your body can burn a small amount of body fat 24 hours a day. It also burns additional body fat after aerobic or anaerobic activities. Aerobic activities, however, have the advantage that you burn sizeable amounts of body fat during and after the activity.

The clearest lay explanation of the metabolic rules for exercise that I have found is Covert Bailey's *Smart Exercise*.[22]

Aerobic activities by definition are activities that require oxygen. Aerobic activities involve contracting muscles many times with little resistance. Aerobic benefits include:
- lowering blood pressure
- increasing blood circulation
- decreasing plaque in blood vessels

- keeping blood vessels flexible
- lessening the risk of cardiovascular diseases
- enhancing the immune system
- enhancing digestion
- increasing energy
- enhancing mental abilities
- keeping tendons and joints strong and elastic
- helping with weight management or weight loss
- increasing High Density Lipids (HDL)–"good cholesterol"
- decreasing the risk of many diseases including adult-onset diabetes
- reducing the risk of cataracts[23]
- enhancing mood
- attenuating depression
- enhancing physical appearance
- enhancing self-esteem
- facilitating sleep

Covert Bailey[24] advises that best aerobic activities involve the whole body. For fit people, walking is not enough of a cardiovascular challenge to be aerobic unless made more difficult; for example, by walking uphill, carrying a backpack, race walking, or power walking. Bicycling can provide a good aerobic workout but primarily involves just the lower half of the body. While swimming is considered an ideal activity, most fit people do not get much aerobic benefit from it. Cross country skiing, racquetball, and running (preferably on a soft surface) provide excellent aerobic benefits. Nordic ski machines, elliptical exercisers, and step machines involve most of the body in aerobic workouts and are gentler on knees and internal organs than jogging or treadmills.

The popular explanation for why physical activity results in feeling better emotionally was that it prompted the body to produce endorphins–natural painkilling hormones. It is questionable, however, whether these large molecules could penetrate the blood brain barrier. Current thinking[25] is that, like the relaxation response (discussed later in this chapter), physical activity gets your mind on a "different wavelength" and off your problems. Both physical exercise and meditating lower blood pressure and in most people lower anxiety.

While these effects only last about twenty to thirty minutes for meditation, they last more than three hours for physical activity.

In one of the most sophisticated studies,[26] over 72,000 female nurses were studied for eight years. The study controlled for factors such as fitness activities, smoking, weight, medical issues, and vitamin use. Brisk walking (at least three miles an hour) for at least three hours a week was as effective at preventing coronary heart disease as vigorous exercise. Thus, cardiovascular fitness does not appear to require extreme efforts or time commitments.

Flexibility, balance, and agility

It is common for top shape athletes who just engage in one sport to be winded and awkward in a sport that uses different muscles. An extreme case is some body builders who can lift hundreds of pounds but have little flexibility or agility. If your fitness activities or sports include flexibility and balance, great. If not, be sure to add some flexibility activities as flexibility and balance are essential to good health–literally and metaphorically. They can be added to a fitness program or sport as the warm up and/or cool down, which also help prevent injuries.

Excellent stretching and flexibility activities include stretching, yoga, tai chi, and Callanetics. Callanetics is a cross between yoga and ballet and is especially popular with women as it tones deep muscles and helps develop a trim figure. It can be learned in classes, book or videotapes.[27]

Even if you prefer to engage in fitness activities later in the day, five minutes of flexibility activities in the morning is a good way to start the day. Spend a few minutes getting the blood flowing well first (e.g., a stationary bicycle). I use a combination of the Yoga "sun salutation," "swimming dragon,"[28] neck rolls, and squats. They are both a good way to loosen up and a good metaphor for being flexible, balanced, and agile the whole day. (I also do a set of pushups to get the blood pumping and as a metaphor for strength.) Tai chi would be an especially good morning flexibility activity. Most of the marital arts offer good flexibility, balance, and agility.

Posture

We wouldn't drive our cars without periodically checking to make sure they are in alignment and the tires are in balance. Yet that is exactly what we do with our posture.

Americans rarely think about their posture–and it shows. Working with computers for hours, sitting in office chairs or in front of television sets, and driving automobiles often contribute to sitting and standing posture problems. Misalignment of posture distorts the alignment of organs in the body and distorts normal body functions. This can impair circulation of blood and lymph and put pressure on various body organs. It can cause herniated discs, stooped postures, shoulder pain, and back pain. Improved posture sometimes is all that is needed to cure headaches, digestive problems, gynecological problems, backache, TMJ, migraine headaches, foot deformities, and many other ailments. Weak or out-of-balance leg, back, abdominal and hip muscles also can cause posture problems and chronic pain. If not corrected, poor posture increasingly takes a toll with age. Posture is the weak link for many people.

Exercise 14-1: Make two mental pictures of yourself when you are 120. Have one with great posture and vitality. Have the other hunched over with poor posture. Memorize the pictures and keep them in mind to motivate yourself.

Some of the most common, easy things to check in posture are:

- Are your feet pointed forward (vs. turned outward)? Turning feet outward distorts your gait, can cause pain, and impairs athletic performance. It can be helped with a conscious effort and exercises. Egoscue's books have several exercises that can help.
- When you walk, do you start with your heel, roll forward to the ball of your foot, and push off from the metatarsal area behind your second and third toes (which automatically spreads your toes apart)? If you are not doing this, you can consciously work on it or do exercises (e.g., Egoscue). If the bottoms of your shoes do not wear evenly, you are not walking correctly.

- When you stand with your hands at your sides, do your palms face the side of your body (vs. your palm turned away from your body and/or in front of your thighs)? If your palms don't face your body, exercises to align your shoulders can help.
- Have someone take a picture of your usual standing and sitting posture and what you think your usual standing and sitting postures should be. Check to see if the standing pictures have your head level and directly over your shoulders, hip joints, knee joints, and ankle joints. Your palms should be against the sides of your body, and your feet pointed forward. Check to see if the sitting posture has your head level and over the shoulders and hips, arm sockets centered (vs. pulled forward), legs not crossed and at a 90-degree angle to the body, and feet flat on the floor.

Good advice on posture can be hard to find. Unfortunately, most podiatrists, orthopedists, and other physicians, with the possible exception of sports physicians, often do not consider posture. They look at bunions, back pain, and other problems often associated with posture, and they see problems in need of pills or surgery. Some of the best sources for posture advice include:
- Feldenkrais practitioners (discussed below)
- Egoscue (discussed below)
- Alexander practitioners (discussed below)
- massage therapists (e.g., polarity therapists)
- movement specialists (kinesthesiologists)
- chiropractors
- some yoga instructors
- some martial arts instructors

The advice you receive should:
- make sense to you
- give you changes you can make or activities you can do
- start giving you results within a few months.

If the advice does not meet these criteria, get a second or even a third opinion.

Moshe Feldenkrais[29] was a brilliant eclectic Russian Israeli who sustained crippling knee injuries. He drew upon his knowledge of biology, cybernetics, neurology, martial arts, linguistics, psychology, and systems theory to teach himself to walk again. His method focuses on making unconscious movements conscious so they can be modified. He was (he died in 1984) especially interested in improving range of motion, flexibility, coordination, and efficient, graceful motion.

While chiropractors focus on bones, and massage therapists on muscles, Feldenkrais practitioners focus on the mental and neurological aspects of movement. Feldenkrais is often taught in classes in which the participants do a variety of non strenuous activities on mats. Individual consultations and therapy are available from certified instructors. If you want a very structured approach, you will find the Feldenkrais approach frustrating. The activities or lessons involve a lot of experiencing and increasing awareness as opposed to checklists and exercises.

The method is particularly popular with artists, musicians, and actors as these professions call for an exquisite understanding of how bodies move. Feldenkrais' books are difficult reading and you would probably find books by his practitioners easier to understand. One Feldenkrais practitioner, Paul Linden, Ph.D., has written specifically on posture for computer users.[30] [31] The Feldenkrais web site is www.Feldenkrais.com. Celebrities who have used Feldenkrais methods include Julius Erving, Norman Cousins, Margaret Mead, David Ben-Gurion, Helen Hayes, Whoopi Goldberg, Yehudi Menuhin, and Yo Yo Ma.

Peter Egoscue, an anatomical physiologist, developed a system for diagnosing and correcting posture problems, including problems of people who have severe disabilities. His program involves performing about a dozen individually selected fitness exercises for an hour a day, several days a week. The frequency is eventually tapered to a maintenance level. The Egoscue exercises use underused muscles and relax overused muscles to restore the balance between opposing muscles and get the body into alignment. Some of the exercises are very relaxing and some are uncomfortable. They do not require special equipment, can be done at home, and do not involve sweating. People with fairly generic problems might get what they need just from his books.[32] [33] [34] For people needing more personalized service, he has a clinic in San Diego.[35] His clinic also has the capacity to diagnose and treat by exchanging videotapes by mail. The web site is www.Egoscue.com. One of the individuals who endorsed Egosuce's program is golfer Jack Nicklaus, who credits the exercises for extending his golf career.

F. Matthias Alexander was an Austrian Shakespearian actor who had difficulty with laryngitis. When physicians could not solve the problem, he intensively studied the problem. He discovered that he tilted his head back each time he started to speak and that this stressed his vocal cords and spine. His studying led to his developing his system of posture training. He died in 1955 after teaching thousands of actors and others. A professional organization certifies Alexander method instructors. It is usually taught on an individual basis in about thirty sessions. As with Feldenkrais training, students are taught to become more aware of what they do with their bodies and students wanting a structured, checklist approach will be frustrated. Alexander teachers place particular emphasis on positioning of the head and "lengthening" the spine. There are several books and videotapes on the method, though each explains that it is difficult to learn the method without live instruction. One of the best web sites for Alexander instruction is www.life.uiuc.edu/jeff/alextech.html.

Breathing

Good breathing is important for:
* a rich supply of oxygen to nourish our cells
* relaxation
* circulating lymph in the lymph system

Most Americans breathe shallowly from their chest as opposed to breathing deeply from their abdomen. Shallow breathing not only limits the amount of oxygen available to your body, but keeps the same stale air in the bottom of your lungs indefinitely. Unlike your blood, which has your heart to circulate it, your lymph has no pump other than your breathing and body movements. Deep breathing helps your immune system by circulating your lymph. Finally, deep breathing is very relaxing. As a psychologist I have worked with several dozen people who have panic attacks. Virtually all of them are shallow breathers whose anxiety causes their chest muscles to further restrict their breathing. They then draw their attention inward, feel like they can't breathe, and start panicking. Deep breathing is the antithesis of the panic attack process and a difficult skill for panicky people to learn. It's bound up in the paradox that you are in more control when you are relaxed and not trying to be in control.

Many fitness regimes include deep breathing. Martial arts, yoga, and meditation in particular emphasize breathing. If you do not obtain good breathing from your fitness activities, you might incorporate them in the cool down phase from physical activities or as a good way to begin or end a day. My personal favorite to get me breathing well in a minute or two is the Swimming Dragon.[36] There are many good yoga books and videos and almost all emphasize breathing. Dharma Singh Khalsa's book and tape *Brain Longevity*[37] also includes breathing activities. Tai chi is an exquisite combination of breathing, coordination, balance, grace, and spiritual harmony.

If your breathing is shallow, your chest will move as you breathe. If you are breathing deeply, most of the movement will be from your abdomen. Americans are self-conscious about their stomachs sticking out and deep breathing causes your stomach to go in and out. Health, however, needs to be the priority. One of the easiest ways to become aware of your breathing is to lie on your back on the floor and place your hand on your stomach. Use your breathing to make your stomach go up and down. Once you have learned the skill lying down, transfer it to sitting and standing postures as well.

Relaxation response

EEG machines measuring our brain waves show that most of our waking time has beta brain waves and most of our sleeping time has delta and theta brain waves. Beta is associated with being very alert and stimulated. With our fast-paced lives, many of us rarely have alpha waves. Alpha waves reflect a mind that is calm, peaceful, and in a trance-like state. With alpha state, your metabolism, blood pressure, heart rate, breathing, and muscle tension decrease. It is a restful time that rejuvenates your body. Your mind is receptive but not consciously thinking and you can access your nonconscious thoughts and creativity. It is the state in which you do your most imaginative thinking and best reading.

If you are old enough to recall the 1970s, you might recall the popularity of alpha wave biofeedback or the Beatles seeking alpha through yoga and transcendental meditation. In 1975 Herbert Benson[38] identified the common denominators for the many approaches seeking the alpha state. They are simply:

* focusing on a repetitive event
  (whether it is verbal, auditory, or motor)
* passively tuning out other stimuli

The relaxation response can be effected with prayer, music (e.g., the Gregorian chant), physical activity (e.g., knitting, repeating a phrase while jogging), or the traditional repetition of a sound or mantra (e.g., ohm, one). The passively tuning out of other stimuli reminds me of watching the scenery from a car or train window when you notice it but don't consciously think about it.

The relaxation response is the opposite of the fight/flight response that puts your body on peak alert for handling emergencies. Benson documents the numerous health benefits of the relaxation response. He believes we are "hard wired"[39] to need the relaxation response. He points out that virtually every culture includes some form of a relaxation response, often in the form of prayer. When the relaxation response is paired with prayer or spiritual states, it often brings a spiritual strength which helps with healing or dealing with stress or traumatic events. You might already engage in relaxation responses. If not, you would be wise to incorporate relaxation responses into your life. You could achieve a relaxation response from something as simple as playing solitaire. The relaxation response can be much more useful to you in trying times, however, if it is associated with prayer or religious ritual.

Sunlight

Light is probably the most overlooked aspect of fitness. Much of the research on light is very well done and has profound implications. Possibly because its commercial applications have not been exploited, we don't hear much about light research. The pioneer in light research was John Ott. He did time lapse photography for Disney studios and conducted fascinating, meticulous research on how different types of light affects plants, animals, and people. His 1976 book[40] is still fascinating reading and includes some of the following research findings:

- Plants only bloom under certain light conditions and/or with certain ratios of daytime to nighttime.
- Mice live twice as long with daylight as opposed to either fluorescent or incandescent lighting.
- Hens live twice as long, lay more eggs with 25% less cholesterol, and are less aggressive in natural or full spectrum light (vs. fluorescent or incandescent light).
- School children are calmer and less hyperactive with full spectrum light (vs. fluorescent or incandescent light).
- Baseball players who switched from pink tinted to medium gray tinted sunglasses became less irritable, more relaxed and confident, and performed better.
- Restaurant workers who worked in a facility with black light ultraviolet lights were especially healthy and congenial.
- Sunglasses, particularly pink tinted ones, increase cancer rates.
- Sunlight or full spectrum light (including ultraviolet light) reduces cancer rates and in some cases reverses cancer.

Ott and his successors found that concerns about ultraviolet light have been overstated. The research on ultraviolet light involved clamping open monkeys' eyes, dilating their pupils, and submitting them to massive amounts of ultraviolet light. It's not surprising that the extreme dosage and the stress caused retinal damage. Similar research concluded that ultraviolet light causes cataracts and cancer. Other research using more natural conditions, however, shows that we need a certain amount of ultraviolet light. There are actually three types of ultraviolet light. UV-A, which is closest to the violet light waves, is responsible for suntans. UV-B activates the synthesis of vitamin D. UV-C, much of which is filtered by the Earth's ozone layer, is effective at killing bacteria, viruses, and infectious agents, e.g., tuberculosis. Ott and Liberman[41] maintain that you need ultraviolet light but that extreme amounts are harmful. So we are back to Aristotle's golden mean.

Natural sunlight has the colors of the spectrum distributed rather evenly and includes some ultraviolet light. Full spectrum light roughly approximates natural sunlight. Sunlight or full spectrum light has many of the same benefits as exercise:[42] decreasing resting heart rate, blood pressure, respiratory rate, blood sugar level, and lactic acid; and increasing energy strength, endurance, tolerance for stress, and the ability of the blood to absorb oxygen.

Incandescent lights (the bulbs found in most homes) overemphasize red/orange/yellow waves, are weak in blue waves, and have almost no ultraviolet waves.[43] Most fluorescent lights emphasize yellow and are particularly weak on red and blue/violet. This is why photographs with regular film often have a yellowish tint when taken under fluorescent lighting.

The research is pretty convincing that you will be healthier and perform better with sunlight or full spectrum light. Full spectrum lights are available for less than $10 a bulb. Brand names include Chromalux and Bulbright for incandescent bulbs and Vita-Lite, True Lite, and Lumichrome for fluorescent bulbs. They are available in many hardware stores, greenhouses, and on numerous Internet sites. Dental offices, certain medical settings, and museums often use full spectrum lights to make precise color decisions and representations. Note that while the Chromolux bulb is considerably closer to natural sunlight than an incandescent bulb, it is still weak on the blue/violet wave length and has virtually no infrared waves. The best source for infrared waves is a "black light."

Liberman discusses how he believes certain colors help with certain illnesses; for example, blue for jaundice or arthritis, red for migraine headaches, ultraviolet light for infections and viruses. He also discusses using pink lights to calm prisoners, and red and blue lights to improve the performance of athletes.

Bears hibernate in the winter and some people have a lot in common with bears. Every fall and winter about ten million Americans who live in temperate climates experience Seasonal Affective Disorder (SAD). Like bears, they crave carbohydrates, become lethargic and irritable, have difficulty waking up, and lose interest in activities including sex. The further north you live, the more likely you are to have significant SAD symptoms.

If you can't be a "snow bird" and spend the winter in Florida, you can make it a point to get sunshine and you can consider a SAD light. SAD lights simulate light waves at dawn (as opposed to a full spectrum light that is simulating light at midday). Being near a SAD light for about half an hour first thing in the morning sends a message to your pineal gland to stop hibernating and stop overproducing melatonin during the day. (Note that SAD lights do not produce ultraviolet light.)

There are several self-help books on SAD and web sites addressing SAD. A good web starting point is the Society for Light Treatment and Biological Rhythms www.websciences.org/sltrb/. SAD lights cost from $200 to $500 and are available from at least a half a dozen companies, all of which are on the Internet. Make sure the light does not have problems with glare or flickering. Personally, I have been pleased with Enviro-Med's biolight and have found one company's inexpensive model creates a harsh glare.

Conclusions

There are plenty of new age books about auras and chakras that are difficult to substantiate with research. I regard these as a "matter of faith." There is a lot of solid research about light that is very important to your fitness. The implications of the solid research are:

- Try to spend at least an hour a day in sunlight, ideally before 10:00 a.m. or after 2:00 p.m.
- Replace many of the lights in your home with full spectrum lights.
- Don't wear sunglasses unless you have to wear them. If you do, chose a neutral gray lens.
- If you wear glasses, special order UV transmitting glasses (that do not block ultraviolet rays).
- It is best not to wear contact lenses, and certainly not contacts with tinted lenses.
- Consider installing UV transmitting windows instead of glass windows in the windows you use the most.
- If you live in a Temperate climate, assess whether you have Season Affective Disorder. If you do, study up on it and use a SAD light in early morning as needed during the late fall and winter.
- Avoid sunburns, excessive tanning, and tanning booths.

- Think of the sun in happy terms as a source of life.

OPTIONAL FITNESS ACTIVITIES

Kegel exercises

Having babies stretches the uterus and pushes the bladder out of its usual position. Kegel exercises tone the muscles that position bladder. Women who don't do Kegel exercises during and for several months after pregnancy are at higher risk of developing urinary stress incontinence. Urinary stress incontinence is the kind of incontinence in which urine leaks out when you exercise, cough, laugh, or sneeze. Kegel exercises are also advisable for many men who have had prostrate surgery.

To locate the muscles, stop urinating in mid stream and start again. The muscles you squeezed around your urethra and anus are the muscles to exercise. Practice squeezing these muscles when you are not urinating. If you are using the right muscles, neither your stomach nor your buttocks should move. Hold and squeeze for three seconds, relax for three seconds, and repeat 10-15 times a day, three times a day.

Massage

Massage is purported to have several benefits:
- **It's immensely enjoyable.** For the most part it requires nothing more of you than showing up, paying the fee, and enjoying it.
- **We all need touching.** In orphanages in which infants' physical needs were taken care of but the infants were not held, the infants became detached, stopped eating, and some even died. Other than a very romantic evening or extended time playing with children, rarely do we get as much touching as when we receive a massage.
- **It is immensely relaxing.** As with the relaxation response, it entrances us with repetitive activity, takes our minds off usual matters, and focuses us on the sensual pleasure.
- **It helps strained muscles.** This is the benefit that usually comes to mind.

- **It stimulates muscles and organs.** Massage increases blood circulation to muscles and body parts in which the blood flow or lymph flow has been restricted. Critics counter that the increased circulation is just to superficial tissues.
- **It releases toxins.** This claim might be true but research data are scant.
- **It realigns and frees energy fields.** Many massage therapies, e.g., polarity, shiatsu, reiki, applied kinesiology, and reflexology, are based on energy fields and stimulating meridian points. Unfortunately there is little research to document the theory.
- **The practitioner might offer health suggestions.** Many massage therapists can offer good advice on what is out of balance and what you can do to achieve better balance or fitness. Ask.

Massages are not essential to health or longevity, but they can help. Not everyone can afford them. But if you can (or have a "handy" good friend or spouse) it certainly is a great way to promote health and longevity.

Better vision

Reading, computer screens and indoor lighting can be hard on our vision. William Bates, a medical school ophthalmology professor, published his radical book, *Better Vision Without Glasses,* in 1921. Bates died in 1931 but his system has been revised and updated by his followers. Janet Goodrich presents an updated version in her book, *Natural Vision Improvement.*[44] It is full of illustrations and visual exercises.

The Bates system and its updates have many physician detractors. Like most alternative health care, research data are scarce. Goodman's book does include summaries of a couple of studies. The most prudent conclusion appears to be that while we cannot presume that all of their teachings are efficacious, many of their recommendations make sense and would do no harm.

The Bates literature claims to reverse visual losses. Even if the program only prevents or slows loss, it is worth considering. Fitness

activities can be slipped in while waiting at a traffic light, waiting in a line, or other down times. Simple activities include:
- moving your eyes in counterclockwise and clockwise directions
- focusing your eyes progressively further away and then closer
- visualizing pictures in your mind's eye
- rubbing the palms of your hands together and placing them over your eyes ("palming")
- relaxing your shoulder and head muscles
- yawning

The most recent update of the Bates method comes from Martin Sussman. He believes that vision is influenced by:
- tension in our body
  - nearsighted people tend to have a lot of tension in their upper back, the base of their neck and around their eyes
  - farsighted people tend to have a lot of tension in their chest, throat, and jaw
  - people with astigmatisms tend to have asymmetries and imbalances in their bodies
- the body's overall health
- subconscious memories and past emotional decisions
- limiting or negative thoughts about vision

He provides data that challenge five commonly held beliefs that limit people from having optimal vision. These *erroneous beliefs* are that poor vision:
- comes with age
- comes with a lot of reading or computer work
- is hereditary
- is caused by weak eye muscles (these muscles are actually 150-200 times stronger than they need to be)
- is caused by eyes being the wrong shape and focusing in front of or behind the retina (causing one to be nearsighted or farsighted)

He offers ten vision habits to reduce physical and mental strain that impair vision:
- blinking frequently (flutter blinking 10-20 times)
- using peripheral vision

- frequently shifting your visual focus (and avoiding staring)
- avoiding day dreaming with your eyes open (as it gives your eyes a double message on where to focus)
- looking with the eyes of a child, i.e., actively looking with awe and wonder vs. just seeing
- nourishing your eyes with sunlight at least fifteen minutes a day, reading with sunlight or full spectrum light, and resting your eyes with total darkness by covering your eyes with the palms of your hands ("palming")
- using an under corrected prescription to challenge your eyes and prompt them to actively look as opposed to passively depend on glasses
- practicing relaxation and good posture
- breathing deeply and regularly to provide the oxygen to nourish your eyes and brain
- looking openly and honestly

Sussman believes that visual problems often stem from unresolved painful emotional experiences, often involving loss, fear, and misunderstanding. To avoid looking at these events, we might adopt limiting beliefs about ourselves. He gives case histories of how dealing with these issues and their subconscious messages resulted in improved vision and creativity. Sussman's program is available in a cassette tape/booklet format or via classes or workshops.[45] Even if you don't follow the full program, there are many tips that can be used in everyday life; for example, blinking your eyes and dong visual activities while waiting in lines or at traffic lights.

Another interesting resource is a pair of cassette tapes by Jacob Liberman.[46] The tapes present his new age holistic view of vision and life.

Facial tone

Even if you feel as young as a child on the inside, people respond to you partly by how you look, especially your face. If your face is a "bag of wrinkles," many people respond to you as an "old person" and experience less pleasure in seeing you. When you look in the mirror, the face looking back can influence how you feel about yourself. If you have a young healthy face looking back in the mirror, great. If not, there might be an alternative to a face lift or just living with it. Cynthia Rowland[47] says that the sagging muscles on our faces and many of our wrinkles are due to facial muscles sagging. She has a set of 18 isometric activities for 15 areas of the face and neck. Her system takes about ten to fifteen minutes a day and, she posits it will, "give you a face lift without surgery." A competitive product[48] stimulates the muscles with mild electrical impulses from a hand-held device powered by a nine-volt battery or wall adaptor. Both approaches involve common sense–that using or stimulating facial muscles improves the tone of facial muscles. Both require a lot of motivation to spend the time and effort–though they can be done while watching television or listening to a radio or music.

Internal cleansing

Rebounders are miniature trampolines that cost about thirty-five dollars. They offer the benefits of jogging with less wear and tear on body joints. Rebounders also are reported to enhance the immune system. The theory is that at the bottom of the bounce, pressure on the body is twice that of gravity, forcing waste out of the cells at twice the normal rate. At the top of the bounce you are at zero gravity and cells take in twice the amount of oxygen.[49] I am not aware of any research support for the purported benefits.

Yogis report that yoga stimulates and cleanses specific organs. They report stimulating and cleansing occurs by increasing the blood flow to specific organs and stimulating the muscles in or around the organs. I am not aware of research verifying the benefits but that does not mean the claims are not valid.

There are hundreds of thousands of people who swear by colonics. In the U.S. John Harvey Kellogg, the founder of Kellogg cereals, was an advocate of colonics and used them extensively in his (Seventh-Day) Adventist Battle Creek Sanitarium. Colonics involve inserting a tube through the rectum and spraying the colon (large intestine) with about forty gallons of filtered water. In theory the colon becomes lined with encrusted fecal material, mucus, and toxins, much like iron water pipes become lined with scale or arteries become lined with plaque. The encrusted material might impede the movement of food through the colon and compromise the action of the colon muscles. In theory the water also stimulates and exercises the muscles. I tried a series of colonics and did not notice any difference–but then I have never had gastrointestinal problems. People whose "weak link" is colon problems or who have a family history of colon cancer might want to look into colonics. A less intrusive alternative to colonics is reflexology, which claims that stimulating pressure points can stimulate the colon or other targeted body organs.

There are many diets and supplements and fasting programs to "get rid of body toxins." Most are just based on testimonials (and possibly placebo responses). There is little if any research supporting them. Fasting can be harmful and dangerous. The fasting products are in a very hyped, buyer beware market.

Boundless energy

Most fitness activities have the paradoxical effect of increasing your energy level. As part of listening to your body, you will want to note what fitness activities or sports and what foods are best at increasing your energy level.

There is a unique book, *Ancient Secret Fountain of Youth,*[50] that describes ten- to fifteen-minute fitness activities designed to effect "boundless energy and spiritual harmony." With a flavor rather like *The Celestine Prophecy,* the book describes how an elderly man went to the Tibetan monks to find the secret of youth. He returned looking many years younger and attributed the change primarily to five activities he learned from the monks. The theory is that the activities get the body's seven vortexes, corresponding with the body's endocrine system, to spin at the same speed. Four of the activities are basically yoga activities. One involves spinning. I didn't experience much success with this one as I did not like spinning. Author Bernie Siegel, M.D. thought enough of the book to write its forward.

Whatever fitness activities you try, ask yourself if the activity is giving you more energy. If not, see if there is a fitness activity that accomplishes the same results but gives you more energy.

ENJOYMENT, FUN, AND POSSIBLY FLOW

Hopefully, the list of fitness outcomes is not oppressive. Often, many outcomes can be met with one activity. For example, if you go rock climbing, you would probably do some stretching and warm up first. During the climb you would periodically engage in aerobic and anaerobic activity. While climbing you would be honing your flexibility, agility, and balance, and possibly using rhythmical deep breathing to maintain concentration. If it is a long climb, the activity might at times take on a relaxation response rhythm and at other times effect a rush of adrenalin. Hopefully the sport gives you a "go for it" sense of energy and inspiration. Finally, it might effect a "flow state" (discussed in Chapter 4). In a flow state you are totally absorbed in the experience, have an optimal level of challenge, and experience great satisfaction in performing the activity. If so, you have covered virtually all of the functions and enjoyed yourself as well. You've even gotten a good dose of sunlight.

Cultivating fitness activities that give you enjoyment and meet your longevity and personal goals makes fitness something you want to do and love doing.

Five keys to motivation

1. Focus on the benefits, not the process. The trick to getting motivated for fitness activities is to focus on the benefits rather than the process. To talk yourself out of exercising, picture yourself exercising and associate into (vividly imagine and feel) the experience. That experience is not very appealing for most people. To motivate yourself to exercise, see the results–yourself looking great and feeling great–and associate into that picture, feeling the benefits in your body. If you find this hard to do, try keeping your head level while your eyes look up when you are visualizing or imaging the benefits and have your eyes look down and to your right when associating into the feelings.

2. Find a good fit with your style. A second key is choosing contexts that fit your style. Ask yourself:
• Do I enjoy exercising more by myself or with other people?

- Do I enjoy competing with others?
- Do I enjoy competing with myself?
- In the past, what has gotten me off track from a fitness program?
- Does music or television make fitness activities more enjoyable for me?
- Do I like working from a videotape (or audiotape)?
- Would I really be more likely to engage in fitness activities on an ongoing, year-around basis at home, outdoors, at a spa, on a team, or some combination of these?

Gregarious people often have much better motivation at the spa or on a team where they can socialize at the same time. Competitive, Type A personalities often do better when there is competition. Homebodies, introverts, and people who like privacy and efficiency usually do better at home. They see a home treadmill or ski machine as safer, practical, convenient, private, and all weather. People who like the outdoors want their fitness activities outside where they can embrace nature.

3. Variety. If you are the kind of person who eats the same breakfast and the same lunch every day at the same time, you do well with habits and would do well with a fitness routine. Many people who try to do the same routine every day, however, reach a point where they are tired of the routine and quit. If that is your style, try a cafeteria approach to fitness. If you are feeling stressed and don't feel up to the ski machine, you might choose yoga. If you are feeling angry or irritable, you might lift weights. If you want to pump yourself up with energy and enthusiasm, you might have a Tae-Bo[51] workout.

If you need a fairly regimented life, you can engage in different activities on different days of the week. Just as people feel a rhythm to the week, with Saturday night being the most entertainment focused, you can design a weekly rhythm to your fitness activities. Jack LaLanne recommends changing your fitness regime every two weeks.

4. Achievable goals. Set goals that are easy to achieve and give yourself bonuses for exceeding them. Many people who exercise are perfectionists. For a perfectionist, planning to exercise every day and missing a day is failure–and failure is a painful experience. Most people do better with modest goals; for example, "I will engage in fitness activities three days a week" (giving yourself bonus "credit" for every additional day). Every time you engage in a fitness activity, you are doing something wonderful for yourself and you should literally thank yourself for doing it and feel gratitude for being able to do it. If you pray, a prayer of gratitude is very appropriate. For most people seeing progress data is very motivating, whether it is how heavy a weight you can lift or waist size. Rather than an "I always have to do more/better" mentality, give yourself credit for maintaining a level of achievement and celebrate when you exceed it. Martial arts instructors are masters at this by awarding different colored belts for different levels of achievement.

How will you celebrate when you achieve a personal best on the number of pushups you do or perform a yoga position you were not able to do previously?

5. Positive self-talk. What you tell yourself about fitness activities is very important. If it is something you "have to do" it is easy to dread doing it. If it is a gift you give yourself and in turn you get fabulous rewards, an internal voice kicks in and says, "let's do it."

Role models

The Greeks understood that mind and body must develop in harmonious proportions to produce a creative intelligence. And so did the most brilliant intelligence of our earliest days–Thomas Jefferson–when he said, 'not less than two hours a day should be devoted to exercise.' If the man who wrote the Declaration of Independence, was Secretary of State, and twice President, could give it two hours, our children can give it ten or fifteen minutes.
–President John F. Kennedy[52]

While there are many role models you could choose, my favorite is Jack LaLanne. His balanced, holistic, practical, optimistic, and spiritual approach to exercise was decades ahead of its time. He started the first health club, invented weight machines, originated exercise videos, and helped millions stay fit with his five-day-a-week television program that aired for 34 years. He also had a gift for showmanship. For his seventieth birthday Jack LaLanne had himself handcuffed and shackled and, fighting strong winds and currents, towed 20 boats with seventy people 1½ miles from the Queen's Way Bridge in Long Beach Harbor to the Queen Mary.[53] Another great role model is Tom Spear, who at 102 plays 18 holes of golf three times a week and drives the ball 200 yards.[54]

Who are some of your longevity role models? If you don't have any yet, start looking for them.

Resources

Edward Jackowski's *Hold it! You're Exercising All Wrong* does a superb job of teaching how to exercise correctly and get the most benefit from your exercise. He convincingly challenges a lot of conventional wisdom and practices in fitness. He prescribes how to tailor your fitness program to your body type and the outcomes you want. Covert Bailey's *Smart Exercise* does a good job of explaining the physiology of losing weight.

People choose exercise videos that have leaders they like and a style and philosophy they like. Another criteria should be whether it meets the other criteria in this chapter–particularly having warm up, stretching, and cool down phases. My personal favorite anaerobic video for men is Gilad Janklowicz's *Arms of Steel.* For aerobic workouts I like Billy Blank's *Tae-Bo. Callanetics,* a cross between yoga and ballet, is especially good at toning deep muscles and increasing flexibility. It is especially popular with women who want to have a better figure. Miriam Nelson's books, *Strong Women Stay Young, Strong Women Stay Slim,* and *Strong Women Strong Bones* are well founded in research. Several resources for posture are suggested earlier in this chapter. If your favorite exercise regime or video does not include all four phases of warming up, stretching, exercising, and cooling down, you can always add the missing step.

Chapter 15

Managing Risks–
A Chain is Only as Strong as its Weakest Link

If at first you don't succeed, don't try skydiving.

To live as long and as healthily as possible we need to intelligently manage risks. That is not to say we shouldn't take risks–that would certainly make for a dull life! The risks we take, however, should be worth the payoff. When Aristotle said "all things in moderation," he did not mean that we should be average. Rather, he was counseling us that most things taken to extremes are problematic. The hallmark of intelligent risk management is pragmatism. Pragmatism asks what gives the most benefit for the least sacrifice.

The Japanese have a long-standing passion and obsession for cleanliness. Indeed, the Japanese word for clean is also the Japanese word for beautiful. Japanese stores are filled with products that are touted as bacteria free. Taxi drivers wear white gloves. Chop sticks are often discarded after one use. Millions of Japanese take pills to remove odor from their perspiration and feces. Are the Japanese healthier? The question is controversial but at least one leading Japanese expert on parasites believes the extreme measures are actually impairing Japanese immune systems by not building resistance to infections. Also, some bacteria perform useful functions and these bacteria are often killed when killing bacteria in general. To support his belief Koichiro Fujita[1] notes that allergic conditions such as bronchial asthma and atopic dermatitis (skin diseases) have a 30% incidence rate in Japan but only 10% incidence rate in the U.S. Certainly, more study is needed. It seems probable, however, that a Felix Unger lifestyle (the obsessive compulsive character in *The Odd Couple*) probably impairs longevity rather than fostering it.

Needless to say, the more risks you take, the more likely you will be burned. I am not saying you have to avoid all risks. If you love driving a sports car or skydiving, you might decide the enjoyment is worth the risk. If you are going to take risks, do your homework so you know how to reduce the risks as much as possible. The goal is to be prudent. If you find yourself becoming a worry wart or obsessive and compulsive about risks, the remedy has become worse than the disease.

Managing risks means becoming your own OSHA (Occupational Safety and Health Administration) investigator. Your "OSHA investigator" should identify the greatest risks in your life and whether the risks are worth the pay offs. Employers spend a lot of time and money meeting safety and accreditation standards. The efforts have saved many lives and prevented millions of injuries. Most large businesses conduct safety inspections periodically (monthly, semiannually, annually). Is risk reduction at work more important than risk reduction in your personal life? You might want to do an initial safety/risk assessment for your own life and then conduct assessments periodically; for example, a year from now, each January 1, or every birthday. The following are some areas that merit your investigative scrutiny.

Athletics

Being physically active is vital to longevity. People who jog ten miles a day outdoors, however, are at high risk for serious health problems and injuries. People who will be fit at 150 are likely to have chosen a combination of sports and exercises that rarely result in serious injuries, do not wear out body parts, and address all their fitness needs (strength, cardiovascular, flexibility, coordination, and enjoyment).

Boxers often develop brain damage from repeated blows to their heads. Professional football is just starting to acknowledge how widespread concussions are among football players. Research is showing that head butting soccer balls can cause subtle brain impairments. The evidence is mounting that even mild head traumas, when repeated, cause brain damage.[2][3] Perhaps one reason women live longer than men is that fewer women play football, hockey, and other contact sports that often cause subtle brain injuries. Think twice before head butting a soccer ball or engaging in sports that involve even mild head trauma.

I heard on National Public Radio that the average life span of a National Football League player is 55. Imagine, teenagers who were some of the healthiest boys in the country, who had plenty of money as adults, having a life span two decades shorter than the rest of U.S. men. Quite a price! A study of more than two thousand Harvard students compared non athletes, major athletes, and minor athletes (who did not earn a letter or participated in a sport that did not award letters). Although presumably major athletes started with the most exceptional health, the minor athletes had the longest life spans and the major athletes the shortest life spans.[4]

Automobile travel

There are 13 million automobile accidents in the U.S. each year[5] (and most other countries have comparable or even higher per mile accident rates). The accidents cause 38,200 fatalities a year and 2.3 million disabling injuries a year. Thus, almost 1% of the population dies or has a disabling injury each year. If accident rates were evenly distributed, you would have about a 50% chance of experiencing a disabling injury (or dying) from an automobile accident by the time you are 60. This is a much bigger risk than heart disease or cancer. Reducing your chances of an automobile accident is one of the most effective actions you can take to foster your longevity.

Whatever you can do to reduce the amount of time you spend driving or riding in cars helps reduce this enormous risk of disability or death. Consolidating trips reduces exposure and gives you more time for more productive things than driving. If you are planning on moving, consider the commuting risks and whether you would be driving into the blinding sunlight when commuting. When you purchase a car, buy one of the safer cars. As a rule of thumb, larger and heavier cars fare better in accidents, though safety features are important too. If you live in an area that has a lot of snow and ice, traction can be a critical safety factor. If you use a car phone while driving, use one that is hands free. Within a few decades auto safety should improve substantially with the introduction of radar devices that warn and protect cars from getting too close to other cars.

Your odds of being in an automobile accident in any given year are one in five. While only 8% of these motorists suffer significant injuries, 90% of motorcyclists suffer significant injuries. Almost 25% of motorcycle accidents are head injuries. In 25% of motorcycle accidents the operator had less than three months experience operating a motorcycle. If you want to live a long, healthy life, don't get on a motorcycle.

Food

Rinsing food reduces the number of chemicals we ingest from pesticides, preservatives, and surface additives to make the food look better. Undercooking meat runs the risk of not killing bacteria. Overcooking meat increases the number of carcinogens. Eating raw seafood increases the risk of disease. Not cooking acidic foods in aluminum or cast iron[6] pans avoids the risk of absorbing the metals through your food.

Choosing foods like raw fruits and vegetables is healthier than choosing processed foods. Having a healthy ratio of carbohydrates, protein, and fat is important to reducing the risk of health problems. I'll leave it to your judgment whether organic foods are worth the premium price. Most people would fail at suddenly trying to follow an ideal diet. Far more effective is gradually improving your diet.

Home safety

If you are choosing a new residence, it is worth playing detective and considering all the risks before you make a down payment or deposit. How much air pollution is in the neighborhood (e.g., smog trapped in valleys, pollution from local industries, auto emissions from freeways and traffic)? What is the water quality in the neighborhood? Is there a problem with radon, lead, or other chemicals in the area or residence? Some of the information is available from the library, some by asking neighbors, and some from hiring an expert for a few hundred dollars to do an inspection.

At home, periodically pretend you have been hired to conduct a safety inspection and advise the owner (yourself) on practical things that could be done to improve home safety. Better yet, arrange with a friend or a professional to do the inspection. The largest cause of home accidents (62%) are due to falls.

Health

Oliver Wendell Holmes, Sr.'s formula for longevity was to have a chronic disease and take care of it.[7]

Most of us have some body systems that are extremely hardy and some that are more vulnerable to illness. You want to focus on what would help your weakest system. For example: If you get a lot of colds, you would want to:

- Perform daily personal hygiene functions such as irrigating your sinuses and scraping your tongue. (Sinus irrigation involves filling a baby syringe or ear syringe with filtered or distilled warm salt water, tilting your head back, squirting the water into your nostrils, and allowing the water to drain into your throat. Tongue scraping involves using a U-shaped instrument to scrape bacteria laden mucus off your tongue. (Scrapers are available in many drug stores and health food stores for about ten dollars.)
- Check your home for proper humidity and for mold and dust.
- Be keenly attuned to how lack of sleep and/or getting depressed might make you vulnerable to colds.
- If you get a lot of colds in winter, determine if you are getting enough sunlight or have problems with Seasonal Affective Disorder (SAD).

If you get a lot of headaches, you want to:
- Explore what contributed to them including the possibility of:
  - certain social situations or stressors
  - poor posture
  - poor breathing
  - certain foods
- Explore what is most helpful in alleviating the headaches including:
  - handling the social situations or stressors differently
  - better posture
  - exercise
  - breathing exercises
  - meditation
  - massage
  - a hot bath

Light

John Ott's[8] classic research showed how we need sunlight to be healthy and how indoor lighting alone leads to health problems. If you cannot obtain at least fifteen to thirty minutes a day of sunlight, consider using light bulbs that more closely mimic the sun's spectrum of light. Spectrum corrected light bulbs, e.g., Chromolux, are available in many hardware stores and by mail and Internet for less than ten dollars a bulb. Another option, particularly if you tend to have depression in late fall and winter, is to get a SAD (Seasonal Affective Disorder) light. There are several SAD light distributors on the Internet. Prices range from $200-$600. (Lights are discussed in more detail in Chapter 14.)

Occupational hazards

Consider whether your job poses health risks and how you can minimize them. If the risks are serious, you might consider other positions or occupations that would be as rewarding and safer.

Shoes

We ask a lot of our feet. The least we can do is to make sure we take good care of our feet. Eventually, custom-made shoes will be affordable and easy to obtain in popular styles. This would involve making a mold of your feet and then ordering shoes to fit the specifications. Once your feet are measured, you could order custom shoes locally or by phone or Internet. Until then most people will settle for what is available in stores.

It is worth the extra money to go to a shoe store that has staff who specialize in orthopedic shoes. They know more about healthy fit than most shoe salespeople and they can better fit each foot's arch, shape, and peculiarities. Once you learn what your feet need and what brands often fit those needs, you will be better at selecting shoes from any store. Women in particular need to find shoes that do not sacrifice comfort for style and to minimize wearing high heels. Fashionable healthy shoes will become more readily available as Baby Boomers insist on them. Loafers do not provide good support and should be worn sparingly. If you wear athletic shoes a lot, select shoes to match your sports and activities (e.g., walking, running, basketball, racquetball). If the bottoms of your shoes wear unevenly, it is a sign of posture or gait problems. Consult someone who is knowledgeable about these problems.

Skin care

Some people take better care of their furniture or car upholstery than their own skin. With people living so much longer, there will be a lot of regrets. Skin needs periodic cleaning, moisturizing, and protection from prolonged exposure to the sun. Skin care isn't just for women.

Surgery and hospitals

Twenty percent of hospital patients leave with a condition they didn't have when they entered the hospital.[9]

At least 44,000 and perhaps as many as 98,000 hospitalized Americans die every year from medical mistakes.
–The Institute of Medicine[10]

If your physician has recommended surgery, investigate options and alternatives, e.g.:
- Explore non surgical alternatives, e.g., exercise, change in diet, body manipulation.
- Research the track record on the surgery using books such as the People's Medical Society's *Good Operations–Bad Operations.*
- Obtain a second opinion.
- Inquire about the specific procedures and whether any of them have less risky alternatives (e.g., is a catheter really needed? depilation vs. shaving a surgical area and risking cuts).
- Check the credentials and experience of the surgeon. Strategies for obtaining this information include:
  - Check to see if the surgeon is Board Certified.
  - Ask the surgeon or hospital how many of these surgeries

he or she has performed in the last two years.
- Ask the hospital Utilization Review Department for data on the surgery.
- Call the Operating Room and asking to speak with a nurse who assists in that type of surgery. Ask the nurse off the record whom he or she would choose if the surgery was on herself/himself.
- Ask your primary care physician to check his/her sources for who has the best reputation for performing that operation.
- Ask a Utilization Review nurse at your insurance company for his/her recommendations.

According to *Consumer Reports*,[11] the most common needless surgeries are inserting tubes in children's ears, removing cataracts, low-back surgeries, gall bladder removals, hysterectomies, Cesarean sections for childbirth, and surgeries to correct sleep apnea, snoring, and jaw pain.

While surgeries are becoming less invasive, many still involve cutting muscle tissue and fascia. It is not unusual for people to have a normal recovery only to develop pain several months later. This can be due to postural changes in adapting to the cut tissue. Most physicians are unaware of this problem. People who are very skilled in body work (e.g., massage therapists, osteopaths, movement specialists, chiropractors) might be able to help.

Water

Our bodies are 75% water and we should be drinking eight glasses of water a day. Most tap water contains chlorine (to kill bacteria) and traces of toxic chemicals. Bottled water is one solution. If you don't want to spend money on bottled water, many water filters are inexpensive and efficient. That doesn't mean never taking a drink from a water fountain or a glass of water when it is served to you. A hassle that extreme is more wearing than occasionally drinking unfiltered water.

Exercise 15-1: Assessing your risks

The following assessment focuses on modest changes to reduce risks. After answering the questions, put a **T** beside items you are willing to take action on starting today. Put a **W** beside the ones you are willing to take action on starting this week. Put an **M** beside items you are willing to take action on later this month. Write this week and this month items on your calendar on a specific date.

1. Without compromising the quality of my life, how can I significantly reduce the number of miles I travel by car?
2. What can I do to make my car safer?
3. The next time I buy a car, what car would meet my needs and be safer than my current car?
4. What changes in my driving habits would make me a safer driver?
5. What could I easily do to lower my exposure to electromagnetic fields (from electrical wires, appliances, electrical equipment, power lines, etc.)?[12]
6. What is the most likely way a fire could start in my residence? What reasonable steps can I take to reduce the risk or contain the fire?
7. What would I be most likely to trip on or slip on at home?
8. If I were to conduct just one health or safety test of my residence (e.g., water, radon, asbestos, wiring, formaldehyde, furnace, gas lines), what would be my priority?
9. What single act would most improve sanitation and reduce the risk of disease in my residence (e.g., removing dust or mold, better cleaning of cutting boards, washing foods, not storing cosmetics and toiletries near the toilet)?
10. Are there any parts of my residence that need better lighting at night (even if just a nightlight)?
11. What could I do to improve the air quality in my home (e.g., change the furnace filter more often, periodically ventilate the home, more house plants)?
12. Could I use fewer insecticides in my home or yard?

13. Do I have an adequate number of functional smoke alarms and fire extinguishers at home?
14. What painless steps could I take to make myself less likely to be a crime victim?
15. What minor change or changes in my eating habits would reduce my risk of health problems?
16. Do I avoid cooking acidic foods in aluminum or iron pots and pans?
17. Are there times when I should wash my hands and don't?
18. Do I brush my teeth at least twice a day and floss my teeth at least once a day?
19. Could I reduce my exposure to chemicals by using less deodorant or using deodorants that do not contain harmful chemicals?
20. What can I do to reduce the frequency or intensity of my most frequent health problems (e.g., colds, pulled muscles, backaches)?
21. When and where would I be willing to engage in better posture when sitting or standing?
22. When and where might I wear healthier shoes?

Chapter 16

Finances for a Long Lifetime

The way to make a man rich is to decrease his wants. [1]
–Ossie Davis

Life begets life. Energy creates energy.
It is only by spending oneself that one becomes rich.
–Sarah Bernhardt

Wake up to a different world

When the U.S. Social Security system started paying benefits in 1937, the average life expectancy was 63. Forty workers were making contributions for every recipient. Most people contributing to the system weren't expected to live long enough to receive benefits. It was not intended to provide a comfortable retirement, but merely a modest financial safety net or as Franklin D. Roosevelt put it, "some measure of protection . . . against poverty-ridden old age." [2] The U.S. life expectancy is at 76.5 years and climbing. In 2012 Social Security starts taking on the 76 million member Baby Boom generation, which turns 66 (the full benefit age for Boomers) between 2011 and 2030. The "Baby Bust" generation that follows only had 44 million members to help fund Social Security for Baby Boomers and earlier generations.

Roosevelt picked age 65 from the German model. Ironically, the German model was based on a political ruse by Otto Bismark. Aspiring to be prime minister, he realized that his rivals were all over 65 and successfully championed legislation to institute a mandatory retirement program. The choice of 65 is that arbitrary.

Social Security will be stretched and stretched and something has to give. One adjustment is the gradual raising of the retirement age to an age more consistent with Americans' health and longevity. Currently, only people born before 1938 are eligible for full Social Security benefits at age 65. For those born between 1943 and 1954 the full benefit age is 66. In 1960 the age becomes 67. Politicians might place a means test on Social Security. With a means test wealthier citizens and possibly middle income Americans would not receive Social Security or would only receive a portion of what is paid to lower income citizens. If this happens, legal definitions of income can be critical to whether you receive Social Security. Currently (1999 taxes) high income workers do not have to make Social Security contributions on earnings over $72,600. Politicians are likely to continue raising this ceiling. This only affects people while they are earning high salaries. Overall, it is best not to count on Social Security.

Congress' repeal of the Social Security earnings penalty in March, 2000 will also encourage workers over 65 to continue working. (The earnings test penalized employment by reducing Social Security benefits by one dollar for every three dollars earned for retirees 65-69. This was in addition to having Social Security contributions deducted from their earnings. Once they turned 70, the earnings limit disincentive no longer applied.)

Of the 76 million Baby Boomers, about a third are investing and saving. Another third live from paycheck to paycheck and will probably have to work well into their seventies. The other third or 25 million have family assets of less than a thousand dollars[3] (excluding asset appreciation on property or stocks). Many Boomers will become financially comfortable from inheritances when their parents die. But many Boomers will be working well past 70 whether they want to or not.

Social Security will still receive contributions from many people over 65 who are still working. As the population gets older, the political power of older people will grow. Politicians know that a much higher portion of citizens over 65 vote than those under 65. Citizens under 40 have an especially low voting rate. The AARP (American Association of Retired Persons) has 32 million members and is growing rapidly. It is second only to the Catholic church in membership. It dwarfs the AFL-CIO with its mere 13.3 million members. *Fortune* magazine ranked the AARP the most powerful lobbying organization in the U.S.[4]

In the U.S. half of the nation's health care dollars are spent on the last six months of people's lives. For Medicare funds, the proportion of funds spent in the last six months is even higher. Often this care is for intrusive treatment, life support equipment, and hospital/nursing home stays that do not promote life but only prolong death. You might want to consider a living will that stipulates that you do not want extreme medical procedures performed if they would not give you a reasonable quality of life but only prolong death. Eventually, Medicare will have to make some tough choices about how to triage these medical expenses.

The plan

Most people spend beyond their means and worry about money. Even many rich people leverage their investments and are vulnerable to bankruptcy if their investments fare poorly. Money is important. Poor people have three times as many physical and mental health problems as people who are not poor. The truly wealthy, regardless of how much or little money they have, do not worry about money. The key to real wealth is to be happy living below your means. The book, *The Millionaire Next Door,* provides hundreds of role models of people who are millionaires but choose to live modestly. These millionaires define material wealth in terms of net worth, not consumption habits. They know a fifty-dollar watch tells time just as well as a Rolex. Sam Walton (of Wal-Mart fame) drove an old pick-up truck. Research[5] in the U.S. and twelve other countries has consistently shown that people who *focus* on material success experience more depression and anxiety and have lower levels of vitality, self-esteem, and self-actualization than those who focus on relationships, self-awareness, and contributing.

Our plan for living long posits that you will probably be earning at least some income in your seventies, eighties and nineties and possibly beyond (this can be passive income). Thus, you don't have to save a hundred years of retirement income by age 65. You do, however, want to have substantial retirement savings by 65 as your funds will need to last a lot longer than most people anticipate. As you continue to earn money and add to your savings, you will be in good shape well before your hundredth birthday. You want to keep your cost of living modest so you don't have to be a workaholic to support your lifestyle and so you can afford to take time off to learn new skills, travel, or just take sabbaticals. You also want to have contingency funds for unexpected problems.

Working past what used to be deemed retirement age isn't just a matter of earning money, it's having new challenges and feeling you are contributing. Living below your means enables you to be wealthy enough to change jobs or careers anytime you no longer find a job interesting and rewarding. If you love your work, you might want to stay with it for decades. If you become bored with your work, however, the price for staying with it is too high. Few things age people faster than plugging away at jobs they don't like. Some highly respected careers tend to foster burn out because of the tedium or repetition. Many attorneys eventually become tired of studying the legal minutiae. I can't imagine being a dentist and filling teeth for a hundred years. On the other hand some careers offer a strong sense of purpose and fulfillment and are less likely to foster burnout, e.g., professors, psychologists, clergy, and artists. It is what you find interesting and makes you want to get out of bed in the morning that is important.

If you need to change careers, it is time to consider what you really want to do. You might be able to capitalize on previous experience so you don't have to start at the bottom of that career ladder. If further education is needed to acquire new skills or credentials, it is worth the investment. Part of the formula for living to be 150 is to be a lifelong learner. People who think of their careers as lasting forty years at the most feel pressure to be constantly advancing their careers. If, however, you believe that you will probably be doing some kind of work for a hundred years, the pace is different. Instead you can believe:

• I will probably want to have several different careers. This will make life interesting and allow me to live what would have been several lives for others.

• I have enough time and financial resources that I can afford to start over with careers and start at the bottom if I think another career path is sufficiently rewarding.

• I'm more interested in personal fulfillment, contributing, and enjoying my career or job than setting new sales records.

• It's like Frank Sinatra sings, "Let's take a trip to Niagara–This time we'll look at the falls."[6]

It will be safest to have your savings and income diversified, e.g., home equity, stocks and bonds, annuities, and retirement programs including Social Security. Interesting financial tools include annuities and reverse home mortgages. Annuities promise to pay you a set amount of money for the rest of your life. They normally are not a good investment as they typically have a large sales charge up front. If you expect to greatly outlive the insurance company's life expectancy tables, however, they can be a great deal. I also like the way the incentives are aligned–the longer you live, the more the benefits exceed your investment. With reverse home mortgages the bank or mortgage company (or individual) pays you a monthly income until what you owe approaches the market value of the home. At that point you would need to negotiate a regular mortgage or sell the home. The arrangement is primarily beneficial for people who only expect to live or at least live in the home for another decade or two at most. When she was 90, Jeanne Calment arranged a variation on this theme that is fairly common in France. An attorney agreed to pay her $500 a month ("en viager") for the rest of her life and he would own her apartment in Arles when she died. She lived to 122. He died at the age of 77 after paying over $184,000 (far more than the apartment's value). His widow continued paying after his death.

Many people live beyond their means and survive from paycheck to paycheck. This fuels stress; for example, fears of what would happen if they lose their job or experience large unexpected expenses. People who want to live long would be wise to live within their means, invest in themselves, and anticipate the unexpected, including the need for periodic educational pursuits for career changes.

The basic tenants of the plan are:
- live below your means
- invest in yourself
- anticipate there will be periodic unexpected expenses
- save for periodic educational pursuits and career changes as the pace of technological and career changes will continue to accelerate

A longevity budget

I would suggest the following financial formula:

- 10% charity
- 10% ongoing education (courses, books, tapes, conferences, etc.)
- 5% fitness and proactive health measures
- 10% "sinking fund" for periods when you do not work due to health, taking a sabbatical, retraining, unemployment, or pursuing avocations
- 15% retirement/savings (taking advantage of tax deferred programs such as IRA, Roth IRA, and 401-K)
- 50% living expenses, paying as you go with possible exceptions for a home mortgage, educational expenses, and/or financing a business

People who know their careers are secure and have no interest in changing careers might not need to set aside as much in funds for retraining, e.g., some college professors, appointed judges, and orchestra conductors.

Investments

Predicting what the stock market will do tomorrow challenges the skills of full-time, highly paid experts. Knowing how to be financially healthy for the next hundred years is even more difficult. Certainly people who are wealthy can diversify their wealth and obtain good advice on how to make sure their money lasts a lifetime. People who plan to live to 150 or longer can take advantage of retirement benefits and annuities which pay for the rest of your life, no matter how long you live. Since the one thing we can count on is change, it is not wise to count on any one institution lasting a hundred years. Instead, have income diversified in case one source becomes defunct. Personally I have always disliked life insurance as you are in effect betting that you won't live long. Annuities and retirement benefits with monthly payments as long as you live, however, reverse the incentive and reward long life.

When it comes to investing, some people are lucky (e.g., their company gave them stock over the years and it did fabulously), some have a knack for investing, and many are lambs ready for slaughter. It's important to know where you are in your evolution as an investor. Not everyone is suited to do well in the stock market for a variety of reasons including lack of interest, lack of technical knowledge, and, most commonly, lack of emotional discipline and fortitude.

Research has consistently shown:

- Mutual funds, advisory newsletters, and professional investors rarely do better than the Standard and Poor's 500 stocks index–and that is before their fees are deducted.[7] Consequently, it is usually wiser to purchase an index fund than most mutual funds. The fees are lower as well. Another option is Stanton's[8] strategy of buying a portfolio of several stocks that are on his list of "America's Finest Companies." Criteria for these 400 companies include at least ten straight years of increased earnings per share. He updates the list each year.

- Over time, no load mutual funds have performed as well as mutual funds that are not no load, making no load funds preferable in most cases.

- Most people who invest in stocks have results that underperform the market. If that is your experience, you would be wiser investing in an index fund or buy and hold blue chip stocks. These strategies also have the advantages of requiring far less of your time studying the market and fewer expenses (stock commissions, books, newsletters and newspapers). Many people, however, cannot resist the temptation to pick the next Microsoft. If this is the case, set aside 10% of your funds for speculation and put the other 90% in an index fund or blue chip stocks.

- A strategy that can limit your losses is to purchase a variety of sound stocks and put a "good until canceled stop loss" order on each at 10% below the purchase price. A stop loss order instructs the brokerage company to sell the stock at the market price if the stock falls to your limit price. This will ensure that if the stock (and possibly the market as a whole) plummets you won't lose more than 10% (actually you also need to subtract commissions and lost interest and add in any dividends you received). If the stock goes up, you can periodically raise your stop loss price so that even if the stock goes down and is automatically sold, you still make a profit.

- Term insurance is a better investment than life insurance. If you believe you will live well over 100 years, the only reason for having a modest amount of term insurance is if you have young children or a dependent spouse or family member and want to allow for the possibility of adversity such as an automobile accident.

To these observations I would add the following advice:
- If your investment strategy works for you, it is probably best to continue that strategy until there is reason to believe that the circumstances have fundamentally changed and invalidate that strategy–and eventually the circumstances will change.
- If you are not willing to make a soul searching examination of your investment psychology and strategies, learn the logistics of investing, and put time into following your strategy, it is probably best to avoid speculative investing and stay with a conservative investment strategy, e.g., a balanced, conservative portfolio.

Resources

The Millionaire Next Door by Thomas Stanley and William Danko provides role models of hundreds of millionaires who earned their wealth and chose to live below their means. Stephen Pollan's *Die Broke* sounds irresponsible but is actually a very conservative call to sanity for Baby Boomers. He advocates working for yourself, paying cash, eschewing credit cards, and working all your life. The die broke part? Well, you can't take it with you. If you are serious about speculative stock market investing, *The Disciplined Trader* makes a convincing case that 80% of investing is psychology and personal discipline and provides a unique insight into the mental discipline it takes to succeed.

Chapter 17

The Evidence for Living 150 Years

The exponential growth in knowledge and technology

When you buy a computer, you discover that in less than a year it has been superseded by faster, better technology. Human knowledge, especially medical knowledge, is doubling every five years.[1] Computer chips for mapping genes double in power every 18 months.[2] CAT scans and MRIs, introduced in the early 1980s, have become as common as X-rays. Twenty years ago, few would have envisioned commonplace use of personal computers or the Internet. In 1977 the President of Digital Equipment Corporation (DEC) told the World Future Society, "There is no reason for any individual to have a computer in their home."[3]

The next twenty years are likely to bring technologies that will profoundly affect our lives in ways that are difficult to imagine now. The question isn't whether but how. Medical researchers, pharmaceutical companies, and computer wizards will continue to dazzle us with new technology. The most profound new technology is likely to come from genetic engineering and gene chips.[4] The other profound technological growth will be in our understanding of how to optimally use and take care of ourselves mentally, physically, and spiritually. As with knowledge and lifestyles today, some people will use these wonderful resources wisely and some will not.

Richard Oliver gives a little perspective. He notes that the agrarian age lasted for about nine thousand years, the industrial revolution for 360 years and the information revolution is about to be superseded after 50 to 60 years. Taking its place will be the biotech revolution which "will last only about 15 to 30 years, but its economic returns will dwarf everything that has come before it."[5]

The coming breakthroughs in genetic engineering

Genetic engineering began in the early 1970s when scientists first learned how to isolate, clone, and "cut and paste" human genes. Genentech launched the first genetically engineered drug, insulin, in

1981. Insulin was created by cloning the human gene code for insulin and transferring it to bacteria which could be grown commercially.[6]

In 1990 and 1991, three National Institute of Science researchers put copies of a missing gene into the white blood cells of a 4-year-old girl and a 9-year-old girl with severe combined immunodeficiency (SCID). With the gene missing, their bodies were not able to produce the adenosine deaminase (ADA), which plays a critical role in the immune system. SCID restricted their lives to a sanitized plastic bubble because they were so susceptible to diseases. The results of the gene implants were dramatic.[7] The girls were restored to health and appeared in press conferences two years later, happy and healthy.

In 1990 the U.S., France, Britain, and Germany agreed to collaborate to map the genetic codes of all human chromosomes. If you think of genes as the bar codes on products we purchase, the Human Genome Project is inventorying each bar code. The project was scheduled for completion in 2005. A working draft is due in spring of 2000 and a highly accurate version by 2003. The ahead-of-schedule pace is due to higher powered computers and a private firm, Celera Genomics, announcing it will have their mapping completed by December 2001. While this is an enormously complex undertaking, human genetic codes are far less complex than the Windows NT operating system in computers.[8] Windows has several million lines of code while humans only have 100,000 chromosomes.

Battelle Memorial Institute, the world's largest nonprofit research laboratory, had its staff predict the top ten technologies of the coming decade. First on their list was the Genome project. They noted that it is not the gene mapping per se, but the enormous commercial applications that make the technology profound.[9] Want to map some genes? While gene mapping equipment costs about $175,000 installed, there is now a do-it-yourself kit for $30,000 that will allow many more researchers to get into the business.[10]

Genes are constantly being turned on and off like lights in a skyscraper. When on, they produce a hormone or enzyme that gives the body instructions. Genetic engineering will result in an inventory of which genes effect which diseases and what treatments are likely to be most effective. Eventually, physicians will use inexpensive disposable biochips to see what your genes are doing and help diagnose and treat your ailments or enhance your health. Daniel

Cohen of the Centre d'Etude du Polymorphisme Humain predicts that by 2010, medicine will be able to genetically treat most serious diseases caused by a single gene defect and that by 2045, most common serious illnesses will be treatable with gene therapy.[11]

IBM plans to spend $100 million to build a computer and software to study human proteins. Dubbed "Blue Gene,"[12] the project includes a computer 500 times faster than 1999 personal computers. Proteins are the building blocks of DNA, its messenger RNA, enzymes, and hormones. The project will be a huge boost to genetic engineering, tissue engineering, and hormone replacement therapies.

Genetic engineering

It is our increasing control over our genes and the deciphering of what certain gene products do that holds the best hope of retarding aging in the near future. –Gerontologist Steven Austad[13]

Genetic engineering involves modifying genes or their protein messengers (hormones or enzymes). Strategies include introducing genetic material that produces a desired protein, or blocks the action of problem genes, or mimics the actions of certain genes. One mechanism is to remove cells with defective genes, alter them, and put them back in the body. (This cut and paste strategy should be familiar to computer users.) Another common mechanism is to put genetic material on a benign virus or bacterium and introduce it into the body.

Companies owned by Novartis (the merged Ciba-Geigy and Sandoz pharmaceutical giants) are developing a TK (thymidine kinase) gene.[14] The TK gene is injected into diseased or cancerous cells. When the patient takes the medication gancyclovir, the gancyclovir kills the cancerous cells. Another application is with organ transplants. Transplants run the risk of the body's immune system rejecting the transplant. TK can be inserted into the transplant organ. After surgery, gancyclovir is only administered if the patient is rejecting the transplant.

Genetic Therapy Inc. (a Sandoz subsidiary) is developing a genetic treatment for glioblastoma brain tumors.[15] The current treatment is surgery and radiation therapy but the tumor usually reemerges in about ten months. After surgery, Genetic Therapy's approach saturates the tumor cavity, where some cancerous cells are almost always left behind, with a solution containing a virus derived from the herpes simplex virus which is encapsulated in a harmless retrovirus. (Retroviruses have RNA rather than DNA and an enzyme that allows them to transform their RNA into DNA.) The retrovirus only attaches itself to cells that are dividing. Hence they attach to the cancer cells. Patients are given an injection of the antiviral drug gancyclovir which interacts with the enzyme produced by the herpes virus and causes the dividing cells to die. Cells which are not dividing are not affected. The genes have been humorously dubbed "suicide genes." The market is large, as 20,000 people in the U.S. and Europe dic of brain cancer each year.

Arthropod-Borne and Colorado State University are working together on "antisense" technology. DNA has a pair of strands–the sense strand that produces RNA and the antisense strand which is a mirror image of the sense strand. (The function of the antisense strand is not understood yet.) With antisense technology the researcher or physician inserts copies of the antisense RNA into the body. The antisense RNA binds to sense RNA and blocks it from carrying out its mission of producing a protein that gives the body instructions. Their research is focusing on yellow fever and dengue fever. The approach is especially appealing because the gene only targets one set of genes and has no effect on other genes. Antisense therapy can also attach the engineered gene to the DNA so the RNA messenger molecules cannot read the DNA. Antisense has been successfully used with animals for problems like asthma.[16]

Ariad Pharmaceuticals has a unique approach to protein deficiencies like diabetes.[17] After a corrective gene is implanted, the gene can be activated by taking a medication. In this way, the medication can activate the gene for a short period of time and produce the desired quantity of protein, e.g., insulin.

Dr. S. Gail Eckhardt is developing a process to treat head and neck tumors by injecting a common cold virus (with part of the genetic material removed) directly into head and neck cancers. The virus only destroys tumor cells with a missing or broken tumor suppressor gene, P-53. The P-53 gene is missing or broken in a high percentage of cancers, and almost universally missing or damaged in head and neck tumors.[18] Clinical trials with humans began in 1996.

Genentech's Herceptin[19] only acts on one gene, the HER2 gene. The HER2 gene prompts cell growth needed to maintain the body. Women with breast cancer, particularly the type that metastasizes, have additional copies of the HER2 genes and the extra copies cause cancerous growth. Herceptin binds to the HER2 cells and prevents the cells from dividing. Thus chemotherapy is often unnecessary.

In 1994 scientists reported they had transplanted a missing "LDL receptor gene" into the liver of a woman with an inherited disorder that caused her to have high cholesterol and rapidly developing heart disease. Her cholesterol level dropped and her arteries became healthier.[20]

Researchers[21] have also found a single gene in humans that suppresses cancer. When either gene of the gene pair is damaged or absent, there is a sharp increase in rates of malignant brain, breast, prostrate, kidney, and skin cancers. Consequently, the gene can help diagnose whether a cancer is benign or malignant. With further research, physicians might be able to replace or mimic the gene when it is missing or damaged.

Eventually physicians will be able to turn off many of the genes causing problems such as cancer or possibly even obesity. Mice whose RII-beta gene was removed were fed a 58% fat diet and remained trim and fit.[22] The gene's effect is to increase metabolism and stimulate brown fat cells to convert calories to heat rather than to stored fat. The mice weighed 10% less than normal but had the same amount of muscle tissue. They ate slightly more than other mice and remained fertile and apparently normal. Other scientists have discovered a gene that they believe will lead to a weight loss medication for humans.[23]

While it is beyond the focus of this book, it is noteworthy that genetic engineering raises many ethical issues, including cloning, choosing the sex of a fetus, trying to design the perfect child ("brains and beauty" genes), whether the technology is universally available, denial of insurance coverage for people with diagnosed "defective" genes, and religious objections to intruding in God's domain.

One of people's biggest fears about aging is Alzheimer's disease. In 1993 Duke University researcher Alan Roses identified four variations of a gene that is associated with Alzheimer's. People with two apo-e4 genes are eight times more likely to develop Alzheimer's and, on the average, their symptoms appear at age 68. People with one e3 gene have an average age of onset at 75. Those with e2 genes have a much lower risk of contracting Alzheimer's. Researchers not only know what genes apparently effect Alzheimer's, they have successfully immunized mice against Alzheimer's disease.[24] [25]   In 1999 researchers began small clinical trials of vaccinating people with mild to moderate levels of Alzheimer's disease.

Historically medicine has focused on curing diseases and has paid far less attention to prevention. Within a few decades, physicians will probably be able to run health checks and identify and disable genes that cause Alzheimer's, Huntington's Chorea and other genetic diseases.

Biochips

Biochips combine computer technology and DNA research. Biochips have microscopic pieces of DNA chemically bonded to a silicon computer chip. When the chip comes in contact with blood or other tissue samples, it identifies patterns in the sample's genes.

Affymetrix and OncorMed are jointly developing a computer chip that can examine a body cell and detect a malfunction in gene P-53, a gene thought to be a key contributor in 60% of human cancers. Research has indicated that women with breast tumors and mutated P-53 genes are in greater danger of metastasis and death than women with normal P-53 genes. The chip could identify which women have these high risk mutations. Physicians would recommend very aggressive cancer treatments for these women and conservative treatment for women with breast tumors and normal P-53 genes.

LeRoy Hood, Ph.D., at the University of Washington, is developing a biochip that distinguishes between slow-growing prostate cancers (that do not need treatment) and aggressive cancers for which surgery is essential.[26] He predicts that by 2010 a biochip will be able to recognize the distinctive gene patterns in the 20 most common types of cancer. Treatment would then be targeted to that particular type of cancer. Also, two researchers independently have identified the PTEN "tumor suppressor" gene that, when absent, contributes to the growth of prostate, breast, and other cancers.[27]

Nanogen is developing diagnostic tests to identify different types of infectious bacteria. It will then track the effectiveness of various antibiotics in treating each type of bacteria.[28] With biochips your physician would test your cells or blood with an inexpensive disposable computer chip to determine the particular type of infection you have (based on which pertinent genes are turned on, turned off, or mutated). The pharmaceutical industry is well aware of the need to tailor medications to biochip diagnoses and is investing billions in joint ventures with biochip firms.

Tissue engineering

In 1995 newspapers and magazines carried a picture of a mouse with a human ear growing out of its back.[29] The mouse graphically illustrated advances in tissue engineering. Tissue engineering combines biological and engineering sciences to culture and transplant human and animal tissues. Tissue engineering closely matches the body's original equipment, requires less surgery and medical care than alternative treatments, and is rapidly becoming the most cost-effective treatment. The initial focus has been on skin and cartilage tissues. Breast, liver, vascular tissues, pancreas, blood cells, heart valves, and other organ tissues are also being developed.[30] Research interest has included stem cells, which are immature cells that have the potential to develop into almost any tissue. Researchers are learning how to insert stem cells into parts of the human body to grow whatever tissue is needed. Chemotherapy kills stem cells that make new blood cells. Physicians are now able to remove stem cells before chemotherapy and grow them in the laboratory for subsequent transplantation.[31]

Skin grafts have been grown and grafted onto burn patients since about 1990. Organogenesis Inc. is working on developing artificial skin from newborn foreskins.[32] The foreskin lacks the immune components that might lead to rejection. Foreskin contains both the dermis and epidermis layers of skin, making it ideal for skin transplants and burn reconstruction. A single foreskin can generate a square meter of skin.

In the U.S. there are 500,000 surgeries a year that require bone substitutes. Physicians often insert biodegradable "scaffolding" and bone cells grown in the laboratory. Carnegie Mellon University is developing a system that grows the cells in the lab and then uses CAT or MRI data to insert layers of custom fitted scaffolding, vessels, and bone tissue into the patient.[33]

Tissue engineering includes encapsulating cells that secrete hormones. CytoTherapeutics Inc., for example, is working on a process that injects encapsulated hormone cells near the spinal cords of individuals with amyotrophic lateral sclerosis (Lou Gehrig's Disease).[34] The technology also might be applicable to diseases such as Parkinson's, epilepsy, multiple sclerosis, and diabetes. It could also be used to replace glands that are removed by surgery or destroyed by cancer, e.g., gall bladders and thyroids. Scientists are working on encapsulated artificial liver cells. Eventually, bone marrow cells might be transplanted into the bones of hemophiliacs.[35] For pain management, cells that produce endorphins could be transplanted next to the source of the pain to counteract the pain.[36]

There are waiting lists for organ transplants. In the U.S. alone eleven people a day die waiting for an organ. Nanotechnology (miniaturization on a microscopic scale) will result in more and more bioreplacement parts.[37] Two biotech firms, Nextram in Princeton, New Jersey and Imutran in Cambridge, England are racing to perfect organ transplants from pigs.[38] Pigs breed and mature quickly, have organs about the same size as human organs, and raise fewer objections from animal rights activists than monkeys would. The biggest concern is making sure the PERV retrovirus is not accidently transmitted to the donor and from the donor to others (c.f. the transmission pattern of the HIV virus).

Genes that control aging

More than 98% of human and chimpanzee genes are comparable but the chimpanzee longevity record is only 39 years. Only about 1,000 genes account for the differences between chimps and people.[39] This is one more indication that it is probably not necessary to alter very many genes to increase longevity.

Southern Methodist University (Dallas) researcher Raj Shoal[40 41] identified the enzyme in fruit flies that helps protect cells from free radicals. He gave fruit fly embryos an extra copy of the gene that produces the enzyme. The result was "super" flies that lived 30% longer than untreated fruit flies and were markedly more active, even in their "old age." (Fruit flies have been a focus of genetic studies because of their large genes.)

Research with yeast, mice, and nematodes have found genes that can lengthen or shorten the aging process by turning them on or off or mutating them. (Nematodes are the phylum of worms that include roundworms, pinworms, hookworms, and the worm that causes trichinosis.) In 1996, geneticists extended the life of nematodes by 500% by removing one gene. Nematodes, which normally have a life span of nine days, lived more than two months.[42] The life span of mice was increased by almost a third by removing one gene.[43 44] The missing gene did not appear to disturb their fertility or other functions.

In 1996, scientists discovered the gene that causes Werner's syndrome, a rare inherited disease that causes premature aging.[45] The disease causes a 20-year-old to have gray hair and the health ailments of someone much older, e.g., cataracts, osteoporosis, and heart disease. Most people with Werner's syndrome die before 50. This gene and the enzyme it triggers appear to play a vital role in how DNA repairs itself and reproduces and is a promising key to how genes program aging.

Telomeres are the extensions on the ends of chromosomes. They are composed of DNA material but do not appear to contain genetic codes. When chromosomes reproduce, the telomeres get shorter. In 1973, Calvin Harley[46] proposed that telomere shortening was the mechanism that limits how many times a chromosome can reproduce. That limit is called the Hayflick effect after Leonard Hayflick, who demonstrated that most types of cells can only reproduce about fifty times. Michael Fossel, a neurobiologist and physician, believes that there are several ways to prevent telomeres from shortening and even ways to restore them to their original size, reversing the aging process and restoring youth.[47] He expects the first human trials by 2005 and widespread telomere therapy by 2015.[48]

In 1997, articles in *Science* and *Nature* indicated that telomeres shrink and lengthen over and over as cells divide, and form a "buffer zone" to protect the DNA.[49] While this questions the simplicity of Fossel's theory, it illustrates how research on telomeres is closing in on exactly how chromosomes work. After Nobel Laureate Thomas Cech identified the human gene that controls the telomerase enzyme, two teams of scientists have introduced the gene into human tissue in the laboratory and found the cells divided indefinitely (while untreated cells all eventually died).[50] Likely initial applications are in helping tissues heal faster.

Brown University researcher John Sedivy[51] has identified a human gene that suppresses the number of times a cell can reproduce (the Hayflick effect). He grew human cells in the laboratory and "knocked out" (removed) the p21 genes. These cells had up to thirty more divisions than cells that still had the p21 gene. Eventually, physicians might be able to remove human cells, knock out the p21 gene and reintroduce the cells into the person's body.

Medical knowledge that improves the quality of life

Advances like hormone replacement therapy go beyond curing disease or letting a person live more years. Hormone replacement has improved the quality of life for women's postmenopausal years. It helps women look and feel younger and avoids the emotional swings, physical symptoms, and memory problems that often accompany menopause. It also reduces the risk of Alzheimer's disease, osteoporosis, heart disease, and colon cancer. New generations of birth control/hormone replacement pills are being developed that will allow treatment to be more individualized to a woman's health history.[52] Harvard scientists[53] have given female mice an implant that keeps their ovaries from dying, thereby blocking the onset of menopause. They think the same method could easily be applied to women to eliminate menopause. Research is also underway to develop "designer" estrogen replacement that will allow men to take estrogen without the feminizing effects (e.g., breast enlargement, increased ratio of fat tissue). This would help reduce men's risk of heart disease and possibly Alzheimer's disease.

Testosterone therapy for men is in an earlier stage of development but is promising. In 1996, *Newsweek* magazine had a cover story on testosterone and DHEA and stories from men who reported these hormones reversed aging and increased their muscle mass, energy, and sexual drive.[54] While more research is needed before such treatments can been regarded as routine, replacing declining hormones appears promising for men as well as women.

In a 1990 landmark study, Daniel Rudman and University of Wisconsin researchers gave healthy men ages 61 to 81 a synthetic Human Growth Hormone (HGH). The injections reversed biological aging by twenty years with a 9% increase in muscle, a 14% decrease in body fat, a 7% increase in skin thickness, and increased strength, improved memory, increased vigor, and enhanced stamina.[55] This was without changes in diet or activities. The control group continued with normal aging. Based on Rudman's results, the National Institute of Aging funded five million dollars of research at nine university medical centers.[56]

Genentech developed recombinant human growth hormone in 1985 for treatment of children whose growth was stunted. A year later Eli Lilly developed a Human Growth Hormone that differed by one amino acid and exactly matched real human growth hormone. After a court battle, the two were given exclusive rights to manufacture human growth hormones under the Orphan Drug Act. The hormone has been used by tens of thousands of children. Khansari and Gustad[57] report that injecting mice with growth hormone has greatly increased the mice's life spans. Swedish researchers administered low doses of human growth hormones to humans and reported improved health with no side effects.[58] Klatz[59] and Cranton and Fryer[60] give several case histories of people who are taking human growth hormones and achieving results similar to the Rudman study. Chein and Terry[61] report using human growth hormone with 800 patients with none of the patients having any major side effects. While Human Growth Hormones are achieving impressive results, they are not likely to be widely used because they have to be injected and are very expensive. In 2000, Human Growth Hormone therapy cost about $10,000 a year, though the price is coming down.

Secretagogues (pronounced suh-CREE-ta-gogs) are chemicals that cause other organs to secrete substances. The term is often used to refer to chemicals which cause the pituitary gland to produce growth hormones. Secretagogues have been used with abnormally short children to prompt more normal growth. Merck (pharmaceutical co.) has commissioned studies of secretagogues with adults. While generally secretive about progress, they do report that elderly people who have used their medication, MK-677, have increased muscle mass, an increased sense of well being, and sleep better.[62] Secretagogues can be taken in a daily pill form, making it more palatable and less expensive. Secretagogues are preferred to HGH as they prompt the body to release HGH in a more natural pattern. Thus, a pill to "turn back the clock" is in human trials with a major pharmaceutical company. Six major pharmaceutical companies are developing secretagogues. The Internet has about a hundred secretagogue products that purportedly prompt the body to produce HGH. Eventually, consumers will have good data on the pros and cons and how to choose the most appropriate secretagogue.

There are a number of commercial products being hyped to improve memory. These have to be viewed very skeptically. Most probably only give placebo benefits unless you happen to have a deficiency the product happens to correct. There is a lot of university and pharmaceutical company research on medications that would enhance memory. Gary Lynch at the University of California–Irvine has identified a class of biochemicals, ampakines, that do appear to improve memory in humans, especially older people.[63] His 54 human subjects showed remarkable improvement in pre/post testing on word games, mazes, and photograph recognition tasks. Young men improved scores by 20% and men over 60 improved their scores by 100%.[64] The change was rapid and short-lived. Cortex Pharmaceuticals has a pill form of the substance under the trade name Ampalex.[65] Genetic engineering has had several examples of enhancing memory and intellectual functioning in animals. Antioxidants have shown considerable promise in preventing the mental deterioration that goes with aging[66] and in improving memory.[67] University of Saskatchewan researchers[68] working with mice have been able to stimulate new nerve growth in the hippocampus (an area deep in the brain that is associated with memory). Two research teams have used genetic engineering to increase the intelligence of mice by inserting a gene.[69]

One of the mechanisms of aging is glucose cross-linking with proteins. Cross-linking makes tissue rigid and gives it a yellowish or brownish color. The process affects our bones, joints, teeth, kidneys, the lenses of our eyes, and, of course, our blood vessels. In our blood vessels the glucose links with cholesterol. This causes a narrowing of the arteries, which increases blood pressure, increases the risk of a stroke, and impedes blood from getting to its destinations. The cross-links were thought to be almost impossible to break. A new drug, Timagedine, however, breaks the cross-links. It is in clinical trials and showing promising results. If it or a comparable medication is successful, it will be possible to undo much of the damage, and stiffness, that at least until now has come with aging.

Another mechanism of aging is cumulative damage caused by free radicals (unattached electrons, usually oxygen, looking for a meaningful relationship with atoms). The 1990s brought a much greater understanding of how certain food, vitamins, and supplements help combat free radical damage. These include: vitamins C, E, and B-12 (folic acid), selenium, Coenzyme Q-10, lipoic acid, phytochemicals, flavonoids, and carotenoids. Researchers have found that excess iron is one of the most pernicious sources of free radical damage. Consequently it is being removed from many multiple vitamins. Many current centenarians did not have the benefit of daily vitamins, much less the more tailored vitamin and supplements available today. Vitamin C supplements, for example, have been found to reduce the incidence of advanced cataracts by 80%.[70] A National Institute of Aging study[71] found vitamin E supplements delayed the progression of Alzheimer's disease by seven months. Vitamin B-12 and B-6 supplements have reduced heart attacks in women by half.[72] The examples could go on and on.

Researchers[73] have identified nitrones–antioxidants that trap free radicals and prevent brain damage–that not only prevent antioxidant damage to brain tissue, but reverse damage in mice. When injected with the chemical, old mice performed as well on mazes as the young mice. The treatment prevents the plaque build up found in Alzheimer's disease. The researchers indicate that the treatment should be applicable to people. While it wouldn't necessarily extend life spans, it would improve the quality of life.

In the early 1990s men who had difficulty getting erections were injecting a vasodilatory drug into their penises. Then Pfizer (pharmaceutical company) introduced Viagra. Now seven million American men are taking sixty million pills a year to help them obtain erections.[74] Viagra is now facing competition from Vasomax and Apomorphine.

Since 1960 death rates from heart disease and stroke have been reduced by more than 50%. Even the common colds and flus might be curtailed by a new medication, Pleconaril,[75] which is showing promise in clinical trials. Plenconaril works by disabling the virus that causes colds and flus and meningitis.

You don't have to look old

Crowns and tooth implants are making it possible for virtually everyone who practices good oral hygiene to have teeth that last a lifetime. Grandmother might have had dentures at 50 but you can have permanent teeth at 150. Millions of people wear contact lenses instead of glasses. Radial keratoplasty and photorefractive keratectomy offers surgical correction for some forms of nearsightedness to 250,000 Americans a year.[76] Cataract surgery and cornea replacement is more than twenty years old. Researchers have successfully transplanted retinal cells into the eyes of rats and are working on developing the technology for people.[77] Scientists are also experimenting with cochlear implants that might eventually help people with hearing impairments hear better.

Plastic surgery was once just for movie stars. Face lifts and abdominal reshaping are becoming increasingly sophisticated, safer, and less intrusive each year. The cost is now within the reach of the middle class. Between 1994 and 1997, 87,000 Americans had face lifts at an average cost of $4,300.[78] In 1997 alone there were two million cosmetic procedures performed in the U.S. Liposuction can excise unwanted fat. Skin care products are helping skin stay resilient longer. Skin cells are being cloned and grown in laboratories for burn victims needing skin transplants. This research will help scientists learn how to help facial skin that has lost its resiliency. Skin creams are in clinical trials that dissipate wrinkles and greatly speed the healing of scars and skin problems.

The obvious hair plugs in hair transplants in the 1970s have been replaced by very sophisticated surgeries. While Minoxidil (Rogaine) and Propecia have only shown modest results in growing hair, pharmaceutical companies know the pay off for a medication to grow hair will be enormous and they are investing millions. Gene researchers have been able to activate resting hair follicles in mice by inserting a gene.[79] [80] [81]   While at a very rudimentary stage, researchers[82] were able to transplant sheaths surrounding hair follicles from the scalp of a man to the arm of a woman who had an incompatible blood and tissue type. Her arm then grew head hair with xy (male) chromosomes. Key to the success was eliminating parts of the tissue that would prompt an immune system rejection, including making sure there were no blood cells in the transplanted sheath. Someday a hair cell, that was transplanted from another person, might make a great plot twist in a murder mystery novel. Meanwhile, good hair pieces can look very real and provide protection from the sun.

Fitness training has become a science. Trainers have become much more sophisticated about how to exercise to obtain the desired strength, aerobic, and flexibility results. Gyms, spas, trainers, home exercise equipment, television programs, and videotapes make very effective exercise within the reach of almost everyone.

Resolving the nutrition puzzle

Common sense says that nutrition plays a significant role in longevity. The literature on nutrition, however, is a tower of Babel. The U.S. government says eggs and red meat are evil and a few years later says they aren't so bad. Even moderate alcohol consumption is blessed by research findings. One author advocates a vegetarian diet while another wants high protein and still another prescribes diets by body types or blood types. Linus Pauling says everyone needs thousands of units of vitamin C each day while the U.S. Government says the recommended daily allowance for adults is 60 mg. Then there are true believers who claim that a particular vitamin or supplement is the critical secret to longevity. Other than avoiding extremes, it's hard to know what to believe. The good news is that research on nutrition is developing a much better understanding of the relationship between nutrition and metabolic processes, hormones, and neural transmitters.

Research on centenarians has found that most lead fairly normal lives and do not follow special diets or take magic pills. They have a wide variety of eating habits and do not go on diets. About the only clear health distinctions between them and people with shorter life spans is that they have kept a stable body weight throughout their life, are physically fit, and do not smoke. Biographies also suggest that most tend to eat a wide variety of foods. Personality traits such as independence, self-reliance, optimism, dealing with problems, using their minds, and having a sense of purpose appear to be more important than what they eat. Reuben Andres' extensive study of mortality patterns challenged conventional wisdom by finding the lowest mortality rates among people who were 10% over ideal body weights and higher mortality among those 10% underweight.[83]

Mind over matter

Drug trials have to include a placebo (sugar pill) because, on the average, one-third of the response to medications is due to expectations (the placebo effect). The "mind-body" literature is replete with case histories of people who had terminal cancer, changed their lives, and lived for many years. Robert Dilts[84] helped his mother achieve this when her physician told her to "get her affairs in order." He relates that he began his research by seeking literature on people who survived cancer. The medical librarians told him they did not have any data on that until he finally came up with the term "remission." *Re-mission* is an apt word as many survivors made major changes in their lifestyles and developed a new *mission* in life. Herbert Benson describes the role beliefs and religion can play in health and healing.[85] Bernie Siegel describes how mental health can be critical in beating cancer.[86] [87] The mind-body literature is also replete with case histories of people who suffer a loss, such as the death of a spouse, lose their "will to live" and die despite good health before the loss. Depression, stress, worry, anger, resentment, and dealing with loss all can take their toll. Effectively dealing with emotions, frustration, and loss are essential to longevity.

Old isn't what it used to be

Our society offers scripts for what to expect as we age. Traditional scripts are to retire at 65, face progressively deteriorating health, and become irrelevant. Traditional scripts do not include living past one hundred or living a vital life much past 70. Challenges to conventional thinking are starting to appear in our culture, like a *New York Times Magazine* special issue titled "Funny We Don't Feel Old."[88] Such articles, however, are still sparse. Unless you have a clear vision of an alternative, it is easy to get sucked into the conventional expectations. Today, to be a centenarian is to be an oddity. The president and Willard Scott send birthday greetings. The newspaper may run an article and ask your "secret" for longevity. In a decade or two it won't be so unusual.

The U.S. Census Bureau estimates for the number of centenarians at:

$$75,000 \text{ in } 2000$$
$$170,000 \text{ in } 2010$$
$$299,000 \text{ in } 2020$$
$$477,000 \text{ in } 1930$$
$$659,000 \text{ in } 2040$$
$$1,208,000 \text{ in } 2050.[89]$$

The aging of our population will create profound shifts in what we think of as old.

People who are centenarians in the 1990s survived very hard times. Only 50% have pension incomes and 12% are on public assistance.[90] More than 60% have less than an eighth grade education. By the year 2015, however, only 10-15% of centenarians will have less than an eighth grade education.[91] Better educated people tend to be more resourceful, have more financial resources, and be more attentive to their nutrition and health. Our increased education, prosperity, and health and beauty products will make for greater stamina and kinder, gentler physical aging. Demographic studies have found that chronic disability rates among Americans over 65 have declined 1-2% a year since 1982, when the surveys began.[92] [93]

Beliefs and expectations are factors too

Everyone knew that no one could run a 4-minute mile because the human body just wasn't capable of doing it. Roger Bannister[94] believed it could be done and used different training regimens, strategies, and beliefs than other runners used. Within a year of his breaking the 4-minute mile barrier in 1954, 37 other runners ran a mile under 4 minutes. New records have been established 17 times and dozens of high school students have run the mile in less than 4 minutes. The current record is 3 minutes and 44.39 seconds. Just wishing something does not make it so and just wishing for a long, vital life doesn't make it happen. Beliefs about what happens to people as they age, however, can become a self-fulfilling prophecy that limits our longevity. Like Roger Bannister, we need to believe it is possible to do something most people don't think can be done–to live to 150 or longer. Like Roger Bannister, we need to develop strategies to achieve new milestones.

Can you really live to be 150? In the late 1950s Leonard Hayflick found that cells appear to have a biological clock that limits the number of times each cell can divide. His research convinced many scientists that human cells had a longevity potential of 115 years. Even when cells stop dividing, they don't necessarily die. Their DNA continues to give instructions and make proteins.[95] Recent research has shown that some cells divide more than others and that genetic engineering can greatly extend the number of cell divisions. As Deepak Chopra[96] points out, Hayflick's studies of aging of cells in test tubes and petri dishes ignore the profound influence that thoughts, feelings, actions, and hormones play in aging vs. longevity. Researchers[97] have been able to add telomerase to human tissue in the laboratory and enable it to reproduce indefinitely (so far 165 times which is more than three times the normal limit). The concern has been that it might prompt cancer but so far the cells are cancer free.

Researchers are skeptical about reports of people in remote areas living over 120 years. Many such claims to longevity are difficult to document because records of the births would be over a hundred years old and hard to locate if records ever existed. Two of the best documented "oldest old" are Jeanne Calment, a French woman who lived 122 years and Izumi Shigichio, a Japanese man who lived 120 years.

Life expectancy tables give extrapolated estimates of the age at which half of the newborns born in the designated year would have died. In the U.S. the life expectancy has risen from 49 in 1900 to over 76 in 1998. The Japanese have a longer life expectancy of 80. Those who have already survived childhood and part of adulthood have even longer life expectancies. Barring a plague worse than AIDS, the average life span is likely to continue to climb. These data are averages and include infant deaths and people who sabotage their longevity with alcoholism, drug abuse, cigarette smoking, obesity, and other self-destructive behaviors.

If you are a reasonably healthy adult who does not engage in these self-destructive behaviors, your life expectancy will be well beyond the 76-year figure. The number of American centenarians has been doubling every ten years. Statistics tell us that the distribution curve for longevity is not likely to abruptly stop at age 115 but have a tapering tail into even older ages. These statistics, however, are like looking in a rear view mirror as they are based on the lifestyles and health resources of previous generations and do not take into account current and future medical advances and other advances that add to longevity.

Assumptions about life expectancy and maximum life span are likely to be blindsided by paradigm shifts and new technology. There have always been scientists who made pronouncements about limits and things that can't be done, e.g.,

- The world won't be able to feed any more people because population increases in a geometric ratio and the ability to produce food only increases in an arithmetic ratio. (Thomas Malthus in 1798 when the world's population was one billion as opposed to six billion two hundred years later.[98])
- Man will never fly.
- Electrons are the smallest particle possible.
  (That is until quarks were discovered.)
- Man is the only animal that uses tools. (Jane Goodall disproved this when she observed chimpanzees using sticks to "fish" for ants.[99])

- Cloning is just science fiction. (Baa says Dolly, the world's first cloned sheep.[100] [101] In 2000 we even had bulls that were clones of cloned bulls.[102])
- Computers can't think. (This one is still open to debate but the computers are closing in on the distinction.)

There are numerous instances of medical "facts" changing. To cite a recent few:[103]

- Stomach ulcers are caused by stress. (While stress contributes to ulcers, medical researchers have determined that ulcers are caused by helicobacter bacteria. Physicians are now successfully treating ulcers with antibiotics.)
- Sugar makes children, especially hyperactive children, hyper. (While there might be some individual cases in which this is true, clinically "blind" studies have convincingly shown no significant increase in activity from sugar.)

Finally, there are beliefs about aging that do not square with current research, e.g.:

- If you live long enough, you will get Alzheimer's disease. (While credible projections from the 1994 Canadian Study of Health and Aging predicted that virtually anyone over 100 would have Alzheimer's, the projection did not square with research on centenarians. Most centenarians do not have Alzheimer's disease.[104] Perls[105] reports that if you make it to 100 you apparently are not at risk for getting Alzheimer's.
- Your brain stops growing after puberty. (Research with mice is clear that stimulating environments effect a flurry of dendrite growth, making new connections in the brain and that physical exercise helps the brain grow blood vessels.[106] Research published in *Nature* in 1996 demonstrated that adult rats in enriched environments developed 15% more neurons in their hippocampal cells.[107])
- IQ declines dramatically starting around age 20. (Many of these conclusions were derived from tests that compared older generations with current generations. Older generations, however, had far less education and stimulation than current generations. Further, many of these studies failed to exclude people who had

health and mental conditions, e.g., Alzheimer's. When these design problems are eliminated, test scores were stable or even improved on many tests until age 60. At 60 researchers started seeing great variance in scores among test takers. Healthy, flexible, better educated individuals continued to do well while less educated individuals were more likely to lose skills. I presume that research would also find that people who continued to read and learn throughout their life did especially well. How good are you at remembering a telephone number you just heard for the first time? Beard[108] had 166 centenarians take a Digit Span test (which is part of the most respected intelligence test). When asked to repeat back a series of numbers, 78% of the centenarians could remember and repeat 4 numbers, 60% 5 numbers, and 38% 6 or more numbers. Two centenarians even remembered and repeated 8 numbers. Generally, older people could do things about as well as they used to but couldn't do things as fast as they used to or couldn't do as many things simultaneously as in the past. On the other hand, they had a much richer knowledge base. To make a comparison with computers, their hard drives had a lot more data and programs but their operating speed (megahertz) was slower than the ever faster new computers. Also keep in mind that pre/post IQ data are pretty old data. Today's health and medical advances might yield much better performance for older people in the future.) In one of the studies, with excellent methodology to control for complicating variables, 70% of participants did not show cognitive decline when retested five or seven years later. These were all individuals over age 65. The 30% who did show decline had atherosclerosis of the carotid arteries (which go to the brain), peripheral vascular disease, diabetes, and/or the APOE e4 gene which is associated with Alzheimer's disease. The e4 gene also appeared to accelerate decline for all of these conditions except for atherosclerosis. The e4 gene, of course, is under intense study for genetic engineering and other interventions.

- You lose 100,000 brain cells a day–never to be replaced, leading to cognitive deterioration with aging. (Even if this were true, the brain has a trillion neurons and in a 150-year life span you would lose less than 1% of your neurons. MRI scans, however, have found that the data were erroneous for people in good health. The earlier studies were flawed by limited instrumentation and by including people with Alzheimer's and other brain diseases. Harvard professor Marilyn Albert[109] followed subjects from their teenage years and found four factors that correlated with good brain functioning: education, physical activity, lung function, and self-efficacy. Research published in *Science* in 1996 reported that while neurons and their myelin coverings might shrink, there is little loss of cortical neurons in normally aging human brains–a much more hopeful state for interventions.[110])

- Japanese and Swedes live longer than Americans. (They have a longer *average* life expectancy because the U.S. has rather high infant mortality rates and somewhat higher death rates until middle age. American adults who reach 80, however, live one or two years longer than Japanese, Swedes, French, and English counterparts.[111])

- Each year you age you are at greater risk of disability or death. (Studies in several countries have found a decline in the mortality rates starting at around age 100, i.e., a person has better odds of making it from 110 to 111 than he or she did of making it from 90 to 91.[112]

- Thin is good, overweight is bad. (As discussed in Chapter 10, Reuben Andres[113] found that the Metropolitan Insurance tables used for ideal weight are too liberal with young adults and too strict with adults over 40. Adults over 40 or 50 who were 10%-20% overweight according to Metropolitan Insurance tables had lower mortality rates than their age counterparts who weighed less. Heymsfield and Allison[114] found that adults over 70 who were 20 pounds, even up to 50 pounds over ideal body weights did not have increased mortality rates while thin adults, even with those with identified diseases excluded, had higher mortality rates.)

- Economists and futurologists lament that centenarians will bankrupt Medicare and Social Security. A U.S. Health Care Financing Administration study found that the average medical expenditures for the last two years of life for centenarians was $8,300 while the average medical expenditures for the last two years of life for people who die at 70 is $22,600.[115] Grim predictions of economic age warfare also ignore that fact that many centenarians continue to contribute to society with paid or volunteer work.

- Getting older is depressing. (To the contrary, studies have found that the older people get, the happier they are.[116] Robert Browning had it right when he said,

> *Grow old along with me! The best is yet to be.*
> *The last of life, for which the first was made.*
> –Robert Browning

Longevity data are a little like autopsies–people have to die before you can gather the data. The data don't take into consideration medical advances and lifestyle. Thus, longevity data are always out of date before the data are issued. Looking at the rapid growth of medical treatments and prevention, great gains in longevity appear inevitable. This leaves you with choices. You can choose to base your assumptions about your longevity on:

- **the technology that is available to you now and will be available to you in the future**
                              -or-
  the state of health and technology of previous generations

- **the lifestyle and mental edge you can live to enhance your longevity**
                              -or-
  average people's lifestyles and thinking

- **reports of healthy, vital, active centenarians**
                              -or-
  conventional "wisdom" about people over 65 losing their memory, not having sex, and "going downhill fast"

The idea of living to 150 years or more used to require a leap of faith, much like a religious person who says she can't prove God exists but has faith. If she were wrong in taking that leap of faith, she would just be dead anyway and had lived a good life. If she is right, she has a heavenly reward. If you believe you will live to 150 and are wrong, you would just die at an earlier age than you hoped (but probably still older than if you had not tried). If you are right, you will live well and long with extra decades to contribute and participate.

With the incredible scientific leaps of knowledge, living to 150 is no longer a leap of faith. The question is not whether, but when and who. You can choose to pretend that science will take a holiday and will not produce any advances to improve longevity and quality of life. Or you can choose to base your life decisions on resources you already have and likely scientific advances that can greatly enhance your life. For those who choose the mental edge and take advantage of resources, the data support the very real possibility of healthy, vital living to 150–and even longer.

Think of all you'd derive just from being alive
And this is the best part, you have a head start
If you are among the very young at heart
–J. Richards and M. Carr's song, *Young at Heart*

Appendix

36 Defy Aging Beliefs

1. My mind is a muscle and I keep it strong and fit my whole life.
2. I can have a sexually fulfilling life my whole life.
3. I practice continuous quality improvement with my mental and physical health.
4. I listen to my body and proactively foster good health.
5. I always have a mission.
6. I search for the smart way to do things.
7. My mind, body, and spirit are constantly renewing themselves.
8. I cultivate my sense of humor.
9. I cultivate a positive vocabulary.
10. I cultivate fond memories and let bad memories wither.
11. Any suggestions of surgery prompt an intense search for alternative solutions.
12. I move like a 20-year-old.
13. I exercise my eyes to improve my vision.
14. I am a lifelong learner.
15. Every age has its benefits.
16. I expect to have an enjoyable, exciting life at 150.
17. I am a trailblazer who leaves behind conventional thinking about longevity.
18. I have a serenity about outliving most people I know.
19. I make new friends all my life.
20. I'm really younger than my chronological age.
21. I pace myself–I'm going to be around a long time.
22. I choose life enhancing risks and reduce risks with little benefit.

23. I use the serenity prayer to give me perspective.

24. I am cheerful.

25. I have a contingency fund.

26. I observe and follow what works for me rather than blindly following generic or expert advice.

27. The resources for living longer are improving every year.

28. There are no accidents in life.

29. I don't need many material things to make me happy and successful.

30. If I intelligently pursue what I love, the money will come.

31. People want to help.

32. I can get everything in life I want if I just help enough other people get what they want.

33. If I lock in my intent, the universe will provide.

34. Anything I need to know is available to me–in a book, library, the Internet, other people, or myself.

35. Most problems are just inconveniences or challenges.

36. We are fortunate to live in a longevity revolution.

Appendix

Example of a Comprehensive Mission Statement
(as of 1/1/00)

1. Vision statement
(for brevity only my vision for defying aging is included)

Vision headline:
live longer, healthier, and better than I ever imagined

An ageless society

Every year the world has become a more magnificent feast of information, activities, and ideas. It's a playground inviting us to gather some playmates and play.

Americans have outgrown the youth cult culture and appreciate people of all ages. We have become an ageless society. With hormone replacements, wrinkle removing, and other medical advances, it's often hard to tell how old someone is anyway. There are centenarians who look, move, and think like 30-year-olds. After childhood age has become meaningless. People are valued for their qualities and contributions rather than their age or color. One hundred is as common as 65 was at the turn of the century. With so much change, people increasingly appreciate the continuity and perspective that experienced people offer. The Mentors for Families Foundation has facilitated many older people "adopting" children and families to be a surrogate grandparent and mentor for struggling families.

Many people pursue serial careers and their cross-pollinating of ideas has become one of the most generative sources of innovation. The very fluid job market rewards workers according to their skills, talent, character, and the services they offer. Many people are self-employed. Most older Americans are financially comfortable enough that they feel they can afford to invest in health, fitness, relationships, helping others, and making a contribution. Centenarians are valued members of society who share their talents and wisdom in profit, nonprofit, and volunteer settings. With so much change people find comfort in leadership by experienced people just as millions were comforted by hearing the evening news by Walter Cronkite, news analysis by Daniel Shore, or leadership by President Reagan.

As the hippie movement in the 1960s and the environmental movement of the 1980s produced a shift in values and consciousness, the whole person movement of the 2010s shifted the focus from materialism to integration of mental, physical, and spiritual health. Brain wave biofeedback devices help people better identify and choose their emotional states and moods. Like dentist visits, most doctor visits are for checkups, monitoring, early detection, and prophylaxis. Telehealth monitoring helps with early identification of problems. Checkups are proactive consultations on how to be as fit and healthy as possible (as opposed to just checking for diseases). Anti-aging medicine is the most common medical specialty. Hearing and vision problems are readily treatable. Genetic engineering corrects a lot of health problems before they are manifested. Cancer, heart problems, and diabetes are as manageable or treatable as tuberculosis. Physicians and the public have a much better understanding of how the mind and body are part of one system.

In the 1990s more and more college students were over thirty. Now half of college students are over fifty. Learning technologies have made it easier to learn information and to understand complex relationships. Brain wave biofeedback devices help people access optimal learning states. The world's best teachers use virtual reality demonstrations to aid learning. Computer chip implants help people supplement their brains with information and information processing skills. Campuses, neighborhoods, and organizations have more of a mix of ages than ever before. With most of the population over 40, television, radio, and the new media formats are offering very diverse and more sophisticated programs at a wide variety of intellectual levels. Information and programs are available on demand 24 hours a day at home.

2. Mission statement:

to learn, practice, and teach how to live healthy, vital, productive lives for 150 years

3. Primary question:

Are you walking your talk?
Alternate: How can you elicit a resourceful state in yourself and in others (now)?

4. Scripts

My parents were at the extreme end of the spectrum on not telling me what to do or giving guidance. Thus I wrote most of my own scripts, often modeling teachers and professors who had a passion for making the world a better place. My mother scripted me for "being more sensitive" (to feelings) than "other men." My father modeled hard work and letting actions speak louder than words. Both modeled very ethical behavior without discussing it or making an issue of it. Both believed in Christian teachings but were not affiliated with a church and did not talk much about religion, other than an interest in Edgar Cayce and Mom attending a Cayce study group on a weekly basis. At 14 I started taking myself to a large interdenominational church. At age 25 I chose to convert to Judaism and to follow a new script.

5. Longevity values

1. My mind is a muscle and I keep it strong and fit my whole life.
2. I can have a sexually fulfilling life my whole life.
3. I practice continuous quality improvement with my mental and physical health
4. I listen to my body and proactively foster good health.
5. I always have a mission.
6. I search for the smart way to do things.

7. My mind, body, and spirit are constantly renewing themselves.
8. I cultivate my sense of humor.
9. I cultivate a positive vocabulary.
10. I cultivate fond memories and let bad memories wither.
11. Any suggestions of surgery prompt an intense search for alternative solutions.
12. I move like a 20-year-old.
13. I exercise my eyes to improve my vision.
14. I am a lifelong learner.
15. Every age has its benefits.
16. I expect to have an enjoyable, exciting life at 150.
17. I am a trailblazer who leaves behind conventional thinking about longevity.
18. I have a serenity about outliving most people I know.
19. I make new friends all my life.
20. I'm really younger than my chronological age.
21. I pace myself–I'm going to be around a long time.
22. I choose life enhancing risks and reduce risks with little benefit.
23. I use the serenity prayer to give me perspective.
24. I am cheerful.
25. I have a contingency fund.
26. I observe and follow what works for me rather than blindly following generic or expert advice.
27. The resources for living longer are improving every year.
28. There are no accidents in life.
29. I don't need many material things to make me happy and successful.
30. If I intelligently pursue what I love, the money will come.
31. People want to help.
32. I can get everything in life I want if I just help enough other people get what they want.
33. If I lock in my intent, the universe will provide.
34. Anything I need to know is available to me–in a book, library, the Internet, other people, or myself.
35. Most problems are just inconveniences or challenges.
36. We are fortunate to live in a longevity revolution.

6. Other values

Affirmations:

- I am called to be an extraordinary parent and husband, and give my family moral guidance and help them develop their talents and skills. *Anytime I have rapport with family members, or realize and help with their needs (not necessarily their wants), or compliment them, or elicit resourceful states from them, or provide guidance or inspiration, I am following my purpose.*

- I walk my talk and foster my own longevity. *Anytime I do something that contributes to my own longevity, I am following my vision and mission.*

- I choose to do the right thing. *Anytime I do the right thing, I am following my values and God's will.*

Beliefs:

- Following Jewish values and traditions enriches my life and gives it continuity and connection. *Anytime I study Jewish literature, pray, observe Jewish traditions, or pass on Jewish traditions I am following my values.*

- Being a lifelong learner is as important as eating each day. *Anytime I learn something new, read, listen to tapes, or listen to informative radio or television programs, I am enriching my mind and following my purpose by sharpening my saw.*

- Being on the cutting edge charges my batteries. *Anytime I pursue cutting edge training or ventures, I am rewarded.*

- I have an obligation to help make the world a better place. *Anytime I do something that contributes to making the world a better place I am following my purpose in life and God's will.*

- Effectively managing finances, earning money, and saving money provides an essential tool for meeting my goals. *Every time I generate more income, or derive more value from purchases, or save money for the future, or learn about successful investing, or make money investing, or learn from my mistakes, I am following my plan.*

- Cultivating optimism makes me and others more successful and happier. *Every time I choose an optimistic interpretation, or make an optimistic reframe, or help others to be optimistic, I am making the world a better place and helping people, including myself, be happier and more successful.*

7. Toward Rules (Included in the beliefs in #6.)

8. Away Rules

I have become much better at not slipping into unresourceful emotional states–particularly depression, anger, embarrassment, and irritation. At the first sign that I am slipping into any of these, I do whatever it takes to get out of them including:
- gaining perspective
- identifying more effective alternatives
- assessing what I learned
- reframing the situation
- imagining myself in the future looking back at the situation
- playing resourceful music
- engaging in resourceful physical activity such as exercise, cleaning, or dancing

9. Capabilities
- good writing skills
- good speaking skills
- good coaching and therapy skills
- creative, innovative thinker
- good leadership skills
- can be very assertive and persistent
- good at perspective and common sense

10. Goals (Behaviors)

BY DECEMBER 31, 2000 and BY DECEMBER 31, 2006		
(omitted for brevity)		
BY 65TH BIRTHDAY (September 25, 2010)		

my speaking/writing/coaching career will be going well, will have several books and/or tapes and free Internet newsletter with more than 100,000 subscribers; David and Rachel will be in college and the twins in fifth grade, and I will be in excellent health and doing 75 uninterrupted pushups each morning	having the time of my life, on top of my game	work the plan and walk my talk . . . etc.

BY 100TH BIRTHDAY (September 25, 2045)		
Cut work down to part-time, excellent health, sharp mind, great friends, lots of grandchildren, and possibly a great grandchild; still writing, speaking, and coaching, periodically take sabbaticals	having the time of my life, on top of my game	−work the plan and walk my talk . . . etc.

BY 150TH BIRTHDAY (September 25, 2095)		
Excellent health, sharp mind, great friends, lots of grandchildren, great grandchildren, & great, great grandchildren; do volunteer work	throughly enjoy the fruits of life and my many blessings, including still being able to give to others	−walk my talk −reassess whether to get an extension on the 150 years . . . etc.

11. Environment

- **Classical music**–when I want to read or write, it usually calms me and helps me have an absorptive mind

- **Fred Astaire**–makes me feel light and breezy, lifts my spirits

- **Opera**–often makes life beautiful but need to be in the right frame of mind

- **Sunshine**–definitely picks up my spirits (and its absence can leave me dragging–use SAD light as needed)

- **Cleaning**–helps me work off irritation

- **Exercise**–gives me energy and leaves me feeling powerful, clean, and renewed (though weight lifting often also requires a nap)

- **Playing with the kids**–brings out my playful side

- **Rapport with my wife**–brings out her affectionate, appreciative, loving side

- **Good talk with friends** like Mike Leahy or Carol Roche–leaves me bubbling with ideas and enthusiasm

Appendix

My Obituary
(sometime after 2095)

The fact that I am giving this speech means that, I am dead. I'm appearing before you through time forward holography. The computer chip tells me that I achieved my goal of living more than 150 years. As you know toward the end of the 21st century it became a custom for centenarians and sesquicentenarians to write their own eulogies to pass on their wisdom. So my purpose today is to share with you what worked in living a vital, fulfilling life for over 150 years.

I was fortunate to have salt of the earth parents who were good people with good values. There was one thing that was very unusual about them. They wouldn't dream of telling their children what to do. I felt that if I told my parents that I was in love with a Martian and wanted to marry her they would have congratulated me and asked when the wedding was. This freedom, which would be a dream come true for many children, provided a great opportunity. It also was a big responsibility. I felt like I had reared myself. I did this by having a lot of role models. Since I was quite shy then, most were models from afar and had no idea they were my role models.

When I graduated from college with a degree in social work, I had a very idealistic mission–to make the world a better place. That mission stuck with me for well over a hundred years and I still believe in it. After college I happened into a rehabilitation counseling program. It was a wonderful happening. The program gave me a budget of about a hundred thousand dollars a year and told me to spend it wisely to help disabled people get their lives back together and get jobs. Back in the sixties, a hundred thousand dollars was a lot of money. It was a real privilege to help people create a new life and often do things that seemed impossible. Eventually, I coordinated a project working with mentally retarded adults. They had lived in an institution almost their whole lives. In those days if you had an IQ less than 60 you might be warehoused in a huge gothic building. We taught the young men to live in apartments or group homes and to work in food service and other jobs. It wasn't supposed to be possible but they did it. It was such a privilege helping them go from such a bleak life to living a normal life.

I was a college professor, an alcoholism counselor, and a clinical psychologist. As with rehabilitation counseling, helping people get their lives together was a great privilege. I discovered an underground movement–Neurolinguistic Programming. I call NLP underground because it was taught in workshops and people had fun–as opposed to college courses where learning was usually dry and dull. NLP practitioners had a lot of insights into how people think and how to make changes [snap finger] very quickly. We did things like curing phobias in twenty minutes. I had been studying hypnosis and getting very good at it. But once I started using NLP and got the quick [snap finger] changes, hypnosis [said very slowly] seemed so plodding and slow. I was hooked on this cutting edge technology and doing the impossible.

My role model in graduate school was professor Henry Leland. He marched to a different drummer and had a vision of what can and should be done to create a normal life for people who had mental retardation. He was very effective in inspiring others to pursue the vision. Probably his only regret in life was that he didn't personally get in a bulldozer and knock down every mental retardation institution in the country. In clinical psychology my role model was psychologist Jim Shulman. He started a one-person private practice and developed it into a four million-dollar practice. He treated staff like family and was more interested in being on the cutting edge than making money–though the money came anyway. Even when he was CEO of a four million-dollar practice, I would often walk into his office and he would be in his hippie beads with the Grateful Dead blaring on the stereo and the incense burning. One of the impossible things he encouraged me to do was to develop a doctoral internship program for future psychologists. The approximately three hundred internship programs were all sponsored by hospitals, universities, government programs, and nonprofit agencies. We became the only private practice to have an accredited internship program.

Managed care took the fun out of private practice. I became captivated with the prospect of people living much, much longer than anyone expected. This was the new frontier. People were talking about living to 100 and it was obvious to me that tens of thousands of people would live to 150 in my lifetime. Longevity experts and advertisements were focused on the physical–do this exercise, take this pill, follow this diet, and eat disgusting sounding stuff like green algae. But I knew that 70% of longevity was mental. (With genetic engineering it is now 90% mental.)

I used my usual strategy of looking for role models. The literature on centenarians was very interesting. Few were vegetarians and not one ate green algae. They only had a few things in common physically. They maintained a constant weight during their adult life, they were very active people, they didn't abuse alcohol, and few smoked–although that Jeanne Calment smoked until she was 117 and set the longevity record at the time at 122 years. What really distinguished them was what was here [gesture to the heart] and here [gesture to the head]. They were extremely resilient people who handled loss, death, and change well. They were eager to learn new things and they always had a sense of purpose. They were very independent people who marched to a different drummer. I thought –that's my script–I can do that.

So I fired my employer and spent the better part of a year writing my first book, *Defy Aging: Develop the Mental and Emotional Vitality to Live Longer, Healthier, and Happier Than You Ever Imagined.* The title was going to be about living to 150 but I found people didn't want to think about being 150 years old. I did personal coaching, radio and TV talk shows, wrote magazine articles and newsletters and had a good time helping people learn what it takes here [heart] and here [head] to live a long vibrant life. Fortunately, I was able to stay close to home and spend a lot of time with my children, David, Rachel, Sharon, and Sonia.

My interest in mental longevity was ahead of the curve and it took awhile for the public to get it. After about ten years it became pop culture just as stress management and self-esteem had in previous decades. With people looking and feeling younger at older ages, they started paying attention to the mental and spiritual aspects of longevity. I wondered whether it would dry up my niche. To the contrary, feeling and looking younger and the spiraling pace of societal and technological change made having a sense of purpose even more poignant.

Colonel Sanders retired at 65. When he saw how paltry his Social Security check was he started hawking his family recipe for chicken. I couldn't imagine retiring. It would be like having a cure for cancer and saying, sorry, I want to play golf. Retiring and the premature aging that often goes with it is caused by losing a sense of purpose and excitement. Besides, I was having too much fun learning, coaching, writing, and being on the cutting edge. Science was helping by helping people look and feel young and healthy and making wrinkles optional. The income was nice too. I did take a lot of sabbaticals.

The challenge was to present my ideas in a way that people would really use them and get great results. Like NLP, it became a collection of strategies. I figured people learn in a lot of different ways so I developed books, workbooks, audio tapes, seminars, and holograms. It was a real coup when Nightingale Conant, the audio/video/holograph company, decided to carry my products. It has been amazing how as I became more "successful" I met more and more "successful" people and it helped my "success" develop more and more momentum.

It wasn't until my 100th birthday that I decided to slow down and forced myself to only work half-time so I could spend more time with my great grandchildren. Paradoxically, the more time I had to think and gain new perspectives, the more I had to write. So the more I slowed down the more I wrote. I wrote more books in my last fifty years than I did in the previous hundred. Throughout my 150 years, I never stopped looking for role models who were marching to a different drum beat, learning new things, or looking for the cutting edge.

I don't know what caused my death. I gather it must have been an acute illness or accident as I don't have any memories of it.

Let me try to summarize the several factors that contributed to my living a long, fulfilling life. I believed I could write my own script and did. I followed different drum beats. I had a passion for being on the cutting edge and doing things that were supposed to be impossible. I was always learning new things and I always had a sense of purpose.

People used to say when you get to age 40 it's all [downhill gesture] downhill. Then it was when you were 65 it's all downhill.

With time it was when you get to be a hundred it's all downhill. Then it was when you get to age 125 it's all downhill. I'm here to tell you that if you take good care of yourself, you take good care of this [heart] and this [head], it just gets better and better.

REFERENCES

Chapter 1: You Are Going to Live Longer- Will You Choose to Live Well?

1. Frost, Robert. (1916). *The road not taken.* New York: Holt, Rinehart, & Winston, pp. 270-171. (This book includes his The Road Not Taken and other poems.)

2. Rowe, John W., & Kahn, Robert L. (1998). *Successful aging.* New York: Pantheon Books, pp. 182-183.

3. *The world almanac and book of facts 1999.* Life expectancy was 47.3 years in 1900 and 76.5 years in 1997 (the latest available data), p. 875.

4. U.S. Census Bureau. Current population reports: Population projections of the United States by age, sex, race, and Hispanic origin: 1993 to 2050. P25-1104.

5. Kolata, Gina. (1996, February 27). New era of robust elderly belies the fears of scientists, *New York Times,* v. 145, pp. A1, C3.

6. Angier, Natalie. (1995, June 11). If you're really ancient, you may be better off, *New York Times,* Sec 4 Week in Review, p. 1.

7. Vita, Anthony. J., Terry, Richard B., Hubert, Helen B., & Fries, James. F. (1998). Aging, health risks and cumulative disability, *New England Journal of Medicine, 338,* 1035-1041.

8. Good health until the last few years is based on the New England Centenarian Study. See: Perls, Thomas T., & Silver, Margery H. (1999). *Living to 100.* New York: Basic Books. Also note the Kolata, Angier, and Vita, *op. cit.*

9. The mental and physical traits were the common denominators that stood out after reviewing hundreds of interviews with centenarians and books such as *Centenarians: The Bonus Years, Living to 100, Centenarians: The New Generation, Centenarians: People over 100: A triumph of will and spirit: The Georgia centenarian study, Centenarians: The story of the 20th century by the Americans who lived it,* and *Jeanne Calment: From Van Gough's time to ours: 122 extraordinary years.* In the last few years there has been a mushrooming of autobiographies and collections of oral histories.

10. The original basis for the 30% figure was a Danish study (discussed in chapter 4) that compared the longevity of fraternal and identical twins. Subsequent research has generally supported this figure and most researchers use the 30% figure. Thomas T. Perls and Margery Silver in *Living to 100* make an interesting case that centenarians may come from a different gene pool. More research is needed on their hypothesis.

11. Edell, Dean. (1999). *Eat, drink and be merry.* New York: HarperCollins.

12. I discovered the term and concept "ageless society" in Klatz, Ronald. (1999). *Ten weeks to a younger you.* Chicago: Sports Tech Labs, Inc.

Chapter 3: Who Will Live to 150 or Longer?

1. Crowley, Susan. (1999, July-August). Live to 100? No thanks, *AARP Bulletin, 40*, pp. 6, 8. This was a phone survey sponsored for the American Association of Retired Persons and conducted April 9-14, 1999 by Market Facts Inc., McLean, VA.

2. Bannister, Roger. (1989). *The four minute mile.* New York: Lyons Press.

3. Seligman, Martin. (1991). *Learned optimism.* New York: Simon & Schuster.

4. Beard, Belle Boone. (1991). *Centenarians: The new generation.* Westport, CN: Greenwood Press, page 1 of the preface.

5. Vaillant, George. (1977). *Adaption to life.* Boston: Little Brown.

6. I took the liberty of translating Vaillant's psychoanalytic terminology into more vernacular terminology.

7. Fiatarone, Maria A., & Garnett, Leah R. (1997, March). Keep on keeping on, *Harvard Health Letter, 22,* 4.

8. Baruch, Bernard. (1954, April 30). Speech to the President's Committee on Employment of the Physically Handicapped (originally said by his father, surgeon, Simon Baruch). As cited in *Gale's Quotations.*

9. Austad, Steven. (1997). *Why we age: What science is discovering about the body's journey through life.* New York: John Wiley & Sons.

10. As cited in Moore, Thomas. (1993). New perspectives on extending human longevity. New York: Simon & Schuster, p. 210.

11. *Ibid.*

12. Perls, Thomas T., & Silver, Margery H. (1999). *Living to 100.* New York: Basic Books.

13. *Ibid.*, pp. 146-151.

14. Kolata, Gina. (1996, February 27). New era of robust elderly belies the fears of scientists, *New York Times, v. 145,* pp. A1, C3.

15. Sorensen, Thorkild, et al. (1988). Genetic and environmental influences on premature death in adult adoptees. *New England Journal of Medicine, 318,* 727-732.

16. Deuteronomy 30:19.

Chapter 4: 36 Beliefs That Foster Your Longevity

1. Esfanidary, F. M. (1973). *Up-wingers: A futurist manifesto.* New York: John Day.

2. The term was coined by Leon Festinger in Festinger, L. (1957). *A theory of cognitive dissonance.* Evanston, IL: Row, Peterson.

3. Cousins, Norman. Interview with Anthony Robbins in *Power talk* cassette tape series (tape #8), (1993) Robbins Research International, 9191 Towne Center Drive, Suite 600, San Diego, CA 92122. [On-line]. www.tonyrobbins.com.

4. Cousins, Norman. (1979). *Anatomy of an illness as perceived by the patient.* New York: Bantam. and Norman Cousins, op cit.

5. Kirsch, I., & Saperstein, G. (1998). Listening to Prozac but hearing placebo: A meta-analysis of antidepressant medication, *Prevention and Treatment, volume 1 issue 1.* [also available On-line by going to: http://members.apa.org/welcome and selecting New Releases: Prevention and Treatment]. The study is also discussed in: Kirsch, I., & Lynn, S. (1999). Automaticity in clinical psychology. *American Psychologist, 54,* 504-515.

6. Morgan, David G. (1997, Fall). The aging of the brain/the aging of the mind. Workshop sponsored by the Institute for CorText Research and Development, P.O. 391480, Mountain View, CA 94039-94039.

7. As cited in Warshofsky, Fred. (1999). *Stealing time.* New York: TV Books, pp. 202-204.

8. Ripley, Kathryn P. (1997, August, 15). The NUN study: Cognitive aging among the very old. In Symposium: Defining normal cognitive aging in the extreme old. (#1106) at the Annual Convention of the American Psychological Association, Chicago, IL.

9. Levy, Becca. (1996). Improving memory in old age through implicit self-stereotyping, *Journal of Personality and Social Psychology, 71,* 1092-1107.

10. Rivers, Joan. (1999). *Don't count the candles just keep the fire lit.* New York: HarperCollins, p. 118.

11. Linkletter, Art. (1988). *Old age is not for sissies.* New York: Viking.

12. *Ibid.,* p. 134.

13. Mahoney, D., & Restak, R. (1988). *The longevity strategy: How to live to 100 using the brain-body connection.* New York: John Wiley.

14. Siegel, Bernie. (1998). *Prescriptions for living.* New York: HarperCollins, p. 88.

15. Mitchell, W. (1993). *The man who would not be defeated.* New York: WRS Group.

16. Reeve, Christopher. (1998). *Still me.* New York: Random House.

17. Csikszentmihalyi, Mihaly. (1999). If we are so rich, why aren't we happy? *American Psychologist, 54,* p. 826.

18. Myers, David G. (1993). *The pursuit of happiness.* New York: Avon.

19. Beard, Belle Boone. (1991). *Centenarians: The new generation.* Westport, CN: Greenwood Press, p. 88.

20. *Ibid.*

21. Data in this section is from Inlander, Charles. (1993). *Good operations –Bad operations: The People's Medical Society's guide to surgery.* New York: Viking Press.

22. Inlander, C. B., Levin, L. S., & Weiner, E. (1988). *Medicine on trial.* New York: Prentice Hall.

23. Egoscue, Peter. (1998). *Pain free: A revolutionary method for stopping chronic pain.* New York: Bantam. Also in: Egoscue, Peter. (1993). *The Egoscue method of health through motion.* New York: HarperCollins.

24. Goodrich, Janet. (1986). *Natural vision improvement.* Berkeley, California: Celestial Arts.

25. Maugham, W. Somerset. (1954). "The summing up" in *The partial view.* London: William Heinmann, p. 172.

26. Hayes, Helen. (1984). *Our best years.* New York: Doubleday.

27. Greer, Germaine. (1992). *The change: Women, aging and menopause.* New York: Alfred A. Knopf.

28. Mroczek, Daniel, & Kolarz, Christian. (1998). The effect of age on positive and negative affect: A developmental perspective on happiness, *Journal of Personality and Social Psychology, 75,* 1333-1349.

29. Beard, Belle Boone. (1991). *Centenarians: The new generation.* Westport, CN: Greenwood Press, p. 12.

30. Lansford, Jennifer E., Sherman, Aurora M., & Antonucci, Toni C. (1998). Satisfaction with social networks: An examination of socioemotional selectivity theory across cohorts, *Psychology and Aging, 13,* 544-552.

31. Rivers, Joan. (1999). *Don't count the candles just keep the fire lit.* New York: HarperCollins, p. 87.

32. Linkletter, Art. (1988). *Old age is not for sissies.* New York: Viking, p. 22.

33. *Ibid.,* p. 32.

34. *Ibid.,* p. 33.

35. As cited in Warshofsky, Steven. (1999). *Stealing time.* New York: TV Books, pp. 59-65.

36. Hamilton, B. (1995). *Getting stared in AA.* Center City, Minnesota: Hazleton, p. 41, 154, 168-169.

37. Brickman, P. Coates, D., & Janoff-Bulman, R. (1978). Lottery winners and accident victims: Is happiness relative? *Journal of Personality and Social Psychology, 36,* 917- 927.

38. Fulgham, Robert. (1991). *Uh-oh.* New York: Ivy, pp. 143-147.

Chapter 5: How to Change Beliefs

1. Based on: Bandler, Richard. (1985). *Using your brain for a change.* Moab, Utah: Real People Press.

2. This Neurolinguistic Programming (NLP) procedure, "kinesthetic belief change" is often taught in advanced NLP workshops. I have not been able to find it described in any books.

3. Anthony Robbins developed this strategy and named it the Dickens pattern. He teaches it in his workshops and includes it in *Personal Power II* cassette tapes (vol. 4) and Compact Discs (CD #8). (1993, 1996), Robbins Research International, 9191 Towne Center Drive Suite 600, San Diego, CA 9212. [On-line]. www.tonyrobbins.com.

4. Chopra, Deepak. (1993). *Ageless body, timeless mind: A quantum alternative to growing old.* New York: Harmony Books, p. 9.

The Chapter 6: The Be-attitudes

1. Seligman, Martin. (1990). *Learned optimism: How to change your mind and your life.* New York: Pocket Books.

2. www.thomasedison.com/edquote.htm.

3. American Psychiatric Association. (1994). *Diagnostic and Statistical Manual of Mental Disorders (Fourth Edition).* Washington, D.C.: American Psychiatric Association, p. 341.

4. Maruta, Toshihiko, et al. (2000, February). Optimists vs pessimists: Survival rate among medical patients over a 30-year period. *Mayo Clinic Proceedings, 75 (2)*, 140-143.

5. Peterson, Christopher. (2000). The future of optimism. *American Psychologist, 55,* 44-55.

6. Seligman, Martin. (1990). *Learned optimism: How to change your mind and your life.* New York: Pocket Books. p. 108.

7. Peabody, Endicott. as cited in *Gale's Quotations.*

8. Baruch, Bernard. (1954). Speech to the President's Committee on Employment of the Physically Handicapped (originally said by his father, Simon Baruch, a surgeon), as cited in *Gale's Quotations.*

9. Robbins, Anthony. (1991). *Awaken the Giant Within,* Summit Books, p. 204. Also in his Unlimited Power Workshops and the accompanying workshop notebook: *Unlimited Power Workshop: The Science of Success Conditioning.*

10. Bandler, Richard. (1987). *Increasing expressiveness,* videotape available from NLP Comprehensive, 1221 Left Hand Canyon Drive, Boulder, Colorado 80302.

11. God grant me the serenity to accept the things I cannot change, the courage to change the things I can, and the wisdom to know the difference.

12. Appearance on the Tonight Show with Jay Leno 9-16-97.

13. Bailey, Roger. (1990). [manual for] *The LAB (Language and Behavior) Profile.* The Language and Behavioral Institute, PO Box 276, West Park, NY 12493, (914) 384-6393.

14. Linkletter, Art. (1988). *Old age is not for sissies.* New York: Viking, p. 33.

15. Fulghum, Robert. *All I really need to know I learned in kindergarten.* New York: Fawcett Books. (Also available on cassette tape.)

Chapter 7: A Lifetime of Mission and Purpose

1. Homer. (circa 750 BCE). *The Odyssey.* Book xv, line 429.

2. Helitzer, Mel. (1992). *Comedy writing secrets.* New York: Writers Digest Books.

3. Adler, Lynn Peters. (1995). *Centenarians: The bonus years.* Santa Fe, New Mexico: Health Press, pp. 169-173.

4. Perls, Thomas, & Sliver, Margery. (1999). *Living to 100.* New York: Basic Books, pp. 35, 55

5. Adler, Lynn Peters. (1995). *Centenarians: The bonus years.* Santa Fe, New Mexico: Health Press, pp. 188-190.

6. *Ibid.,* pp. 200-203.

7. *Ibid.*, pp. 265-268.

8. *Ibid.*, p. 289.

9. *Ibid.*, p. 295.

10. Burney, Melanie. (1999, October 6). Woman to be minister at 81. www.infobeat.com/stories/cgi/story.cgi?id=2561514661-7ea.

11. Adler, Lynn Peters. (1995). *Centenarians: The bonus years.* Santa Fe, New Mexico: Health Press, pp. 260-263.

12. Shuman, Susan. (1999, November). Back to school: Campus communities beckon retirees. *AARP Bulletin, 40,* 9-11.

13. Lewis, Robert. (1999, October). Older workers vow to stay on the job, *AARP Bulletin, 40,* p. 4.

14. Perls, Thomas, & Sliver, Margery. (1999). *Living to 100.* New York: Basic Books, p. 153.

15. Fisher, Mark. (1990). *The instant millionaire.* San Rafael, CA: New World Library, pp. 93-96.

16. Dilts, Robert. (1990). *Changing belief systems with NLP.* Cupertino, CA: Meta Publications, 153-155.

17. Siegel, Bernie. (1989). *Peace, love and healing: Bodymind communication and the path to self-healing: An exploration.* New York: Harper & Row. And in Siegel, Bernie. (1986). *Love, medicine and miracles: Lessons learned about self-healing from a surgeon's experience with exceptional patients.* New York: Harper & Row.

18. Lewitzky, Bella. (1992). In Phillip L. Berman & Connie Goldman (Eds.), *The ageless spirit,* (p. 159). New York: Ballantine.

19. Dilts explains the concept in all of his books including: Dilts, Robert, Hallbom, Tim, & Smith, Suzi. (1990). *Beliefs: Pathways to health and well-being.* Portland, Oregon: Metamorphous Press. and Dilts, Robert. (1990). *Changing belief systems with NLP.* Cupertino, CA: Meta Publications.

20. Dilts, Robert. (1990). *Changing belief systems with NLP.* Cupertino, CA: Meta Publications, p. 210.

21. Adapted from: Dilts, Robert. (1990). *Changing belief systems with NLP.* Cupertino, CA: Meta Publications, pp. 210-211.

22. Allen, James. (1987). *As you think.* New York: New World Library, pp. 39-40.

23. Jones, Laurie Beth. (1996). *The path: Creating your mission statement for work and for life.* New York: Hyperion, p. 3.

24. Humbert, Phillip E. (1999). The JoyFULL Professional Practice. Cassette tape series (tape #1, side #A) available from www.PhillipHumbert.com.

25. Leider, Richard J. (1997). *The power of purpose: Creating meaning in your life and work.* San Francisco: Berrett-Koehler.

26. These concepts come from transactional analysis theory, which is neo-Freudian. The popular version is "I'm OK, You're OK." Probably the best book on the subject is Claude Steiner's 1974 book, *Scripts people live.*

27. Robbins, Anthony. (1997). *O.P.A. life planner.* Robbins Research International, 9191 Towne Center Drive, Suite 600, San Diego, CA 92122. [On-line]. www.tonyrobbins.com..

28. Robbins, Anthony. (1997). *Life Mastery* (manual) which accompanies his Mastery University seminar. Section on O.P.A.–Philosophy, p. 7.

29. Dilts, Robert. (1994). *Strategies of genius: Volume 1: Aristotle, Sherlock Holmes, Walt Disney, Wolfgang Amadeus Mozart.* Capitola, CA: Meta Publications. In this book Dilts models the cognitive processes of Disney and three other seminal minds.

30. Robbins, Anthony. (1997). *O.P.A. life planner* (manual). Robbins Research International, 9191 Towne Center Drive, Suite 600, San Diego, CA 92122. [On-line]. www.tonyrobbins.com.

Chapter 8: Married for a Hundred Years?

1. Franklin, Benjamin. (1738). *Poor Richard's almanac.*

2. Collins, Marva. (1982). *The Marva Collins way.* Los Angeles: J. P. Tarcher, pp. 78, 139.

3. Gottman, John. (1999). *The seven principles for making marriage work.* New York: Crown Publishers, p. 2.

4. Gottman, John. (1994). *Why marriages succeed or fail.* New York: Simon & Schuster. He also is a frequent contributor to professional journals and it is worth watching to see if he comes out with any new or revised books.

5. Gottman, John. (1999). *The seven principles for making marriage work.* New York: Crown Publishers.

6. *Ibid.*, p. 81.

7. Covey, Stephen. (1997). *The 7 habits of highly effective families.* New York: Golden Books. The philosophy is in all of his 7 habits books.

8. Gottman, John. (1999). *The seven principles for making marriage work.* New York: Crown Publishers, pp. 83-84. The couples' observations were compared with the research staff's observations. Some of the differences are due to unhappily married couples questioning the intentions behind positive actions. Assuming either positive or negative intentions contributes to a self-fulfilling prophecy about the intentions, i.e., partner's tend to fulfill your beliefs and expectations.

9. Gottman, John. (1994). *Why marriages succeed or fail.* New York: Simon & Schuster, p. 129.

10. *Ibid.,* p. 129.

11. As cited in Gottman, John. (1999). *The seven principles for making marriage work.* New York: Crown Publishers, p. 49.

12. Kreidman, Ellen. (1989). *Light his fire.* New York: Villard Books, p. 44.

13. Gottman, John. (1999). *The seven principles for making marriage work.* New York: Crown Publishers, p. 130.

14. *Ibid.,* p. 140.

15. The concept of active listening and I-messages was developed by psychologist Haim Ginott in the 1960s.

16. Gigy, Lynn, & Kelly, Joan. As cited in Gottman, John. (1999). *The seven principles for making marriage work.* New York: Crown Publishers, p. 16.

17. Gottman, John. (1994). *Why marriages succeed or fail.* New York: Simon & Schuster, p. 45.

18. Carstensen, Laura L., Gottman, John M., & Levenson, Robert W. (1995). Emotional behavior in long-term marriage. *Psychology and Aging, 10,* 140-149.

19. Gottman, John. (1994). *Why marriages succeed or fail.* New York: Simon & Schuster, p. 61.

20. Baucom, Don. As cited in Gottman, John. (1999). *The seven principles for making marriage work.* New York: Crown Publishers, p. 262.

21. Robbins, Anthony. (1988, 1993, 1996). Love strategies. This strategy is taught in his *Unleash the Power Within* and *Date with Destiny* seminars and in his audio tape (or compact disc) series, *Unleash the power within* and *Personal power.* Robbins Research International, 9191 Towne Center Drive Suite 600 , San Diego, CA 92122 or [On-line]. www.tonyrobbins.com.

22. Based on Robbins, *Ibid.*

23. Sher, Barbara. (1998). *It's only too late if you don't start now: How to create your second life after 40.* New York: Delacorte Press, Chapter 6.

24. Heschel, Abraham Joshua. (1955). *God in search of man: A philosophy of Judaism.* New York: Farrar, Straus, and Giroux.

25. Kreidman, Ellen. (1998). *The 10-second kiss.* New York: Dell.

26. Cronyn, Hume, & Tandy, Jessica. (1992). In Phillip L Berman & Connie Goldman (Eds.), *The ageless spirit,* (p. 56). New York: Ballantine.

27. Fincham, Frank, & Beach, Steven. (1999). Conflict in marriage: Implications for working with couples, *Annual Review of Psychology, 50,* 47-77. The 35% more illness figure was cited in Gottman, John. (1999). *The seven principles for making marriage work.* New York: Crown Publishers, p. 4.

28. Anthony Robbins developed this strategy and named it the Dickens pattern and teaches it in his workshops. The Dickens pattern is also on Robbins' *Personal Power II* cassette tapes (vol. 4) and Compact Discs (CD #8). (1993, 1996), Robbins Research International. 9191 Towne Center Drive Suite 600 , San Diego, CA 92122 or [On-line]. www.tonyrobbins.com.

29. Gottman, John. (1994). *Why marriages succeed or fail.* New York: Simon & Schuster.

30. Gottman, John. (1999). *The seven principles for making marriage work.* New York: Crown Publishers.

31. Kreidman, Ellen. (1991). *Light his fire: How to keep your man passionately and hopelessly in love with you.* New York: Dell Paperback. *Light her fire: How to ignite passion, joy, and excitement in the woman you love.* New York: Dell Paperback. (Both are also available in cassette tapes.)

32. E.g., Mental health: Does anything help? (1990, November). *Consumer Reports, 60,* 734-739.

33. Weiner-Davis, Michele. (1992). *Divorce Busting.* New York: Fireside Book.

34. The Gottman Institute, P.O. 15644, Seattle, WA 98115, 888-523-9042, [On-line]. www.gottmanmarriage.com.

Chapter 9: Sex

1. Medina, John. (1996). *The clock of ages.* Cambridge, Massachusetts: Cambridge Massachusetts Press.

2. Seratonin Selective Uptake Reinhibitors (SSRIs) are a family of antidepressants that became popular in the 1990s because they had fewer side effects than the tricyclic family of antidepressants.

3. Masters, W., & Johnson, V. (1970). *Human sexual inadequacy.* Boston: Little Brown.

4. Nicol, John. (1999, March 22). Sex at $15 a tablet, *McClean's, 112,* 58-59. (Note the $15 is Canadian dollars.)

5. Chiang, H., Wu, C., & Wen, T. (2000). 10 years of experience with penile prosthesis implantation in Taiwanese patients, *Journal of Urology, 163,* 476-480.

6. Wallace, Irving, Wallace, Amy, Walleschinsky, David, & Wallace, Sylvia. (1981). *The intimate sex lives of famous people.* New York: Dell Publishing (paperback), p. 40.

7. Berek, Jonathan (Ed.). (1996). Novak's gynecology 12th ed. Baltimore: Williams & Wilkins, p. 288.

8. Wallace, Irving, Wallace, Amy, Walleschinsky, David, & Wallace, Sylvia. (1981). *The intimate sex lives of famous people.* New York: Dell Publishing (paperback), p. 40.

9. *Ibid.*

10. *Ibid*, p. 42.

Chapter 10: Outliving Family and Friends

1. Siegel, Bernie. (1986). *Love, medicine, and miracles.* New York: Harper & Row, p. 5.

2. Wagner, Harald. (1996). Catholic theology on death. In Howard Spiro, Mary McCrea Curnen, & Lee Palmer Wandel, (Eds.), *Facing Death.* New Haven: Yale University Press, p. 141.

3. Albom, Mitch. (1997). *Tuesdays with Morrie: An old man, a young man, and life's great lesson.* New York: Doubleday. (It is also a television movie and on cassette tape.)

4. Samuel II Chapter 12.

5. Linkletter, Art. (1992). In Phillip L. Berman & Connie Goldman (Eds.), *The ageless spirit,* p. 59. New York: Ballantine.

6. Examples include Neurolinguistic Programming (NLP), Eye Movement Desensitization Reprocessing (EMDR), and Thought Field Therapy (TFT).

7. Coffee, Gerald. (1990). *Beyond survival.* New York: Putnam.

8. Berg, Art. (1995). *Some miracles take time: A love story, a tragedy, a triumph.* Highland, Utah: Invictus Communications. And in *Finding peace in troubled waters: Ten life preservers for when your ship springs a leak.* Hesperia, California: Desert Book.

9. Frankl, Victor. (1984). *Man's search for meaning.* New York: Simon & Schuster.

10. Graves, Sandra. As quoted in Shaw, Eva. (1994). *What to do when a loved one dies.* Irvine, CA: Dickens Press, p. 157.

11. Akner, Lois. (1993). *How to survive the loss of a parent: A guide for adults.* New York: William Morrow, pp. 58-60.

12. Jones, Doris Moreland. (1997). *And not one bird stopped singing.* Nashville, TN: Upper Room Books.

13. Chopra, Deepak. (1993). *Ageless body, timeless mind: The quantum alternative to growing old.* New York: Harmony Books.

14. Foos-Graber, Anya. (1989). *Deathing: An intelligent alternative for the final moments of life.* York Beach, Maine: Nicolas-Hays.

15. The classic documentation of these experiences are the interviews reported in Moody, Raymond. (1976, 1980). Life after life: A scientific investigation of the near-death experience. New York: McCann & Goghegan. And in (1978). *Reflections on life after death.* New York: Bantam. Also note Ring, Kenneth. (1984). *Heading toward omega: In search of the meaning of near-death experience.* New York: William Morrow.

16. Kushner, Harold. (1982). *When bad things happen to good people.* New York: Schocken Books.

17. Siegel, Bernie. (1998). *Prescriptions for living.* New York: HarperCollins, p. 20.

18. Bryant, Robert Jean. (1991). *Stop improving yourself and start living.* San Rafael, CA: New World Library.

Chapter 11: Time and Change

1. Rivers, Joan. (1999). *Don't count the candles just keep the fire lit.* New York: HarperCollins, p. 152.

2. Gordon, Ruth. (1976, 1986). *My side.* New York: Primus–Donald I Fine, Inc., Introduction in 1986 edition (by her husband Garson Kanin).

3. Siegel, Bernie. (1998). *Prescriptions for living.* New York: HarperCollins, p. 23.

4. Dilts, Robert. (1990). *Changing belief systems with NLP.* Cupertino, California: Meta Publications.

5. Another reason appears to be how people are neurologically "wired." When making a mental image of something people have seen before (the past), most people look up and to their left. Thus looking to the left for a visual representation of time fits best with the way most people think. Similarly, when constructing visual images of things we have not seen before (including the future) most people look up and to their right, where most people have the future on their time lines.

6. Siegel, Bernie. (1986). *Love, medicine & miracles.* New York: Harper & Row. And in (1989). *Peace, love & healing.* New York: Harper and Row.

7. Benson, Herbert. (1996). *Timeless healing: The power and biology of belief.* New York: Fireside.

8. *Ibid.*, p. 267.

9. Siegel, Bernie. (1986). *Love, medicine & miracles.* New York: Harper & Row, p. 47.

10. *Ibid*, p. 54.

11. Horowitz, R. I., et al. (1990). Treatment adherence and risk of death after a myocardial infarction, *Lancet, 336,* 542-545.

12. Phillips, D. P., Van Voorhees, C. A., & Ruth, T. E. (1992). The birthday: Lifeline or deadline?, *Psychosomatic Medicine, 54,* 532-542.

13. Levinson, Daniel J. (1978). *The seasons of a man's life.* New York: Ballantine Books, p. 322.

14. Gail Sheehy. (1974). *Passages: Predictable crises of adult life.* New York: E. P. Dutton, p. 20.

15. Her thesis finding was cited in Friedan, Betty. (1993). *The fountain of age.* New York: Simon & Schuster, p. 159.

16. Prochaska, James, Norcross, John, & DiClemente, Carlo. (1994). *Changing for good.* New York: William Morrow.

17. Barker, Joel. (1992). *Paradigms: The business of discovering the future.* New York: Harper Business.

18. As cited in: Cerf, Christopher, & Navasky, Victor. (1998). *The experts speak.* New York: Villard, p. 230.

19. *Ibid.*, p. 231.

20. *Ibid.*

Chapter 12: Eating and Drinking and Common Sense

1. Yutang, Lin. *The importance of living.* Chapter 9, Section 7. As cited in *Gale's Quotations.*

2. Davis, Adelle. (1954). *Let's eat right to keep fit.* Chapter 1.

3. As cited in Edell, Dean. (1999). *Eat, drink and be merry.* New York: HarperCollins, p. 62.

4. Krumholz, Harlan, et al. (1994). Lack of association between cholesterol and coronary heart disease mortality and morbidity and all-cause mortality in person older than 70 years, *Journal of the American Medical Association, 272,* 1335-1340.

5. Fried, Linda, et al. (1998). Risk factors for 5-year mortality in older adults: The cardiovascular health study, *Journal of the American Medical Association, 279,* 585-592.

6. Hulley, Stephen, & Newman, Thomas. (1994). Editorial: Cholesterol in the elderly: Is it important? *Journal of the American Medical Association, 272,* 373.

7. As cited in Edell, Dean. (1999). *Eat, drink and be merry.* New York: HarperCollins, p. 63.

8. *Ibid.*

9. *Ibid.,* p. 64.

10. *Ibid.,* pp. 63-64.

11. As cited in Edell, Dean. (1999). *Eat, drink, and be merry.* New York: HarperCollins, p. 54; 170.

12. Sears, Barry. (1995). *The zone.* New York: ReganBooks, pp. 107-108.

13. Sears, Barry. (1999). *The anti-aging zone.* New York: ReganBooks, pp. 41-42.

14. It's amazing how the placebo effect holds true with both medical and psychological phenomenon. While the magnitude of the placebo effect varies from study to study, on the average it clusters around 33%. Some of the better citations of the placebo effect include: Kirsch, I., & Lynn, S. (1999). Automaticity in clinical psychology. *American Psychologist, 54,* 504-515., Chopra, Deepak. (1993). *Ageless body, timeless mind.* New York: Harmony

Books, p. 18., and Benson, Herbert. (1996). *Timeless healing: The power and biology of belief.* New York: Fireside, pp. 20-21; 27-39; 117.

15. Ikemi, Y., & Nakagawa, S. (1962). A psychosomatic study of contagious dermatitis. *Kyoshu Journal of Medical Science, 13,* 335-350.

16. Kirsch, I., & Saperstein, G. (1999). Listening to Prozac but hearing placebo: A meta-analysis of antidepressant medication. In I. Kirsch (Ed.), *How expectancies shape experience* (pp. 303-320). Washington, DC: American Psychological Association.

17. Kirsch, I., & Lynn, S. (1999). Automaticity in clinical psychology. *American Psychologist, 54,* 504-515.

18. Beard, Belle Boone. (1991). *Centenarians: The new generation.* Westport, CN: Greenwood Press, p. 44.

19. *Ibid.,* p. 46.

20. Perls, Thomas T., & Silver, Margery H. (1999). *Living to 100.* New York: Basic Books, p. 58.

21. Fine, Jennifer, et al. (1999). A prospective study of weight change and health-related quality of life in women, *Journal of the American Medical Association, 282,* 2136-2142.

22. *Ibid.*

23. Diamond, Harvey, & Diamond, Marilyn. (1985). *Fit for life.* New York: Warner Books.

24. D'Adamo, Peter. (1996). *Eat right for your type.* New York: Putnam.

25. Ullis, Karlis. (1999). *Age right: Turn back the clock with a proven personalized antiaging program.* New York: Simon & Schuster.

26. Sears, Barry. (1995). *The zone.* New York: ReganBooks.

27. *Ibid.,* pp. 19-20.

28. Levine, James, Baukol, Paulette, & Pavlidis, Ioannis. (1999). The energy expended in chewing gum (letter to the editor), *New England Journal of Medicine, 341,* 2100.

29. Dilts, Robert, Hallbom, Tim, & Smith, Suzi. (1990). *Beliefs: Pathways to health and well-being.* Metamorphous Press: Portland Oregon.

30. Anderson, John. (1999, September). Just my (metabolic) type. *Alternative Medicine,* issue 31, 52-54. [Online]. www.bloodph.com.

31. Ingram, Donald, Lane, Mark, & Roth, George. (1998). Calorie restriction in monkeys, *Life Extension, 4,* pp. 36-43.

32. Warshofsky, Fred. (1999). *Stealing Time: The new science of aging.* (The book is a companion to a Public Broadcasting Service 3-hour television program.)

33. Walford, Ray. (1998). Caloric restriction: Eat less, eat better, live longer, *Life Extension, 4,* 19-22.

34. Weindruch, Richard. (1996). Caloric restriction and aging, *Scientific American, 274,* 46-52.

35. Walford, Ray. (1995). *The anti-aging plan: Strategies and recipes for extending your healthy years.*

36. Best, Ben. (1998). Making the choice: Can calorie restriction work in humans?, *Life Extension, 4,* 29-35.

37. As cited in Warshofsky, Fred. (1999). *Stealing time.* New York: TV Books, p. 109.

38. Hayflick developed his theory in the 1970s. The most complete statement of his work is in: Hayflick, Leonard. (1994). *How and why we age.* New York: Ballantine.

39. Andres, Reuben, Elahi, D., Tobin, J. D., Muller, D. C., & Brant, L. (1985). Impact of age on weight goals, *Annals of Internal Medicine, 103,* 1030-1033.

40. Allison, D. B., et al. (1997). Body mass index and all-cause mortality among people age 70 and over: The longitudinal study of aging, *International Journal of Obesity, 21,* 424-431

41. Associated Press. (1995, October 18). For elderly, thinner isn't better, researchers say, *New York Times on disc* (access #9300048546).

42. Fine, Jennifer, et al. (1999). A prospective study of weight change and health-related quality of life in women, *Journal of the American Medical Association, 282,* 2136-2142.

43. National Resource Defense Council. (1999, March). Bottled water: Pure drink or pure hype? (Attachment to the NRDC citizen petition to the U.S. Food and Drug Administration for improvements in FDA's bottled water program), Chapter 3: Bottled water contamination: An overview of NRDC's and others' surveys. [On-line]. www.nrdc.org/nrdcpo/bw/chap3.html.

44. Tardy, Marcella. (1999, January 20). Are health claims for bottle water all wet? *News-Star/Booster.* [On-line]. www.intheloop.net/newsstand/newsstar/012099/water.html.

45. Tasting shows tap water is up there with Evian. (1997, August 17). *Sunday Times (London).* [On-line]. www.clo2.com/reading/archive/taste.html.

46. Pure Earth Technologies, Inc., 352 Friendship Court West, Marietta, GA 30064, 1-800-669-1376 [On-line]. www.pureearth.com.

47. Shiu, Garmen. (1997, November 12). Don't re-use your plastic water bottle, *Channel 2000 News (a Los Angeles TV station).* [On-line]. www.channel2000.com/news/stories/news-971111-211014.html.

48. Paolini, Kenneth, & Paolini, Talita. (1999). Special report: How to make absolutely sure you are drinking pure water. [On-line]. http://www.factsource.com/srwater.html.

49. Sears, Barry. (1995). *The zone.* New York: ReganBooks, p. 148.

Chapter 13: Supplemental Vitamins, Minerals, and Hormones

1. Carper, Jean. (1995). *Stop aging now: The ultimate plan for staying young and reversing the aging process.* New York: HarperCollins, p. 16, and Harper Audio (cassette tape).

2. Weil, Andrew. (1999). *Self Healing, "premier issue," of his newsletter,* 1-3.

3. Life Extension Foundation, PO Box 229120, Hollywood, Florida 33022-9120, 1-800-841-5433. Current annual dues are $75, which includes their monthly journal. [On line]. www.lef.org.

4. Farnsworth, Norman. (1999, March 17). Herbal Medicines. Presentation to Mount Carmel East Hospital Medical Staff. He is a research professor of Pharmacognosy in the College of Pharmacy at the University of Illinois at Chicago and a leading researcher in herbal medicines.

5. Robbers, James, & Tyler, Varro. (1999). *Tyler's herbs choice: The therapeutic use of phytomedicinals* (2nd ed.). New York: Haworth.

6. Foster, Steven, & Tyler, Varro. (1999). *Tyler's honest, herbal: A sensible guide to the use of herbals and related remedies* (4th ed.). New York: Haworth.

7. Life Extension Foundation. (1998). *The directory of life extension nutrients and drugs.* PO Box 229120, Hollywood, Florida 33022-9120, 1-800-841-5433, [On-line]. www.lef.org.

8. Rudman, Daniel. (1990). The effects of Human Growth Hormone in men over 60 years old, *New England Journal of Medicine, 323,* 1-6.

9. As cited in Klatz, Ronald. (1997). *Grow young with HGH.* New York: HarperCollins, pp. 30-35.

10. Ullis, Karlis. (1999). *Age right: Turn back the clock with a proven personalized antiaging program.* New York: Simon & Schuster, pp. 58-59.

11. Klatz, Ronald. (1997). *Grow young with HGH.* New York: HarperCollins.

12. Klatz, Ronald. (1999). *Ten weeks to a younger you.* Chicago: Sports Tech Labs, Inc.

13. *Ibid.*

14. Ullis, Karlis. (1999). *Age right: Turn back the clock with a proven personalized antiaging program.* New York: Simon & Schuster, p. 62.

15. Klatz, Ronald. (1997). *Grow young with HGH.* New York: HarperCollins, pp. 228-248.

16. Ullis, Karlis. (1999). *Age right: Turn back the clock with a proven personalized antiaging program.* New York: Simon & Schuster, pp. 58; 63.

17. *Ibid.*, p. 63.

18. Klatz, Ronald. (1999). *Ten weeks to a younger you.* Chicago: Sports Tech Labs, Inc., pp. 76-77.

19. Bhasin, Shalender, et al. (1996). The effects of supraphysicologic doses of testosterone on muscle size and strength in normal men, *New England Journal of Medicine, 335,* 1-7.

20. Klatz, Ronald. (1999). *Ten weeks to a younger you.* Chicago: Sports Tech Labs, Inc., p. 132.

21. Ullis, Karlis. (1999). *Age right: Turn back the clock with a proven personalized antiaging program.* New York: Simon & Schuster, pp. 165-166.

22. Replenish testosterone naturally: Plant extracts favorably alter hormone metabolism and improve sexual desire in men. (2000). *Life Extension, 6,* 25-30.

23. Ullis, Karlis. (1999). *Super T: The complete guide to creating an effective, safe, and natural testosterone enhancement program for men and women.* New York: Simon & Schuster, pp. 72-73.

24. Ullis, Karlis. (1999). *Super T: The complete guide to creating an effective, safe, and natural testosterone enhancement program for men and women.* New York: Simon & Schuster.

25. King, Douglas S., et al. Effect of oral androstenedione on serum testosterone and adaptions to resistance training in young men, *Journal of the American Medical Association, 281,* 2020-2028.

26. Roberts, Bill. (1999, June 28). Ask Bill Roberts: None so blind: The JAMA study on androstenedione, Vol. 2 (12) [On-line]. www.thinkmuscle.com/nonmembers/roberts/990628.htm.

27. Estrogen therapy? Don't worry! (1999, October). *Life Extension, 5,* 37-38.

28. Ullis, Karlis. (1999). *Super T: The complete guide to creating an effective, safe, and natural testosterone enhancement program for men and women.* New York: Simon & Schuster, pp. 73-75.

29. As cited in: Weakened bones can afflict men, too. (1999, August). *Focus on Healthy Aging (newsletter), 2 (8),* p. 7.

30. Ullis, Karlis. (1999). *Age right: Turn back the clock with a proven personalized antiaging program.* New York: Simon & Schuster, p 168.

31. Life Extension Foundation, PO Box 229120, Hollywood, Florida 33022-9120, 1-800-841-5433. Current annual dues are $75, which includes their monthly journal and a 25% discount on their supplements. [On-line]. www.lef.org.

32. American Academy of Anti-Aging Medicine, 1341 W. Fullerton, Suite 111, Chicago, IL 60614, 773-528-8500. [On-line]. www.worldhealth.net.

Chapter 14: Fitness: Emotional vs. Outcome-based Choices

1. Jackowski, Edward. (1995). *Hold it! You're exercising all wrong.* New York: Simon & Schuster Fireside, p. 27.

2. As cited in Rivers, Joan. (1999). *Don't count the candles just keep the fire lit.* New York: HarperCollins, p. 40.

3. As cited in Edel, Dean. (1999). *Eat, drink, and be merry.* New York: HarperCollins, pp. 110-111, 113-114.

4. Bailey, Covert. (1994). *Smart exercise.* New York: Houghton Mifflin, pp. 82-85.

5. Hopkins, Tom. (1994) *Low impact selling.* Tom Hopkins International Publisher. (He also discusses the theme in most of his books, tapes and seminars.)

6. Nyad, Diana. (1998, June 12). Post football life, National Public Radio Morning Edition Broadcast, [On-line]. www.npr.com.

7. Bailey, Covert. (1994). *Smart exercise.* New York: Houghton Mifflin, pp. 39-41.

8. Asken, Michael, & Schwartz R. (1998). Heading the ball in soccer: What's the risk of brain injury? *The Physician and Sportsmedicine, 11,* 37-45.

9. Kelly, James P. (1999). Traumatic brain injury and concussion in sports, *Journal of the American Medical Association, 282,* 989-991.

10. Jackowski, Edward. (1995). *Hold it! You're exercising all wrong.* New York: Simon & Schuster Fireside, p. 70.

11. Hipprocrates (circa 400 BCE). While the dictum to first do no harm is widely believed to be in the Hippocratic oath, it is not in the most commonly quoted ones (there are many versions). Rather the oath admonishes physician's to only act to cure patients. Hippocrates does gives the do no harm admonition in *Epidemics.* The Hippocratic oath apparently predated Hippocrates and originated with a Pythagorean sect in the fourth century BCE.

12. Jackowski, Edward. (1995). *Hold it! You're exercising all wrong.* New York: Simon & Schuster Fireside.

13. Fiatarone, Maria, & Garnett, Leah R. (1997, March). Keeping on keeping on. *Harvard Health Letter, volume 22.*

14. Liebman, Bonnie. (1995, December). Use it or lose it (interview with William Evans, Director of the Noll Physiological Research Center, Pennsylvania State University). *Nutrition Action Healthletter, 22 (10)*, 1-5. Also available on the Infotrac database.

15. Raloff, Janet. (1996). Vanishing flesh: Muscle loss in the elderly finally gets some respect. *Science News, 150,* 90-91.

16. Nelson, Miriam E. (1997). *Strong women stay young.* New York: Bantam Books.

17. Frontera, W. R., Meredith, C. N., O'Reilly, K. P., Knuttgen, H. G., & Evans, W. J. (1988). Strength condition in older men: Skeletal muscle hypertrophy and improved function, *Journal of Applied Physiology, 64,* 1038-1044

18. Nelson, Miriam. (1996). As cited in *Science News, 150,* 90-91.

19. Fiatarone, M. A., Marks, E. C., Ryan, N. D., Meredith, C. N., Lipsitz, Lewis, & Evans, W. J. (1990). High-intensity strength training in nonagenarians, *Journal of the American Medical Association, 263,* 3029-3034.

20. Fiatrone, Maria, & Evans, William. (1990). *Journal of the American Medical Association, 263,* 3029-3034.

21. Liebman, Bonnie. (1995, December). Use it or lose it (interview with William Evans, Director of the Noll Physiological Research Center, Pennsylvania State University). *Nutrition Action Healthletter, 22 (10)*, 1-5. Also available on the Infotrac database.

22. Bailey, Covert. (1994). *Smart exercise.* New York: Houghton Mifflin.

23. Liebman, Bonnie. (1995, December). Use it or lose it (interview with William Evans, Director of the Noll Physiological Research Center, Pennsylvania State University). *Nutrition Action Healthletter, 22 (10)*, 1-5. Also available on the Infotrac database.

24. Bailey, Covert. (1994). *Smart exercise.* New York: Houghton Mifflin.

25. McDonald, Kim. (1998, August 14). Scientists consider new explanations for the impact of exercise on mood, *Chronicle of Higher Education,* pp. A-15-16.

26. Manson, JoAnn, et al. (1999). A prospective study of walking as compared with vigorous exercise in the prevention of coronary heart disease in women. *The New England Journal of Medicine, 341,* 650-658.

27. Pinckney, Callan. (1984). *Callanetics.* New York: William Morrow. There are several videotapes. I think the best is the original one, *Callanetics,* an MCA Home Video, www.callanetics.com.

28. Shih, T. K. (1989). *Swimming Dragon: A Chinese way to fitness, beautiful skin, weight loss and high energy.* Barrytown, NY: Station Hill Press. There is also a video of the exercise: Shih, Tzu Kuo, *Swimming dragon form.* New Age Products, P.O. Box 2591, Church Street Station, New York City, NY 10008-2591.

29. Feldenkrais movement is based on Moshe Feldenkrais' teaching. Feldenkrais has several books which are theoretical and difficult reading. His practitioners have written less theoretical books. Feldenkrais practitioners are listed on the web site: www.Feldenkrais.com.

30. Linden, Paul. (1999). *Compute in comfort: Body awareness training: A day-to-day guide to pain-free computing.* Berkeley, CA: North Atlantic Books.

31. *Ibid.*

32. Egoscue, Pete. (1993). *The Egoscue method of health through motion.* New York: Harperperennial.

24. Egoscue, Pete. (1999). *Pain free at your PC.* New York: Bantam Doubleday Dell.

34. Egoscue, Pete. (1998). *Pain free: A revolutionary method for stopping chronic pain.* New York: Bantam Doubleday Dell.

35. The Egoscue Method, 12707 High Bluff Drive, Suite 150, San Diego, California 92130, 1-800-995-8434, [On-line]. www.egoscue.com.

36. Shih, T. K. (1989). *Swimming Dragon: A Chinese way to fitness, beautiful skin, weight loss and high energy.* Barrytown, NY: Station Hill Press. There is also a video of the exercise: Shih, Tzu Kuo, *Swimming dragon form.* New Age Products, P.O. Box 2591, Church Street Station, New York City, NY 10008-2591.

37. Khalsa, Dharma Singh. (1997). *Brain Longevity.* New York: Warner Books. Also available on cassette tape from Time Warner Audio Books.

38. Benson, Herbert. (1975). *The relaxation response.* New York: William Morrow.

39. Benson, Herbert. (1996). *Timeless healing: The power and biology of belief.* New York: Fireside.

40. Ott, John. (1973, 1976). *Health and light.* Columbus, OH: Ariel Press.

41. Liberman, Jacob. (1991). *Light medicine of the future.* Santa Fe, NM: Bear & Co.

42. *Ibid.,* p. 10.

43. *Ibid.*, p. 66.

44. Goodrich, Janet. (1986). *Natural vision improvement.* Berkeley, CA: Celestial Arts, [On-line]. www.ozemail.com.au/~good4nvi/.

45. Sussman, Martin. (1990). *The program for better vision.* (three cassette tapes and instructional booklets). The Cambridge Institute for Better Vision, 65 Wenham Rd., Topsfield, MA 01983. 1-800-372-3937, [On-line]. www.asia-view.com/nvi.html.

46. Liberman, Jacob. (1994). *Light: A new paradigm for health and healing.* (two cassette tapes). Sound Horizons Audio-Video, 250 West 57th St., Ste. 1527, New York City, NY 10107.

47. Rowland, Cynthia. (1997). *Facial magic success program* (booklet and videotape). New Vision and Marketing & Communications, [On-line]. www.facialmagic.com.

48. Dermal-Tone, 2500 Chandler Ave. #10, Las Vegas, Nevada 89120. 1-800-750-0070, [On-line]. www.dermaltone.com.

49. Morton Walker, M.D., preventive medicine specialist as cited by Goulart, Frances S. (1987). In *Staying young: How to look good, feel better, and live longer.* West Nyack, New York: Parker Publishing Co., p. 182.

50. Kelder, Peter. (1998). *Ancient secret of the fountain of youth.* New York: Doubleday.

51. Tae-Bo is a high energy marital arts routine that is fast, upbeat, and enthusiastic. It is good for flexibility, agility, aerobics, confidence building, and posture. Blanks, Billy. (1998). *Tae-Bo* (videotapes). 1-877-228-2326,[On-line]. www.taebo.com.

52. Kennedy, John F. (1961, December 5). Address to the National Football Foundation. As cited in *Gale's Quotations.*

53. LaLanne, Jack. (1995). *Revitalize your life after 50.* Mamaroneck, NY: Hastings House.

54. Perls, Thomas, & Silver, M. H. (1999). *Living to 100.* New York: Basic Books, his picture is on p. 153 and some commentary on p. 109.

Chapter 15: Managing Risks

1. Weiner, Eric. (2000, February 17). Is cleanliness dangerous? National Public Radio *Morning Edition.* [On-line]. www.npr.com.

2. Asken, Michael, & Schwartz R. (1998). Heading the ball in soccer: What's the risk of brain injury? *The Physician and Sportsmedicine, 11,* 37-45.

3. Kelly, James P. (1999). Traumatic brain injury and concussion in sports, *Journal of the American Medical Association, 282,* 989-991.

4. Polednak, Anthony, & Damon, Albert. (1970). College athletics, longevity, and cause of death, *Human Biology, 42,* 28-46.

5. National Safety Council. (1998). *Accident facts.* National Safety Council. (Data cited is for 1997.)

6. Current thinking is that most adults have too much iron and that iron is one of the nastiest oxidants. Many multiple vitamins for men have removed iron from the formula. Some fanatics even recommend donating blood to lower the iron content of your blood. Women who menstruate, however, might need extra iron as iron is essential to making new blood. The principle sources of iron in people's diets are red meats, seafood, soybeans, liver, and greens.

7. As cited in *Gale's Quotations.*

8. Ott, John. (1973). *Health and light.* Columbus, OH: Ariel Press.

9. Inlander, C. B., Levin, L. S., & Weiner, E. (1988). *Medicine on trial.* New York: Prentice Hall.

10. Neegaard, Lauran. (1999, November 30). Clinton urges war on medical errors. Associated Press [On-line]. www.infobear.com/stories/cgi/story.cgi?id=2562333201-bb3.

11. *Consumer Reports on Health.* (1998, March). Needless surgery, needless drugs, 1-5.

12. Most research has not supported electromagnetic fields causing disease. The famous study of electromagnetic fields in Denver had serious methodological flaws, e.g., it was a phone survey conducted during the day time and respondents were limited to people who were home during the day. Nevertheless, research has shown that our bodies have electromagnetic fields and it seems prudent to avoid undue exposure to electromagnetic fields. See: Austad, Steven. (1997). *Why we age: What science is discovering about the body's journey through life.* New York: John Wiley & Sons, p. 169.

Chapter 16: Finances for a Lifetime

1. Davis, Ossie. (1992). In Phillip L. Berman & Connie Goldman (Eds.), *The ageless spirit,* (pp. 66-67). New York: Ballantine.

2. Roosevelt, Franklin. (1935, August 14). President Roosevelt's statement when signing the Social Security Act of 1935.

3. Research and Policy Committee for Economic Development. (1995). *Who will pay for your retirement: The looming crisis.* Edited by the Committee for Economic Development.

4. Birnbaum, Jeffrey. (1998, December 7). The influence merchants, *Fortune, 138,* 134-152.

5. Kohn, Alfie (New York Times News Service). (1999, February 7). Psychologists prove adage: Wealth can't buy happiness, *Columbus Dispatch,* Insight section. (The article was based on numerous studies by psychology professors Richard Ryan and Tim Kasser.)

6. Adair, Tom, & Dennis, Matt. (1941). *Let's get away from it all.*

7. Stanton, Bill. (1998). *The America's finest companies investment plan.* New York: Hyperion, pp. 63-66.

8. Stanton, Bill. (1998). *The America's finest companies investment plan.* New York: Hyperion.

Chapter 17: The Evidence for Living 150 Years

1. Bradbury, Robert. (1994). Issues involving lifespan extension: What is the maximum lifespan? [On-line]. Bradbury@aeiveos.wa.com.

2. Stipp, David. (1997). Gene chip breakthrough, *Fortune, 135*, 56-73.

3. Olson, Ken. As cited it Cerf, Chriswtopher, & Navasky, Victor. (1998). *The experts speak.* New York: Villard, p. 231.

4. *Ibid.*

5. Oliver, Richard W. (2000). *The coming biotech age.* New York: McGraw-Hill, p.21.

6. Engineering health. (1994*).* *The Economist, 330*, F13-15.

7. *Ibid.*

8. Bradbury, Robert. (1994). Issues involving lifespan extension: What is the maximum lifespan? [On-line]. Bradbury@aeiveos.wa.com.

9. Davis, Bennett. (1995). Battelle's best guesses: The top ten technologies that will significantly influence our lives in the next decade, *Omni, 17*, 42ff.

10. Marshall, Eliot. (1999). Do-it-yourself gene watching, *Science, 286*, 444-446.

11. Engineering health, *op. cit.*

12. Svensson, Peter (Associated Press). (1999, December 6). IBM plans computer to study body. AP Wire Story on Internet.

13. Austad, Steven. (1997). *Why we age: What science is discovering about the body's journey through life.* New York: John Wiley & Sons, p. 219.

14. Freundlich, Naomi. (1997, January 20). A booster shot for gene therapy, *Business Week,* pp. 92-94.

15. Guidera, Mark. (1996, Sept. 19). Genetic therapy tests new treatment, *The Baltimore Sun,* 1C.

16. Nyce, Jonathan, & Metzger, W. James. (1997). DNA antisense therapy for asthma in an animal model, *Nature, 385*, 721-725.

17. Freundlich, Naomi. (1996, January 20). One giant leap for gene therapy? *Business Week,* p. 119.

18. Finley, Don. (1996, Aug. 25). Gene therapy treatment for diseases now available in San Antonio, *San Antonio Express-News.*

19. Ma, Lybi. (1998, October 28). Molecular attack on malignancy: Herceptin offers new hope for victims of breast cancer. [On-line]. www.discover.com/science_news/biology/attack.html.

20. Bishop, Jerry E. (1994, April 1). One of first successful cases of gene put permanently in person is described, *The Wall Street Journal,* p. B4 (W), p.B2 (E).

21. Sternberg, S. (1997). Newfound gene linked to several cancers, *Science News, 151,* 191.

22. Lose a gene, lose some weight–in mice. (1996). *Science News, 150,* 125.

23. Rundle, Rhonda. (1996, May 30). Scientists discover genetic switch that may lead to weight-loss drug, *The Wall Street Journal, Europe, 14,* 4.

24. Barinaga, Marcia. (1999). An immunization against Alzheimer's?, *Science, 285,* 175-177.

25. Travis, J. (1999). A vaccine for Alzheimer's disease?, *Science News, 156,* 20.

26. Cookson, Clive. (1997, Feb. 16). Scientists developing chip to diagnose cancers, *The Financial Times,* (Scripps Howard News Service #01245*19970216*00064).

27. Pennisi, Elizabeth. (1997). New tumor suppressor found–twice, *Science, 275,* 1876-1879.

28. Travis, John. (1997). Chips ahoy: Microchips covered with DNA emerge as powerful research tools, *Science News, 151,* 144-145.

29. Toufexis, Anastasia. (1995). An eary tale, *Time, 146,* 60.

30. SoRelle, Ruth. (1996, Sept. 16). Building blocks of tissue engineering/growing human ears on mice just the beginning, experts say, *The Houston Chronicle,* p. 7-Discovery.

382   References

31. Blood-producing stem cells thrive in vitro. (1999, July 12). *Chemical & Engineering News, 77,* 26.

32. *Ibid.*

33. Carnegie Mellon University's Bone Tissue Engineering Initiative. [On-line]. www.cs.cmu.edu/People/tissue/front_page.html.

34. Blood-producing stem cells thrive in vitro. (1999, July 12). *Chemical & Engineering News, 77,* 26.

35. *Ibid.*

36. *Ibid.*

37. Davis, Bennett. Battelle's best guesses: The top ten technologies that will significantly influence our lives in the next decade, *Omni, 17,* p. 42ff.

38. Stolberg, Sheryl. (1999, October 3). Could this pig save your life? *New York Times Magazine.* [On-line]. www.nytimes.com/library/magazine/home/19991003mag-pig-transplants.html.

39. Bradbury, Robert. (1994). Issues involving lifespan extension: What is the maximum lifespan? [On-line]. Bradbury@aeiveos.wa.com.

40. Warshofsky, Fred. (1999). *Stealing time.* New York: TV Books, pp. 125-126.

41. Allen, Jane E. (Associated Press). (1998, June 7). New gene extends lifespan of flies, *Columbus Dispatch,* p. B6.

42. Hewitt, Duane. (1996, June 24). Geneticists extend worm life span by five times! [On-line]. duane@immortality.org.

43. Guarente, Leonard. Mutant mice live longer, *Nature, 402,* 243-244.

44. Migliaccio, E., et al. (1999). The p66shc adaptor protein control oxidative stress response and life span in mammals, *Nature, 402,* 309-313.

45. Yu, Chang-En, et al. (1996, April 12). Positional cloning of the Werner's syndrome gene, *Science,* pp. 258-262.

46. Hayflick, Leonard. (1994). *How and why we age.* New York: Ballentine Books, p. 135.

47. Fossel, Michael. (1996). *Reversing human aging,* New York: William Morrow & Co.

48. Fossel, *op. cit.,* p. 177.

49. Kolata, Gina. (1997, Feb. 25). Scientists rethinking the role of chromosomal 'leader tape,' *New York Times,* Sec. C Science Desk, p. 3.

50. Warshofsky, Fred. (1999). *Stealing time.* New York: TV Books, p. 163.

51. Warshofsky, Fred. (1999). *Stealing time.* New York: TV Books, pp. 76-77.

52. Mestel, Rosie. (1997). Redesigning women, *Health, 11,* 70-76.

53. Menopause blocker shows promise. (1997, November 16). *The Columbus Dispatch, p.* B6.

54. Cowley, Geoffrey. (1996, September 16). Super-hormone therapy: Can it keep men young? *Newsweek, 128,* 69-77.

55. Rudman, Daniel, et al. (1990). Effect of human growth hormone in men over 60 years old, *The New England Journal of Medicine, 323,* 1-6.

56. Ronald Klatz, (1997). *Grow young with HGH.* New York: HarperCollins, p. 95.

57. Ronald Klatz, (1997). *Grow young with HGH.* New York: HarperCollins, pp. 60-62.

58. Jorgensen J. O. L., et al. (1994). Three years of growth hormone treatment in growth hormone-deficient adults: Near normalization of body composition and physical performance, *European Journal of Endocrinology, 130,* 224-228. (As cited in Klatz, *op cit.*)

59. Klatz, *op cit.*

60. Cranton, Elmer, & Fryer, William. (1996). *Resetting the clock: 5 anti-aging hormones that are revolutionizing the quality and length of life.* New York: M. Evans and Co.

61. Klatz, *op cit.,* p. 37.

62. Ricks, Delthia. (1996, December 27). Age-old question: Can youth be preserved, restored? *The Orlando Sentinel,* C-1.

63. Hotz, Robert Lee. (1996, November 18). New drug found to improve memory, *Los Angeles Times,* A-1.

64. Geary, James. (1999, May 5). Should we just say no to smart drugs? [On-line]. http://pathfinder.com/time/magazine/1997/int/970505/science.should_we_jus.html.

65. Hotz, *op. cit.*

66. Raloff, J. (1997). Novel antioxidants may slow brain's aging, *Science News, 151*, 53.

67. Warshofsky, Fred. (1999). *Stealing time.* New York: TV Books, p. 131.

68. NeoTherapeutics News Release. (1998, May 21). Neotrofin reported to stimulate nerve regeneration. [On-line]. http://gaston.infowest.com/hypernews/get/cpn/research/152.html.

69. Travis, J. (1999). Gene tinkering makes memorable mice, *Science News, 156,* 149.

70. Warshofsky, Fred. (1999). *Stealing time.* New York: TV Books, p. 130.

71. *Ibid.*

72. *Ibid.,* pp. 131-132.

73. Raloff, J. (1997). Novel antioxidants may slow brain's aging, *Science News, 151,* 53.

74. Nicol, John. (1999, March 22). Sex at $15 a tablet, *McClean's, 112,* 58-59. (Note the $15 is Canadian dollars.)

75. Haney, Daniel Q. (1999, January 16). Anti-viral drug stops colds and other ills, *Columbus Dispatch* (AP Wire story), 8B.

76. Follow-up: Surgery for the near sighted. (1995, January). *Consumer Reports, 60,* 6-7.

77. Keeton, (1992). *Longevity: The science of staying young.* New York: Viking Press, p. 241.

78. Seligson, Susan V. (1997). The changing face of cosmetic surgery, *Health, 11,* 85-90.

79. Associated Press. (1999, October 5). Men may bid "hairwell" to baldness. [On-line]. www.infobeat.com/stories/cgi/story.cgi?id=2561498814-e4b.

80. Travis, J. (1999). Gene therapy tackles hair loss, *Science News, 156,* 283.

81. World Health Network. (1999). Move over Rogaine? Protein sheds light on tumor formation. [On-line]. www.worldhealth.net/news/99070504.html.

82. Reynolds, Amanda, et al. (1999). Trans-gender induction of hair follicles: Human follicle cells can be induced to grow in an incompatible host of the other sex, *Nature, 402,* 33-34.

83. Andres, Reuben, Elahi, J. D., Tobin, D. C., Muller, D. C., &, Brant, L. (1985). Impact of age on weight goals. *Annals of Internal Medicine, 103,* 1030-1033.

84. Dilts, Robert, Hallbom, Tim, & Smith, Suzi.(1990*). Beliefs: Pathways to health & well-being,* Portland, Oregon: Metamorphous Press.

85. Benson, Herbert. (1996). *Timeless healing: The power and biology of belief,* New York: Simon and Schuster Fireside Book.

86. Siegel, Bernie. (1989). P*eace, love, and healing.* New York: Harper & Row.

87. Siegel, Bernie. (1986). *Love, medicine, and miracles.* New York: Harper & Row.

88. Funny, we don't feel old. (1997, March 9). *New York Times*–Magazine section. This was the caption on the cover of the issue, which contained several articles on aging.

89. The Census report listed low, medium and high projections. These data are from the medium series. U.S. Commerce Dept., Bureau of the Census, Current Population Reports: Population Projections of the United State, by Age, Sex, Race, and Hispanic Origin: 1993 to 2050, P25-1104, p. xvi.

90. Smith, David W. E. (1993). *Human longevity.* New York: Oxford University Press, p. 127.

91. Kolata, Gina. (1996, February 27). New era of robust elderly belies the fears of scientists, *New York Times, 145,* A1, C3.

92. *Ibid.*

386   References

93. Angier, Natalie. (1995, June 11). If you're really ancient, you may be better off, *New York Times,* Sec 4 Week in Review, p. 1.

94. Bannister, Roger. (1955). *The four-minute mile.* New York: Lyons & Burford.

95. Keeton, Kathy. (1992). *Longevity: The science of staying young.* New York: Viking Press, p. 59.

96. Chopra, Deepak. (1993). *Ageless body, timeless mind.* New York: Harmony Books.

97. Ferber, Diane. (1999). Immortalized cells seem cancer free so far, *Science, 283,* 154-155.

98. Malthus, Thomas. (1798). An essay on the principle of population.

99. Goodall, Jane. (1971). *In the shadow of man,* Boston: Houghton Mifflin.

100. Wilmut, I., Schieke, A. E. McWhir, J., Kind, A. J., & Campbell, K. H. S. (1997). Viable offspring derived from fetal and adult mammalian cells, *Nature, 385,* 810-813.

101. Kolata, Gina. (1997, February 23). Scientists reports first cloning ever of adult mammal, *New York Times,* section 1, p. 1.

102. Goto, Shihoko. (2000, January 24). Clone of cloned cow bred in Japan, (AP Wire story on Infobeat News), www.infobeat.com/stories/cgi/story.cgi?id=2563592797-485.

103. Medical myths stand the test of time: Even physicians buy into ages-old explanations. (1996, May 12). *The Columbus Dispatch,* via *New York Times* News Service.

104. As cited in Perls, Thomas, & Silver, Margery. (1999). *Living to 100.* New York: Basic Books, p. 27.

105. Perls, Thomas, & Silver, Margery. (1999). *Living to 100.* New York: Basic Books, p. 28.

106. As cited in Warshofsky, Fred. (1999). *Stealing time.* New York: TV Books, pp. 175-178.

107. Kempermann, Gerald, Kuhn, George, & Gage, Fred H. (1997). More hippocampal neurons in adult mice living in an enriched environment, *Nature, 386*, 493-495.

108. Beard, Belle Boone. (1968). Some characteristics of recent memory of centenarians. *Journal of Gerontology, 23,* 23-30.

109. As cited in Warshofsky, Fred. (1999). *Stealing time.* New York: TV Books, pp. 201-202.

110. Widkelgren, Ingrid. (1997). For the cortex, neuron loss may be less than thought, *Science, 273,* 48-50.

111. Manton, K. G., & Vaupel, James W. (1995). Survival after the age of 80 in the United States, Sweden, France, England, and Japan, *New England Journal of Medicine, 333,* 1232-1235. Also reported in Kolata, Gina, After 80 Americans live longer than others, *New York Times,* Nov. 2, 1995, p. B14.

112. Manton, Kenneth G.(1992). In Richard M. Suzman, David P. Willis and Kenneth Manton, (Eds.) *The oldest old.* New York: Oxford University Press, pp. 160-161.

113. Andres, Reuben, Elahi, J. D., Tobin, D. C., Muller, D. C. & Brant, L. (1985). Impact of age on weight goals. *Annals of Internal Medicine, 103,* 1030.

114. Associated Press. (1995, October 18). For elderly, thinner isn't better, researchers say, *New York Times,* 18. (New York Times ondisc access #9300048546).

115. Warshofsky, Fred. (1999). *Stealing time.* New York: TV Books, p. 10.

116. Mroczek, Daniel, & Kolarz, Christian. (1998). The effect of age on positive and negative affect: A developmental perspective on happiness, *Journal of Personality and Social Psychology, 75,* 1333-1349.

Index

The American
Academy of
Anti-Aging
Medicine

Join the Ageless Society
Application for New Membership

Name: _____

Title: _____

Organization:_____

Address:_____

_____

Phone: _____

FAX: _____

E-mail:_____

I would like to receive the A4M
free e-newsletter ___yes ___ no

Membership Category:

___Physician Member (M.D.,
   D.O.) $150 per year

___Scientific/Healthcare $95 per year, ___General Public $65 per year,
___Student/Intern/Resident/Retired $50 per year

I wish to be accepted as a member of the American Academy of Anti-
Aging Medicine and agree to abide by its By Laws and Code of Ethics.
Signed: _____

Please Select a Voluntary Contribution Level (not required):
___US $50 ___US $100 ___US $150 ___(other) $_____ [as
unrestricted funds] ___ US $250 (for participation the Consumer
Education and Research Council)

___Check enclosed OR I authorize payment in the amount of US$_____
to my credit card: ___ VISA ___ MASTERCARD ___ AMEX
Card No.:_____ Expiration date:_____
Name (as appears on card): _____
Signature:_____
Please select a membership premium: ___ *Ten Week to a Younger You*
(retail value $15.95) ___ *Seven Anti-Aging Secrets* by (retail value
$18.95) ___ One year Basic Listing on www.worldhealth.net
Physician's and Supplier's Directory (retail value $59.95) *Mail to:*
A4M, 1510 West Montana, Chicago, IL 60614 or FAX to 773-528-5390

Benefits of Membership:
- Discounts on all A4M
  publications
- Discounts for conference
  registrations
- Complimentary sub-
  scription to *Anti-Aging
  Medical News*
- *Select a **premium** (see list
  below)*

*For an Organizational Mem-
bership offering extended
benefits, call 773-528-4333*

Visit A4M's award-winning web site: http://www.worldhealth.net

Quick Order Form for Autographed Books

You can order autographed copies of *Defy Aging* from the web site www.DrBrickey.com or by copying and mailing or FAXing this page to New Resources Press, 865 College Ave., Columbus, OH 43209, FAX: 614-237-5333.

Please send me ____ copies of *Defy Aging.* I understand that I may return any of the books for a full refund–for any reason, no questions asked. *Defy Aging* is $24.95+ shipping. There is a 20% discount for orders of three or more books. Shipping is $4 in U.S. or Canada for first the first book and $2 for each additional book. International shipping is $9 for the first book and $5 for each additional book. Ohio residents add 5.75% sales tax ($1.44 per book). Payment method: Mail a check, or order by Master Card or VISA. Payment type: ____check enclosed
____VISA Card   ____Master Card
Card Number: _____
Expiration Date: _____
I authorize payment of $_____ from my credit card
Name as it appears on the card:_____
Signature:_____Today's date:_____

____Check here is you would like the book(s) autographed.
____Check here to also receive the free E-mail Newsletter, *Defy Aging*
My E-mail address is:_____
Mail my book(s) to:

_____
_____
_____

Quick Order Form for Autographed Books

You can order autographed copies of *Defy Aging* from the web site www.DrBrickey.com or by copying and mailing or FAXing this page to New Resources Press, 865 College Ave., Columbus, OH 43209, FAX: 614-237-5333.

Please send me ___ copies of *Defy Aging.* I understand that I may return any of the books for a full refund–for any reason, no questions asked. *Defy Aging* is $24.95+ shipping. There is a 20% discount for orders of three or more books. Shipping is $4 in U.S. or Canada for first the first book and $2 for each additional book. International shipping is $9 for the first book and $5 for each additional book. Ohio residents add 5.75% sales tax ($1.44 per book). Payment method: Mail a check, or order by Master Card or VISA. Payment type: ___check enclosed
    ___VISA Card   ___Master Card
Card Number: _____
Expiration Date: _____
I authorize payment of $_____ from my credit card
Name as it appears on the card:_____
Signature:_____ Today's date:_____

___Check here is you would like the book(s) autographed.
___Check here to also receive the free E-mail Newsletter,
    Defy Aging
    My E-mail address is:_____
Mail my book(s) to:

_____
_____
_____

Free E-mail Newsletter

The free E-mail newsletter, *Defy Aging,* is available by subscribing on-line at www.DrBrickey.com.

Life Coaching

Remember how Merlin coached and mentored King Arthur? He helped Arthur sort out life's challenges, gain perspective, and develop vision, goals, and strategies. He was Arthur's personal advocate who was solely interested in Arthur's needs and success. Life has become even more complex than in Arthur's time. Life coaching gives you your own Merlin. Like Merlin's coaching and mentoring, the emphasis is on what you are thinking and doing now and what you want to be thinking and doing in the future.

Life coaching helps you forge your own path in life and take your life to a higher level. It capitalizes on three decades of professional experience helping people determine and achieve their goals. It's like having a partner in life who is only interested in your well-being. Life coaching usually is conducted by phone several times a month. More information on Dr. Brickey's life coaching services is on his web site www.DrBrickey.com or you can listen to a recording about life coaching by calling 212-461-2797 anytime. To arrange a personal consultation, E-mail DrBrickey@DrBrickey.com or call 614-237-4556.

To Contact the Author

Dr. Mike Brickey is interested in your comments and feedback. He is available for public speaking, seminars, and personal life coaching. He can be reached by

web site: www.DrBrickey.com
E-mail: DrBrickey@DrBrickey.com
writing: Mike Brickey, 865 College Ave., Columbus, OH 43209
calling: 614-237-4556